I0050978

6G-Enabled IoT and AI for Smart Healthcare

In today's era, there is a need for a system that can automate the process of treatment for the patient if medical facilities are out of reach. Smart healthcare can step in to make the patient more self-dependent. 6G with its features can be seen as the future of smart healthcare with IoT and AI.

6G-Enabled IoT and AI for Smart Healthcare: Challenges, Impact, and Analysis offers the fundamentals, history, reality, and challenges faced in the smart healthcare industry today. It discusses the concepts, tools, and techniques of smart healthcare as well as the analysis used. The book details the role that machine learning-based deep learning and 6G-enabled IoT concepts play in the automation of smart healthcare systems. The book goes on to present applications of smart healthcare through various real-world examples and includes chapters on security and privacy in the 6G-enabled and IoT environment, as well as research on the future prospects of the smart healthcare industry.

This book:

- Offers the fundamentals, history, reality, and the challenges faced in the smart healthcare industry
- Discusses the concepts, tools, and techniques of smart healthcare as well as the analysis used
- Details the role that machine learning-based deep learning and 6G-enabled IoT concepts play in the automation of smart healthcare systems
- Presents applications of smart healthcare through various real-world examples
- Includes topics on security and privacy in 6G-enabled IoT, as well as research and future prospectus of the smart healthcare industry

Interested readers of this book will include anyone working in or involved in smart healthcare research which includes, but is not limited to, healthcare specialists, computer science engineers, electronics engineers, systems engineers, and pharmaceutical practitioners.

Artificial Intelligence in Smart Healthcare Systems

Series Editors: Vishal Jain and Jyotir Moy Chatterjee

The progress of the healthcare sector is incremental as it learns from associations between data over time through the application of suitable Big Data and IoT frameworks and patterns. Many healthcare service providers are employing IoT-enabled devices for monitoring patient healthcare, but their diagnosis and prescriptions are instance-specific only. However, these IoT-enabled healthcare devices are generating volumes of data (Big-IoT Data) that can be analyzed for more accurate diagnosis and prescriptions. A major challenge in the above realm is the effective and accurate learning of unstructured clinical data through the application of precise algorithms. Incorrect input data leading to erroneous outputs with false positives shall be intolerable in healthcare as patient's lives are at stake. This new book series addresses various aspects of how smart healthcare can be used to detect and analyze diseases, the underlying methodologies, and related security concerns. Healthcare is a multidisciplinary field that involves a range of factors like the financial system, social factors, health technologies, and organizational structures that affect the healthcare provided to individuals, families, institutions, organizations, and populations. The goals of healthcare services include patient safety, timeliness, effectiveness, efficiency, and equity. Smart healthcare consists of m-health, e-health, electronic resource management, smart and intelligent home services, and medical devices. The Internet of Things (IoT) is a system comprising real-world things that interact and communicate with each other via networking technologies. The wide range of potential applications of IoT includes healthcare services. IoT-enabled healthcare technologies are suitable for remote health monitoring, including rehabilitation, assisted ambient living, etc. In turn, healthcare analytics can be applied to the data gathered from different areas to improve healthcare at a minimum expense.

This new book series is designed to be a first-choice reference at university libraries, academic institutions, research and development centers, information technology centers, and any institutions interested in using, design, modelling, and analyzing intelligent healthcare services. Successful application of deep-learning frameworks to enable meaningful, cost-effective personalized healthcare services is the primary aim of the healthcare industry in the present scenario. However, realizing this goal requires effective understanding, application, and amalgamation of IoT, Big Data, and several other computing technologies to deploy such systems in an effective manner. This series shall help clarify the understanding of certain key mechanisms and technologies helpful in realizing such systems.

Designing Intelligent Healthcare Systems, Products, and Services Using Disruptive Technologies and Health Informatics
Teena Bagga, Kamal Upreti, Nishant Kumar, Amirul Hasan Ansari, and Danish Nadeem

Next Generation Healthcare Systems Using Soft Computing Techniques
D. Rekh Ram Janghel, Rohit Raja, and Korhan Cengiz

6G-Enabled IoT and AI for Smart Healthcare
Challenges, Impact, and Analysis

Edited by
Ashish Kumar
Rachna Jain
Meenu Gupta
Sardar M.N. Islam

CRC Press
Taylor & Francis Group
Boca Raton London New York

CRC Press is an imprint of the
Taylor & Francis Group, an **informa** business

Designed cover image: Shutterstock

First edition published 2023
by CRC Press
6000 Broken Sound Parkway NW, Suite 300, Boca Raton, FL 33487-2742

and by CRC Press
4 Park Square, Milton Park, Abingdon, Oxon, OX14 4RN

CRC Press is an imprint of Taylor & Francis Group, LLC

© 2023 selection and editorial matter, Ashish Kumar, Rachna Jain, Meenu Gupta and Sardar Islam; individual chapters, the contributors

Reasonable efforts have been made to publish reliable data and information, but the author and publisher cannot assume responsibility for the validity of all materials or the consequences of their use. The authors and publishers have attempted to trace the copyright holders of all material reproduced in this publication and apologize to copyright holders if permission to publish in this form has not been obtained. If any copyright material has not been acknowledged please write and let us know so we may rectify in any future reprint.

Except as permitted under U.S. Copyright Law, no part of this book may be reprinted, reproduced, transmitted, or utilized in any form by any electronic, mechanical, or other means, now known or hereafter invented, including photocopying, microfilming, and recording, or in any information storage or retrieval system, without written permission from the publishers.

For permission to photocopy or use material electronically from this work, access www.copyright.com or contact the Copyright Clearance Center, Inc. (CCC), 222 Rosewood Drive, Danvers, MA 01923, 978-750-8400. For works that are not available on CCC please contact mpkbookspermissions@tandf.co.uk

Trademark notice: Product or corporate names may be trademarks or registered trademarks and are used only for identification and explanation without intent to infringe.

Library of Congress Cataloging-in-Publication Data

Names: Kumar, Ashish (Professor of computer science), editor. | Jain, Rachna (Professor of information technology), editor. | Gupta, Meenu, (Professor of computer science), editor. | Islam, Sardar M. N., 1950- editor.
Title: 6G-enabled IoT and AI for smart healthcare : challenges, impact, and analysis / edited by Ashish Kumar, Rachna Jain, Meenu Gupta, Sardar M.N. Islam.
Description: Boca Raton : CRC Press, 2023. | Series: Artificial intelligence in smart healthcare systems | Includes bibliographical references and index.
Identifiers: LCCN 2022060565 (print) | LCCN 2022060566 (ebook) | ISBN 9781032343457 (hardback) | ISBN 9781032343549 (paperback) | ISBN 9781003321668 (ebook)
Subjects: LCSH: Medical informatics--Technological innovations. | Wireless communication systems in medical care. | Artificial intelligence--Medical applications. | Internet in medicine. | Internet of things.
Classification: LCC R858.A3 A165 2023 (print) | LCC R858.A3 (ebook) | DDC 610.285--dc23/eng/20230406
LC record available at https://lccn.loc.gov/2022060565
LC ebook record available at https://lccn.loc.gov/2022060566

ISBN: 9781032343457 (hbk)
ISBN: 9781032343549 (pbk)
ISBN: 9781003321668 (ebk)

DOI: 10.1201/9781003321668

Typeset in Times
by KnowledgeWorks Global Ltd.

Contents

Preface...vii

Editors...ix

Contributors xi

Chapter 1 Introduction to Smart Healthcare: Healthcare Digitization 1

Sai Dhakshan Y. and Amit Kumar Tyagi

Chapter 2 AI and IoT for Smart Healthcare: Background and
Preliminaries 23

*Prabhjot Kaur, Sharad Chauhan, Meenu Gupta,
and Ashish Kumar*

Chapter 3 Security and Privacy Issues in Smart Healthcare Using
Machine-Learning Perspectives...41

*Ashish Kumar, Neha Gupta, Paarth Bhasin, Sharad Chauhan,
and Imane Bachri*

Chapter 4 A Framework for Virtual Reality in Healthcare: Insight for
Disaster Preparation 57

*Tina Dudeja, Akanksha Dhamija, Tanisha Madan,
Richa Sharma, Narina Thakur, and Zarqua Neyaz*

Chapter 5 Mobile Healthcare Applications: Critical Privacy and
Security Issues, Challenges, and Solutions 69

*Sunita Kumari, Arush Sachdeva, Anant Bansal,
and Deepanshu Pal*

Chapter 6 6G-Enabled IoT for e-Healthcare Systems: Emergence and
Upgradation 121

Richa Gupta and Deepshikha Yadav

Chapter 7 Machine Learning in Healthcare Cybersecurity: Role of
Human Activity Recognition and Impact of 6G in Smart
Healthcare 143

Neha Gupta, Suneet Kumar Gupta, and Vanita Jain

Chapter 8   6G-Enabled IoT Wearable Devices for Elderly Healthcare 157

Shubham Gargrish, Sharad Chauhan, Meenu Gupta,
and Ahmed J. Obaid

Chapter 9   6G-Based Smart Healthcare Solutions: Beyond Industry 4.0
Trends and Products 171

Chander Prabha and Deepak Kumar Jain

Chapter 10   Influence of AI and 6G-Enabled IoT in Smart Healthcare:
Challenges and Solutions 183

Kritika Upadhyay and Manisha Bharti

Chapter 11   Success Stories for IoT-Enabled 6G for Prediction and
Monitoring of Infectious Diseases with Artificial
Intelligence 199

S. Chandrakala and G. Revathy

Chapter 12   Emerging Internet of Things (IoTs) Scenarios Using
Machine Learning for 6G Over 5G-Based
Communications 215

Raghav Dangey, Arjun Tandon, and Amit Kumar Tyagi

Chapter 13   6G: Technology, Advancement, Barriers, and the Future............... 239

Meghna Manoj Nair and Amit Kumar Tyagi

Index 251

Preface

With the development of information technology, smart healthcare has become imperative for the new generation. Smart healthcare incorporated technologies like IoT, machine learning, and deep learning to transform the traditional medical system. Smart healthcare aims to make the healthcare system more efficient, convenient, and personalized for each user. The key to success is addressing the existing system's problems and providing a solution that can be implemented in real-time scenarios. Enhancing healthcare quality and improving access to health records while maintaining reasonable costs is challenging for healthcare organizations globally. An aging population implies an increase in chronic diseases requiring frequent visits to healthcare providers and increased hospitalization needs. The rise in the number of patients requiring constant care significantly increases medical treatment costs. Over the past few decades, Information and Communication Technologies (ICT) have been widely adopted in the healthcare environment to make healthcare access and delivery more accessible and cost-effective. The use of ICT has led to the development of electronic health record (EHR) systems. EHRs contain complete patient health history (current medications, immunizations, laboratory results, current diagnosis, and so on) and can be easily shared among various providers. The adoption of ICT in the health sector is generally referred to as digital healthcare.

Over the years, digital healthcare has extended from maintaining electronic patient data and providing patient web portals to allowing further flexibility and convenience in healthcare management. It is commonly referred to as connected health, such as smartphones, mobile applications, and wireless technologies, allowing patients to connect readily with their providers without visiting them frequently. Conventional mobile devices (such as smartphones) are used together with wearable medical devices (such as blood pressure monitors, glucometers, smart watches) and Internet of Things (IoT) gadgets to enable continuous patient monitoring and treatment at their homes. Smart health is expected to keep hospitalization expenses low and provide timely treatment for various medical ailments by placing IoT sensors on health monitoring equipment. The information collected by these microchips can then be sent to any remote destination. The collected data are then forwarded to a local gateway server via a Wi-Fi network so end systems (such as a physician's laptop) can retrieve the collected data from the gateway server. Regular server updates allow physicians access to real-time patient data. These devices work together to create a unified medical report that various providers can access.

This book aims to publish original and innovative research works focusing on smart healthcare challenges using 6G and IoT. This book discusses the 6G-enabled IoT with AI and machine learning-based medical facilities to provide a solution that can be implemented in real-time scenarios. Also, the sensors can be integrated with 6G to give the regular server update, allowing physicians access to real-time patient data is incorporated. These devices will create a unified medical report that various providers can access. Smart healthcare aims to make the healthcare system more efficient, convenient, and personalized for each user. Smart healthcare incorporated technologies like IoT, machine learning, and deep learning to transform the traditional medical system. This book is a result of the handwork of many researchers around the globe. The book contains theoretical and practical knowledge of state-of-the-art IoT, 6G technologies, and their applications that introduce the readers to how these applications can apply to smart healthcare.

Ashish Kumar, Rachna Jain, Meenu Gupta,
and Sardar M.N. Islam

Editors

Dr. Ashish Kumar is an assistant professor with Bennett University, Greater Noida, UP, India. He completed his PhD in computer science and engineering from Delhi Technological University (formerly DCE), New Delhi, India in 2020. He received a best researcher award from the Delhi Technological University for his contribution in the computer vision domain. He has completed a MTech in computer science and engineering from GGS Indraprastha University, New Delhi. He has published many research papers in various reputed national and international journals and conferences. His current research interests include object tracking, image processing, artificial intelligence, and medical imaging analysis.

Dr. Rachna Jain is an associate professor (IT Department) in Bhagwan Parshuram Institute of Technology (GGSIPU) since August 2021. She worked as an assistant professor (Computer Science Department) in Bharati Vidyapeeth's College of Engineering (GGSIPU) from August 2007 to August 2021. She completed her PhD from Banasthali Vidyapith (Computer Science) in 2017. She received her ME in 2011 from Delhi College of Engineering with a specialization in Computer Technology and Applications. She received her BTech in 2006 from NC College of Engineering, Kurukshetra University. Her current research interests are cloud computing, information security, deep learning and machine learning. She has contributed more than 20 book chapters in various books. She has also served as Session Chair in various international conferences. She completed DST project titled "Design an Autonomous Intelligent Drone for City Surveillance" as CO-PI. Dr. Jain has a total of 16+ years of academic experience with more than 100+ publications in international conferences and international journals (Scopus/ISI/SCI) of high repute.

Dr. Meenu Gupta is an associate professor at the UIE-CSE Department, Chandigarh University, India. She has completed her PhD degree in Computer Science and Engineering with an emphasis on traffic accident severity problems from Ansal University, Gurgaon, India, in 2020. She has more than 13 years of teaching experience. Her research areas cover machine learning, intelligent systems, data mining, artificial intelligence, image processing and analysis, smart cities, data analysis, and human/brain-machine interaction (BMI). She has edited two books on healthcare and cancer diseases and authored four engineering books. She is a reviewer for several journals, including Big Data, CMC, scientific reports, and TSP. She is a life member of ISTE and IAENG. She has authored or co-authored more than 20 book chapters and over 50 papers in refereed international journals and conferences. She has four filed patents and was recently awarded the best faculty and researcher of the department.

Dr. Sardar M.N. Islam is a professor at Victoria University, Melbourne, Australia. He has lived, studied, worked, and travelled (extensively) to different countries over a long period. He adopts a global and humanistic approach in his research and academic works. His research has attracted international acclaim, leading to several appointments as a distinguished visiting professor, or adjunct professor. Dr. Islam has also received many invitations to address international conferences as a keynote speaker. He has published 31 authored research books (published by reputed publishers) and about 250 articles. He is also a distinguished visiting professor of Artificial Intelligence, UnSri; adjunct professor of IT and Business, Armstrong Institute, Melbourne; and editor-in-chief of *International Transactions on Artificial Intelligence*.

Contributors

Imane Bachri
Laboratory of Applied Geology,
  Geomatics and Environment
Hassan II University, Faculty of Science
  Ben m'sik
Casablanca, Morocco

Anant Bansal
G.B. Pant DSEU, Okhla I Campus
New Delhi, India

Manisha Bharti
Department of Electronics and
  Communication Engineering
National Institute of Technology
Delhi, India

Paarth Bhasin
Bharati Vidyapeeth's College of
  Engineering
New Delhi, India

S. Chandrakala
Intelligent Systems Group, School of
  Computing
SASTRA University
Thanjavur, India

Sharad Chauhan
Chitkara University Institute of
  Engineering and Technology
Chitkara University
Punjab, India

Raghav Dangey
School of Computer Science and
  Engineering
Vellore Institute of Technology
Chennai, Tamil Nadu, India

Sai Dhakshan Y.
School of Computer Science and
  Engineering
Vellore Institute of Technology
Chennai, Tamil Nadu, India

Akanksha Dhamija
Department of Computer Science and
  Engineering
Bhagwan Parshuram Institute of
  Technology
Delhi, India

Tina Dudeja
Department of Computer Science and
  Engineering
Bhagwan Parshuram Institute of
  Technology
Delhi, India

Shubham Gargrish
Chitkara University Institute of
  Engineering and Technology
Chitkara University
Punjab, India

Meenu Gupta
Department of Computer Science and
  Engineering
Chandigarh University
Punjab, India

Neha Gupta
Bharati Vidyapeeth's College of
  Engineering
New Delhi, India
and
CSE Department
Bennett University
Greater Noida, UP, India

Richa Gupta
Maharaja Surajmal Institute of
  Technology
Delhi, India

Suneet Kumar Gupta
CSE Department
Bennett University
Greater Noida, UP, India

Deepak Kumar Jain
Chongqing University of Posts and
  Telecommunications
Chongqing, China

Vanita Jain
ECE Department
Bharati Vidyapeeth's College of
  Engineering
New Delhi, India

Prabhjot Kaur
Chitkara University Institute of
  Engineering and Technology
Chitkara University
Punjab, India

Ashish Kumar
Bennett University
Greater Noida, India

Sunita Kumari
G.B. Pant DSEU, Okhla I Campus
New Delhi, India

Tanisha Madan
Department of Computer Science and
  Engineering
Bhagwan Parshuram Institute of
  Technology
Delhi, India

Meghna Manoj Nair
Vellore Institute of Technology
Chennai, Tamil Nadu, India

Zarqua Neyaz
Department of ECE
Bharati Vidyapeeth's College of
  Engineering
New Delhi, India

Ahmed J. Obaid
Department of Computer Science,
  Faculty of Computer Science and
  Mathematics
University of Kufa
Najaf, Iraq

Deepanshu Pal
G.B. Pant DSEU, Okhla I Campus
New Delhi, India

Chander Prabha
Chitkara University Institute of
  Engineering and Technology
Chitkara University
Punjab, India

G. Revathy
Intelligent Systems Group, School of
  Computing
SASTRA University
Thanjavur, India

Arush Sachdeva
G.B. Pant DSEU, Okhla I Campus
New Delhi, India

Richa Sharma
Department of Computer Science and
  Engineering
Bhagwan Parshuram Institute of
  Technology
Delhi, India

Arjun Tandon
School of Computer Science and
  Engineering
Vellore Institute of Technology
Chennai, Tamil Nadu, India

Narina Thakur
Department of Computer Science and
  Engineering
Bhagwan Parshuram Institute of
  Technology
Delhi, India

Amit Kumar Tyagi
Department of Fashion Technology
National Institute of Fashion
  Technology
New Delhi, India

Kritika Upadhyay
Department of Electronics &
  Communication Engineering
National Institute of Technology
Delhi, India

Deepshikha Yadav
Maharaja Surajmal Institute of
  Technology
Delhi, India

1 Introduction to Smart Healthcare

Healthcare Digitization

Sai Dhakshan Y. and Amit Kumar Tyagi

CONTENTS

1.1 Introduction 1
1.2 Motivation..4
    1.2.1 Aspects of Smart Healthcare 5
1.3 Progress towards Smart Healthcare...6
    1.3.1 Healthcare – Pre-COVID 2019...6
    1.3.2 Healthcare during COVID-19 Era..7
    1.3.3 Healthcare Post-COVID-19 Era 9
1.4 Internet of Things-Based Healthcare... 10
1.5 Blockchain and Its Benefit in Healthcare 11
1.6 Artificial Intelligence and Its Benefit in Healthcare................................... 13
1.7 Problems with Access to Present Healthcare System.................................. 15
1.8 Challenges in Healthcare Digitalization.. 16
1.9 Future Research in Smart Healthcare... 18
1.10 Conclusion 20
References..20

1.1 INTRODUCTION

Smart healthcare is the ability of cyber-physical systems (CPS) to integrate with AI, ML, IoT and blockchain to cater the needs of telemedicine for the users. The rapid increase in the world population renders a critical challenge to the existing medical and healthcare services [1, 2]. Although the healthcare infrastructure and cutting-edge technologies are improving, the medical system still faces three critical issues: AI in smart healthcare, its ability to recreate intelligence and intellectual actions of human according to the specific situation. AI is aiding many sectors such as smart environment particularly in smart grid, robotics, etc. AI is a combination of algorithms from mathematics and computer science which process the algorithms. Topics used are linear algebra, statistics, probability and calculus. There are three types of AI such as artificial narrow intelligence, artificial general intelligence and artificial super intelligence. Artificial narrow intelligence works where the machines are already given a predefined decision by humans and process it; in this stage the AI will not think on its own and it is the simplest level of AI.

DOI: 10.1201/9781003321668-1

1

Artificial general intelligence is employed when the AI is used in the machines as the freedom to think but only at a human level. Artificial super intelligence is applied when the intelligence of the in-built AI exceeds the intelligence of humans. IoT is the artificial intelligence that is put into action in the IoT devices. After the AI has taken a decision, it is now the task of the IoT devices to fulfill the decision and produce the desired output. IoT connects all the devices working in the internet to the cloud and access them from one place. Blockchain is a public ledger technology for peer-to-peer transactions (started for finance applications) and finding its best use in many modern-day applications. Blockchain (usually) are of two types: private and public. Blockchain offers a data storage system which is more secure, has high efficiency, privacy and stability. Current uses of blockchain are in cryptocurrency public ledger, financial services, supply chain management, etc. As the name suggests, 'Big Data' represents large amounts of data that is unmanageable using traditional software or internet-based platforms [3]. Big Data can be classified as data having aspects such as:

- *Volume:* It refers to the size of the data occupying the user's environment created from different sources.
- *Velocity:* It refers to Big Data being transmitted and available in real time, e.g., vital signs, and often arriving in bursts rather than at a constant rate [4].
- *Variety:* It refers to the different types of data which are generated or processed like whether the data is grouped or ungrouped and raw or clean, etc.
- *Value:* The value of the data means what the impact of the particular data will have on the organization in business analytical part.
- *Veracity:* The veracity of the data refers to the accuracy, truthfulness and meaningfulness of the data generated for the particular program to be run by the organization. It also refers to the meaningfulness of the analysed data from the generated data, and whether it is being helpful for the study or not. Big Data will help to maintain all the transactional records, financial details and will keep the track of Electronic Healthcare Records (EHRs) of patients, feedback and schedule of doctors and nurses and help administration to make decisions [5]. This concept is being used in many facets of healthcare, ranging from predicting patterns in the health of the people like disease prediction, symptom prediction and predicting physical exercise to improve health [6]. Edge-of-Things (EoT) is a new computing paradigm that represents a middle computing layer between IoT devices and cloud computing, bringing computing power (e.g., IoT gateways) closer to IoT devices. The EoT layer is not only useful for basic transmitted functionality but can also perform real-time analytic services and smart decision-making within a local smart community domain [7]. In this chapter, we will be studying the integration of these technology in action.

Types of healthcare systems are:

- **Remote patient monitoring:** Remote patient monitoring is a common application of IoT device. It is most commonly available as a wearable IoT device that tracks the heart rate, calories, blood pressure, body temperature and more.

Once the data has been collected, it forwards the data to another software application. Designing sensors for medical equipment to collect data is a well-known research area of electronic healthcare. Notwithstanding, that equipment is very specific and are mostly located in hospitals and similar healthcare facilities [8]. The heartbeat sensor is developed based on the plethysmography theory. It measures the change in blood volume through a person's organ that causes the light intensity to move through that organ [9]. After it tracks if there is any emergency situation or something is wrong with the vitals of the person, it sends the result to the relatives of the person and also the doctor. New researchers developed a smart healthcare system that monitored patients' health using five sensors: two sensors (heart rate sensor and body temperature sensor [LM35]) for patient condition monitoring and three sensors (room temperature sensor [DHT11], CO sensor [MQ-9], and CO_2 sensor [MQ-135]) for detection of the living [10].

- **Glucose monitoring:** There is a problem in glucose monitoring device that it is not able to get the correct results since the glucose of the patient fluctuates widely; therefore, periodic testing is not enough to detect a problem. IoT devices can solve this problem by automatic monitoring of glucose level in a patient and keeping a record and whenever there are continuous peaks in the glucose consistently, it will conclude the patient's glucose level is problematic. Challenges in setting up this device include that it should be small enough to be set in a watch and not consume too much charge in a small period of time. Future research in glucose-monitoring devices must address these challenges and find alternatives.
- **Hand hygiene monitoring:** In a place like hospitals or food-preparing stations, hygiene should be ensured at all times. The spreading of any bacteria, fungus, or dirt to the objects should be minimized; therefore, in order to ensure the employees in the hospital are sanitized, there is a hygiene-monitoring device setup. The device can give instructions on how to sanitize for a particular surgery for a particular patient. Research shows that these devices reduce infection rates in the patient post-surgery by more than 60%.
- **Depression and mood monitoring**: It is sometimes difficult for patients to visit their psychologist or the healthcare provider to describe their feeling every week. There is mood-monitoring IoT devices which address the challenge by monitoring the patient's heart rate and blood pressure which can, in turn, tell about the patient's mental well-being. This is the best device which tells the patient that he/she is depressed before the patient is admitting it. Future research in these areas include accurate prediction of the depression symptoms from a dataset of the blood pressure and heart rate collected and check in accordance with the user using it now and get a complete accuracy result.
- **Parkinson's disease monitoring:** People with age above 50 or 60 years or more prone to Parkinson's disease resources that the early onset of Parkinson's can be cured using drugs but later stages of Parkinson cannot be cured. IoT solve these challenges by continuously collecting data about the Parkinson symptoms from the patient so that it can be cured in the early stages.

- **Connected inhalers**: Asthma and COPD attacks come suddenly with only a little warning. Persons experiencing attacks need help from other people; therefore, the respected members to the patient will be informed of the asthma attack. The connected inhalers can also monitor the frequency of the asthmatic attack and it can find the reasons behind the attack by collecting the data from the environment on what triggers the attack. The connected inhalers can also alert patients when they leave home without taking inhalers.
- **Ingestible sensors:** The ingestible devices in the body, which are called biosensors sauce, go inside the body and collect the data from the digestive and other systems and provide data about the stomach pH level, etc. Therefore, it must be small enough to be swallowed easily and must be able to pass through the esophagus. Nanoparticle biosensors have been designed in a way that they are fully implantable on patient's body. These sensors act as a 'fuel gauge' transmitting internal measurements of physiological function in a step towards digitizing the human body [11].
- **Connected contact lenses**: Contact lens is another healthcare device which provides data in a passive way. It includes a micro camera with which the user takes pictures at a snap of his finger, and Google is the first company to have patented connected contact lenses. Connected contact lenses are equipped with zoom in and zoom out features.
- **Robotic surgery:** As discussed earlier, usage of robots in smart surgery can help the doctors to make micro-size incisions in human blood vessels so that it can lead to accurate cut and the surgery would be infectionless and it promotes faster healing for patients. Challenges of this device is that it must be micro-sized and reliable enough to perform micro inclusions without any disruption in the process. Robotic sensors are already used in the surgery but the research of micro-robot hands is in development stage.

1.2   MOTIVATION

In a vast country like India or the United States of America, the number of doctors per 100,000 people is very low and not everyone can get access to the best healthcare; therefore, there is no option of choosing the best doctors in the world, the patients seem to be fine if there is at least a doctor available for the treatment. Therefore, telemedicine is very much ignored by the patients due to the lack of knowledge to the access of telemedicine. In this chapter, it is discussed about how the healthcare digitization can take place and the end users can benefit from it and become knowledgable to telemedicine; the smart helathcare devices are also discussed in this chapter. In the year 2020, corona virus has changed the world's existing healthcare system and the transformation of the healthcare digitization was at a very slow pace. But after the corona virus hit us in 2019, there was a rapid digitization which has not happened in the previous decade. The governments which could not adapt to the digitization or ignored digitization faced an increasing number of COVID-19 cases during the pandemic.

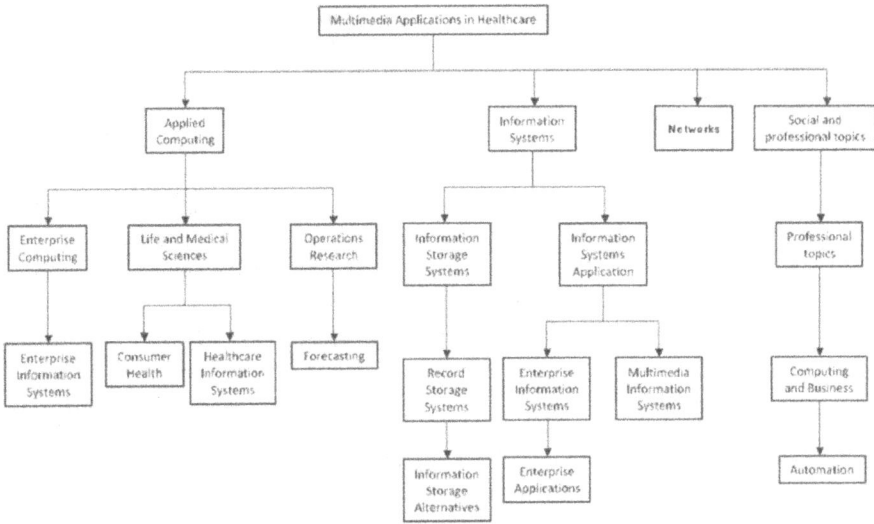

FIGURE 1.1 Multimedia applications in healthcare.

One such example is South Korea which did not adapt to digitization due to its stringent measures imposed in the smart healthcare sector which increased the COVID-19 cases in the country. In this chapter, we have analysed the healthcare sector before, during and after the COVID-19 pandemic. The purpose of this chapter is to connect different technologies such as AI, IoT, Big Data and blockchain analysing about its intcroperability and also the technical challenges faced while connecting these technology. There is an under-utilization of blockchain in smart healthcare sector; therefore, in the chapter, the used cases of all the technologies in the smart healthcare, the barriers in the way of smart healthcare which the patients feel difficult and the telemedicine benefits which removes the following said barriers are also discussed.

On the other hand, we can see (in Figure 1.1) the role of multimedia application and its importance in healthcare and smart healthcare.

1.2.1 ASPECTS OF SMART HEALTHCARE

Digitization of healthcare is not only technological advancement but it's an all-round development of smart healthcare facilities that is information-based. The healthcare hospitals and the primary health centres are in the process of developing to an information-based system but it is also the time for the healthcare ecosystem in homes and community to adapt to information-based system. It makes the information-based system more efficient and can be easily personalized and convenient for the larger scale healthcare systems to access it. Hence, there are few requirements for smart healthcare which can be listed here as:

- **Patient-centred care:** The traditional healthcare model followed was a disease-centric approach where the focus was shifted through diagnosing the symptoms patients have and it wasn't treated according to the doctors-prescribed treatment protocols. If the patient had a previous history of other diseases or allergies and if it is not treated in accordance to the disease-centric approach, it can pose a serious challenge; therefore, in this chapter, usage of electronic health records is discussed in detail. If the patient's past health history is ignored and is given a wrong treatment, it can result in a dangerous situation. The main focus of the patient-centric approach lies in the health history of the patient needs and the beliefs of the patient. The patient's preference is given a high value in a patient-centred care.
- **Personalized management:** Healthcare in today's generation provided healthcare system hospitals. The service is never customizable or changed according to the patient's needs. In building a patient-centric smart health-care environment, the needs and preferences of patients must be respected and the system takes the patients' opinions into consideration.
- **Prevention is better than cure:** This model focuses on the preventive measures rather than treating a disease after it occurs. This is made possible by continuously monitoring the user behaviour of their body conditions, symptoms, environment, lifestyle choices which are the most important factors causing illnesses. Analysing these factors can help in making the people more health conscious and prevent ailments and alleviate diseases in the future.

1.3   PROGRESS TOWARDS SMART HEALTHCARE

1.3.1   Healthcare – Pre-COVID 2019

In the 1970s, AI was introduced to healthcare sector to solve existing problems in bio-medical engineering. Advances in AI in emerging technologies such as Big Data, machine learning and cloud computing has also been an integral part of evolving smart healthcare before 2019. The Watson for oncology is an AI smart health-care application created by IBM; it is a product trained by the oncologists for the users to get an opinion on diagnosis for cancer and gives a good accuracy of 90% e-solutions by the oncologists. The AI has developed an algorithm for accurate diagnosis of diseases, predication of response from the user, improving efficiency in the workflow operations in the hospital, increasing the overall procedure accuracy. In the 1950–1970s era, an industrial robotic arm was built by the General Motors in 1961 and was used in the assembly line for predefined die casting. Shakey, the flakey robot, was developed by the Stanford Research International (SRI), but for the smart healthcare field AI was very slow to be adopted.

The 1970s era was a period referred to as AI winter as it had low fundings for any technology to be developed, but yet there was an official adaptation of AI in health-care in 1971 by the SUMEX-AIM for the biomedical researchers across the world to connect to each other. Later in 1975, there was a conference in the Rutgers University about the topic AI in medicine.

In 1987, DXplain was developed by the University of Massachusetts that proposed to generate differential diagnosis to provide information of about 500 diseases. In the recent era, pharma Bot was developed in 2015 to assist in medicine education. Using AI, the healthcare system was transformed more into patient-centric approach and helped in increasing the efficiency of staff in the hospital. As of now, there are many hospitals and health centres equipped with smart healthcare system. Additionally, wearable scanners or medical devices are used for patient health management after treatment, and apps that are developed exclusively for certain hospitals can check patients' conditions 24/7.

In the pre-COVID period, in addition to telemedicine, there were a number of contactless healthcare systems in use. In the pre-COVID era, there were medical personnel tracking systems checking vital signs using the technology radio frequency identification known as RFID. In the recent era, there was employability of AI-based robots in the healthcare industry to assist in in-patient rounds, writing and modification of medical records, administerial work in the reception and assisting in providing information about the treatment. Before the COVID era, there was no emphasis on the mental health of a person and not much importance was given to the mental health monitoring.

1.3.2 Healthcare during COVID-19 Era

Even after our world seeing many epidemics like the swine flu, SARS, COVID-2019, etc., the whole world was shocked and was not prepared for the corona virus. People in India already having less medical knowledge became more scared and insecure due to the fake news spreading around the world due to the virus. But from the doctor's side there was no fear as the virus seemed similar to the SARS Cov-2 pandemic in the 2000s, but the doctors feared the patients having other complications like diabetes millets, chronic kidney disease, lung disease, etc. are at a greater risk since the death in corona was very minimal but the persons with other complications were more likely to be affected.

The immediate effects of corona virus on the person in the world are listed next:

- Decreased financial security: For the people without valid medical insurance in India or the USA feared of the high-cost of medical treatment for the corona virus.
- Increased stress on informal caregivers: Since the virus is communicable, even the informal caregivers such as parents or relatives to virus-affected person fear to give the unconditional help to the affected person.
- Challenges with protections of individuals with disabilities: Not all persons with disabilities have a caretaking member with them, it was difficult for the people with disabilities not having a caretaker.
- Absenteeism of home care workers: The pandemic has largely affected the home care workers' profession since the person hiring employees for the home workers profession feared that the home care workers working in different houses have the chance to spread the virus to the ones who is hiring. There was also a fear among the primary workers to work in the public places due to the chances of catching the virus.

- Delay in the procedure for the chronic conditions apart from corona virus: There was non-availability and poor management of doctors in the city by the hospital management due to the pressure created by the spreading virus, for the other treatment for the chronic conditions were delayed.
- Ignorance to visit healthcare centres in person: During the time of virus spreading, the patients having other problems other than corona virus started looking for inaccurate home remedies specified in different health-care websites. If there is a fever or common cold, the reason for its cause can be many, but the remedies given in the website will not work for all the causes, therefore a doctor's diagnosis is the best.
- Impacts on mobility due to confinement: Due to some areas being marked as red zone which means it is affected highly by the virus, those sorts of places or the road leading to those places are blocked, therefore the primary health-care facility or the hospital or pharmacy in that area cannot be reached.
- Concerns about medicine shortages: During the early stages of the pandemic, due to the less awareness of the virus or not following the protocols which are needed to be followed in the work environment, some of the pharma industries were closed fearing the spread of virus among its employees, resulting in drug shortage in the country. Also, during the initial stages of the pandemic, there was a block of import/export of drug in the industry leading to the shortage of drugs.
- Problems about using masks and face coverings for those having breathing difficulty: The people who had past history of breathing difficulties, such as asthma, wheezing, etc., felt the strain in using the mask in public places during the pandemic.
- Distress and burnout of healthcare workforce: As discussed earlier, there was poor management of the workforce during the pandemic including the healthcare staffs, nurses and doctor. There was also poor management of different wards in the society. The lessons learnt during the pandemic was to involve a patient-centric treatment approach and innovative smart health-care methods needed to be adopted.

During the pandemic, many hospitals in the country have shut down its health-care facility for treatments such as diabetes, hypertension by at least 50%, and also more than 60% of the country's rehabilitation facilities have been closed during the pandemic in order for the doctors to avoid face-to-face counselling. Also, during the pandemic, many people preferred online diagnosis instead of the traditional way of meeting the doctor. There was a rapid development of the telemedicine sector of the smart medicine sector during the pandemic which reduced the interaction of the patient with the third person and now they can directly be diagnosed by the doctor. The amount of usage of the smart healthcare systems by the patients before the pandemic was 10% but after the impact of the virus it grew to 50% facilitating more people to use innovative and contactless healthcare systems. In the interview with the team of Stanford Institute of Health and Medicine, it was mentioned that 76% of the outpatient causalities were dealt online.

Such telemedicine services can reduce the risk of infection during the spread of an epidemic disease by delivering care through ICT while the patient practices social distancing. The AI in healthcare was proved and doing greater achievements in reducing the problems in healthcare industry such as shortage of healthcare personnel, abolished the token system being followed in the hospitals and healthcare centres. During the pandemic, there was many research showing the accurate test of the corona virus such as the one like X-ray of lungs and using the concepts of convolutional neural networks in testing for the corona virus in the individual. The AI foundation in basis of healthcare setup now will also be helpful in the future to predict the growth of virus, prevent the spread of virus in smart environment. It uses IoT and AI to get the things needed to be done by the user.

1.3.3 HEALTHCARE POST-COVID-19 ERA

The World Health Organization, in 2019, defines telemedicine as 'the delivery of healthcare services, where distance is a critical factor, by all healthcare professionals using information and communication technologies for the exchange of valid information for diagnosis, treatment and prevention of disease and injuries, research and evaluation, and for the continuing education of healthcare providers, all in the interests of advancing the health of individuals and their communities'.

COVID-19 proved to be a great macroeconomic shock: the stock prices in April 2020 fell down to great margins like Nifty crashed to its low 8,000 rupees and in October 2022 regained momentum and clinched 16,000 rupees. Not only in India but also in the United States and in the European Union, there was a massive hit in the stock market that reflected in the country's economic downfall. But due to the adaption of modern-day technologies during the COVID-19 and the post-COVID-19, the companies were able to manage itself to run with the profit margin instead of a loss. Those companies which could not update themselves to modern-day technology suffered a loss. For a smooth functioning of the government, the government ensured to change its policies and priorities. Due to this change in priority and policy, the growth of IoT in smart environment could be achieved particularly in the smart healthcare. Most of the leading experts and researchers believe that there will be a greater influence of technology in the life of humans in the post-COVID era too.

Telemedicine market was 45.5 billion dollars in 2019 and suspected to reach 175 billion by 2026. This determines the demand of IoT in smart healthcare sector. Modern-day researchers and engineers need to come up with new research products for smart healthcare. Healthcare companies should dedicate smart healthcare division as the research division due to the rise in market demand for smart healthcare products. The growth of the smart healthcare products owes to the government's regulation with respect to telemedicine to minimize the spread of COVID-19 by contactless treatment. The telemedicine products directly impacted the other industries because using of telemedicine products ensured contactless treatments which reduce COVID cases which in turn made the government to remove new regulations that made the other industries to recover. Countries such as South Korea under-utilized smart healthcare products by imposing rigid regulations on smart healthcare sector which fuelled the spread of COVID-19 and industry loss in their country;

therefore, without the help of government healthcare, the development of telemedicine cannot take place. Information and Communication Technology (ICT) will play a greater role in the healthcare domain such as in the treatment of disease, prevention and analysis, etc. In the future, smart healthcare products will develop an effective disease treatment measure and prevention and spontaneous action to healthcare personal shortage or equipment shortage and innovative methods to create smart healthcare environment.

1.4   INTERNET OF THINGS-BASED HEALTHCARE

The definition of IoT based on IoT European Research Cluster (IECR) project it as a dynamic network infrastructure which has the capability of self-configuration on the bases of interoperable and standard communication protocols. IoT is about integration of the 'things' that form the life of people into software applications, leveraging benefits from the information continuity. IoT technology is a recent component of ICT, looking into the potential of combining wireless sensor networks, beacons, radio-frequency identification (RFID), data processing and security in healthcare services [12–18].

- **IoT for patients:** The modern-day IoT smart healthcare devices enable the use for person of any age and can also wear the device. Example of few devices are fitness bands that monitor blood pressure, heart rate, oxygen level SpO_2. It also monitors the calorie count, exercise monitoring and the blood pressure during the exercise. In this way, the patients and the patients' relatives can monitor their family members. On any disturbance in the regular activity or the body vitals of the patient, the IoT device will send an alarm to the family members mentioning the emergency of the patient; this, in turn, effectively enables better tracking system for the elderly patients and even a small disturbance noticed and treated can prevent a major incident.
- **IoT for physicians:** As mentioned, wearing IoT devices and monitoring equipment helps in a way where the physician can track the patient's data and keep a track of their record in a digital format and can also be ready for a procedure in case of immediate medical attention. This helps healthcare professionals to be more watchful and connect to the patients immediately, and this in turn achieve the goal of patient-centric healthcare systems.
- **IoT for hospitals:** Apart from the advantage of monitoring patients' healthcare using smart IoT devices, the hospital also gets IoT devices tag with location sensors to track their medical equipment like surgery instruments, wheelchairs, oxygen cylinders, etc. In India, due to the COVID-19, there was a shortage of oxygen cylinders. By implementing the IoT sensors for the location tracking, the hospitals could track the medical equipment instead of leaving it to the third-party members who in turn would sell the oxygen cylinder for money in the private market. Blockchain supply chain management technology could also be used in this process (this we will discuss later in the chapter). Deployment of medical staff at different locations in the hospital can also be virtualized and analysed using IoT devices using technology such as AI and machine-learning algorithms.

In the hospitals, IoT devices can also be used in monitoring devices from preventing patients getting infected. Another use of IoT devices hospitals include inventory, temperature monitoring, humidity monitoring and environmental monitoring.

- **IoT for insurance company:** Insurance companies using IoT-enabled devices reduce fraudulent claim of insurance. The recent development of IoT devices allowed insurance companies to keep track of patients' health by accessing to their exercise routine. This information will be helpful in either reducing or increasing the insurance premium.

1.5 BLOCKCHAIN AND ITS BENEFIT IN HEALTHCARE

There are few benefits of using decentralized and distributed concept using healthcare, which can be listed here as:

- Securing patient data: Confidentiality of patients' data is the most important part of healthcare sector. There are many instances where the patient's record is tampered with, and the same data is replaced by another data submitted to the doctors and hospital. Between 2010 and 2022, there are more than 200 million patient records which are breached. They not only get to manipulate the data of patient but also misuse their account information. The better alternative to securing patient record is blockchain as it is already used for application such as supply chain management in tracking of goods and transactions peer to peer, blockchain can ensure tamper-proof distribution in correcting patient records and can be used to store patients' records in a secure way.
- Supply chain management of healthcare drugs and equipment: Medical drugs or surgical equipment are not directly made in the hospital; they are imported from labs and pharmaceutical industries worldwide and are further supplied from the industries to the other countries according to their needs; therefore, due to the long, tedious process of drug import, blockchain can be used in the supply chain management of medical drugs to ensure tamper-free distribution and transparency.
- Single longitudinal patient records: Blockchain is a chain of blocks and all the attributes of the patients' record with the hospital is noted and will be entered into the blockchain ledger. The attributes can be lab test results, treatment, fees or past diseases. This can be used by the hospital physicians and workers to analyse the patient's disease based on the lab test from a single record and offering incentives to regular patients.
- Supply chain optimization: As discussed previously, the authenticity of the medical goods such as medical drugs and surgery equipment need to be ensured of their authenticity. The previous use of blockchain in supply chain management can be used in the supply chain management of the medical drugs and products. This enables the hospital or the buyer to view the visibility and transparency of the goods that was bought. This also increases the confidence of the customers to buy from the same company again.

- Decentralized storage of medical records: The InterPlanetary file storage system in the blockchain enables the industry to store data in the decentralized storage environment.
- Improves electronic health record systems: Not only the patients record system can be stored under the blockchain, the medical drugs available in the healthcare facilities and the medical equipment can also be stored in the blockchain decentralized storage which can be later be viewed to see the availability and can be edited.

In the last, few key features of Blockchain Technology can be found in Table 1.1. Hence, few other benefits are:

- **Patients predictions for improved staffing:** To reduce the labour cost during a shift in the hospital and to avoid unnecessary labour cost, it is necessary to have the correct number of workers to be present at the hospital unit for a good customer service. Applications of healthcare data analytics can be used in this scenario to predict the number of patients for a good customer service outcome. Use cases of healthcare analytics are applied in many domains, such as medical expenses, clinical data, patient behaviour and the pharmaceutical industries. It is used in both the macro- and micro-level work. Analytics facilitates both administrative and financial data analysis. Data analytics healthcare is used to ease the doctors in making the decisions faster using the data available and enhance the treatment of patients. This is used for the patients having medical histories and suffering from multiple conditions. Help in examining the data of the patient and medicines prescribed by the doctor and dosage level check to see if it is the correct treatment and then revert to the patient and make amends in case of any errors.
- **Electronic health records (EHRs):** Electronic health records is one of the important applications of Big Data in smart healthcare. Health records are stored for each person which includes the demographics, medical history,

TABLE 1.1
Key Elements of Blockchain Technology

Features	Provided by Blockchain (Y/N)
Decentralized	Y
Transparent	Y
Immutable	Y
Autonomy	Y
Open source	Y
Anonymity	Y
Trusted	Y

allergies and laboratory test results. Records are shared with the health-care person to the information system in a secure way. Every record has one modifiable file where doctors can change data in the record. Electronic health records can also alert and remind the patient when they should get a new lab test or visit a doctor for a follow-up. Many countries apart from the USA are struggling to implement electronic health record in their system. European Union are left behind and the United States digitized health-care using electronic health record with 94% of the hospitals adopting it. McKinsey report states that the electronic health record has improved outcomes in treating cardiovascular ailments and saved $1 billion due to reduced office receipts and lab tests. EHRs may empower patients to play more active roles in caring for their health by directly delivering information to these individuals. Patients not only can know specific details about their health parameters and illnesses but can also present medical records to other healthcare professionals when needed [19].

- **Enhancing patient engagement:** Many patients are becoming interested in smart healthcare device that record the heart rate, blood pressure, calorie count and oxygen level in the body and that information can be coupled with other datasets available to identify similarities between the two data-sets and if identified it would display if they are at a risk of that particular disease. Person suffering from chronic insomnia and higher heart rate can signal risk for cardiovascular diseases in the future. Patients become health conscious and get incentive from insurance companies and lower their insurance amount. Use case of the said product is suitable for person suffering from asthma or high blood pressure and can reduce unnecessary visits to the hospital.
- **Track mass diseases:** COVID-19 pandemic has impacted humans around the world physically, mentally and socially. Its ability to spread and mutate to strong form challenged the healthcare industry which tried to learn from it and control the spread of the disease. With the help of the Big Data technologies, the healthcare professionals were able to track in real time the spread of corona virus, how fast it is able to mutate to other virus and its effect on the country's economy. This is only done by analysing massive amounts of datasets coming from different medical sources. Technologies such as AI, medical imaging and analytics allowed to detect corona virus in the patient from chest X-ray, tomography, ultrasounds, etc. It was in 2022 that the EU patented the research 'analyses images of the lungs taken by a CT scanner, identify the signs of coronavirus, and assesses the lesions' to identify the signs of corona virus. This level of technology helped the EU to flatten the corona virus curve.

1.6 ARTIFICIAL INTELLIGENCE AND ITS BENEFIT IN HEALTHCARE

An example comes from the world of chess, which was the first real test of human intellect versus the machine. In 1997, IBM's Deep Blue beat the reigning chess grandmaster Garry Kasparov, a tremendous feat of computational capability for the time [20].

- **Increased efficiency of the diagnostic process**: A lack of the existing medical data history can increase the chances of errors of the physicians in the diagnostic process. The use of AI in smart healthcare will be able to predict and diagnose the disease origin faster than the lab testing by the clinic with a very minimal percentage of error, that is, lower than the human error. For example, in 2017, there was a research published for detecting and diagnosing breast cancer using deep learning, AML models, which proved to be a percentage higher in accuracy than pathologist testing technology. Not only AI and ML are needed to provide accurate solutions, the vast amount of data, which is the Big Data, is needed to write efficient algorithm to get accurate solutions.
- **Reduced overall costs of running the business:** As discussed earlier, using AI the process of manual testing makes the diagnosis and the treatment more efficient but it also cuts the cost required to do it manually. The technology is developed using image processing and analytics. AI can analyse images of CT scan, X-ray etc., and can reduce the manual work involved and also reduce the percentage of error. In smart healthcare, patients are treated faster and there are no tedious waiting times, no admission fees, etc. Implication of AI-IoT in surgery has cut the cost up to 40 billion dollars.
- **Safer surgeries:** AI, IoT devices in the smart healthcare can provide assistance in surgery and reduce the manual error during the surgery. Robots or the devices can be more cautious when working around sensitive organs tissues and reduce the risk of infection and unnecessary blood loss. Treatment of very minute blood vessels or nerves in the body that is a study with shows robot hands are much more efficient than manual hands to treat the sensitive places. The advantage of robot hands over manual hands is that it can reduce tremor during the surgery and as a result it reduces the error due to manual human tremor.
- **Enhanced patient care:** Healthcare facilities before COVID-19 pandemic were not well managed and was chaotic. The hospital did not make any effort to manage the mess and patient care was not patient-centric. A study showed that 80% of the patients feel poor communication is the worst part in the treatment process. AI can rapidly scan data reports using image analytics and faster processing of data could be used to avoid the tedious process for the patients to be followed [3, 13, 20–22].
- **Easy information sharing:** As said before, the use of blockchain in smart healthcare integrated with AI and IoT device can increase the efficiency of the transfer and storage of data. It tracks the data of the patient and can do it in seconds, whereas traditional tracking of data is more time-consuming, which in turn allows doctors to focus on treatments rather than the data tracking. The device called freestyle liber glucose monitoring system helps patients to track their glucose levels and transfer the glucose-level reports to the doctor or the professional in the hospital for efficient treatment.

- **Better prevention care:** Aarogya Setu app developed by the Indian government in collaboration with the National Informatics Centre is one such AI ML integrated device application which tracks the user with COVID-19 symptoms. It proved to be of great help in reducing the infection in the country. Intelligent platform called Blue Dart analysed the spread of COVID-19 using airline ticket and flight path and accurately predicted that the spread was from Wuhan to Bangkok and Taipei.

1.7   PROBLEMS WITH ACCESS TO PRESENT HEALTHCARE SYSTEM

Few problems with access to present healthcare system are:

- **Limited appointment availability office hours:** Mini healthcare hospitals and primary health centres are open when the working-class people work, which is between 8:00 a.m. and 6:00 p.m. Therefore, the timing is not always useful. Timings should benefit the working-class people as well as the non-working-class people in order to avoid a rush or a queue. Extending the healthcare centers working hours will be one of the most important tasks in building a patient- centric medical treatment. The alternative of this is allowing patients to receive medical treatment without their physical presence in the hospital, that is, their virtual presence in the video call or conference call with which is directly connected to the doctor. Due to a smaller number of doctors per area of 10,000 people is an important factor for the limited appointment availability in many countries such as United States and India. There must be an efficient relocation of the doctors from different centres in the time of work to fulfill the appointments of the patient.
- **Geographic, clinician shortage issues:** Due to higher pay in urban areas, doctors are most likely to shift their centres to urban areas and people living in rural areas cannot get the same quality of the healthcare facility. The rural residents can also encounter social and various communication barriers in their process of access to the healthcare that limit their ability to get the best of treatment. In order for them to receive the best healthcare, there must be access to necessary healthcare services available in a timely manner. Study shows that rural people have to travel 40 miles for a radiation treatment and the urban residents travel only 15 miles for the same treatment. Due to the boom of access to telemedicine or smart healthcare after the pandemic and also during the pandemic, it reduced the gap between the patients and the doctor living in both urban and rural areas so that they get the same quality of the treatment from the city doctors. It was only for the lab test that patients had to go to the nearest lab centre. The telemedicine services also connect smaller hospitals or healthcare centres with the larger government academic medical centres. A study shows that in the United States there are 40 physicians per 100,000 people in rural areas and 53 physicians per 100,000 people in the urban areas.

- **High healthcare costs:** The main barrier in the way of accessing the best healthcare system by the user is the high healthcare cost. In a study by the best health and Gallup poll, it was found that three out of ten Americans reasoned the high cost of healthcare as a barrier for them, as a result they skipped medical care at least once in three months. One more study tells that a person making more than \$120,000 annually, out of which 20% said that they could not access the healthcare due to its high cost. The cost of the healthcare treatment is increased by around 10% which is higher than pre-COVID-19. Nearly 40% of the US citizens skip treatment or regular follow-up to the doctor due to the high cost of healthcare, in which 30% were from high-income group and 50% of the low-income patients skip care because of the high healthcare cost.
- **Social determinants:** In addition to the barriers of the healthcare industry, there are also social determinants of patients which play a major role in their access to the healthcare which makes it harder for them to get into the doctor's office. Some social determinants already discussed in the chapter include geographical location, income and transportation access. In addition, race or racial discrimination also resulted in problems related to access of healthcare by the patient. Red lining policy introduced back in 1938 to separate desirable and undesirable created racial discrimination. Therefore, there needs to be healthcare digitalization. Traditional healthcare organizations have realized that they need to change the way they work; for example, over the past two years, most of the large pharmaceutical companies have started to employ a chief digital officer [23].

1.8   CHALLENGES IN HEALTHCARE DIGITALIZATION

Popular challenges faced in implementing/building a smart healthcare system are:

- **Old habits of employees and customers:** The process of digital transformation is itself a long process that too in the healthcare domain. The employees or the customers might feel anxious to use or adapt to new solutions; instead, they often stick to the old solution because of their old habits which restrict in improving the patient-centric treatment approach. The new enterprise software domain is widely being accepted by many healthcare organizations thinking that without change the competition is very tough. Healthcare digitalization is not only implementing new software and developing mobile and web applications, it is also changing the way the employees and users think and work. The entire process will need a huge amount of funding but once the technology is developed, it always works for a lifetime sparing only few developments on upgrade which is at a less cost.
- **Lack of software interoperability:** Interoperability is defined as a connection of different CPS device and application to access exchange integrated and cooperatively used data in a coordinator manner within and across regional and national boundaries to provide timely and seamless portability

of information and optimize the health of individuals and populations globally. Exchanging information between two or many systems involving their respective technologies can be a desirable feature in healthcare digitalization, for example, the data of the patient stored in blockchain must be transferred to the IoT device to check if the patient is eligible for a discount in the treatment based on their previous entries. The absence of interoperability between the software makes the communication between the company and the patients less efficient and more time-consuming.

- **Data protection:** Some of the goals of information security systems are:
  - Confidentiality: It implies securing the information from the unauthorized user to see.
  - Integrity: It implies that patient's data will not be changed by a third-party user.
  - Authentication: It means that identification of the person who is trying to access the data in the system.
  - Availability: It means that authorized users can anytime access their data when in need.

Hence, respecting the user's data in the process of smart healthcare digitalization transformation is very important. If the data of the patient is breached, it can be misused by the third party. As discussed earlier, it can also be used for fraudulent purposes by hacking banking number information so that miscreants can steal money from the innocent users.

- **Costs of digitalization:** Cost of healthcare digitalization is not cheap. It needs IT infrastructure to build a new smart healthcare product for the healthcare company and the work is not over after developing the product. The product must be maintained, developed, upgraded and updated by the IT company; therefore, more funds will be needed for building it. But looking at the advantages, the healthcare company would generate income and save funds by offering new medical services to their customers.
- **Data processing:** A huge amount of data is needed for the machine-learning algorithm to work efficiently and give accurate solution to the users. But in the reality, only a small amount of data are collected by hospitals, clinic and professional. Without huge amount of data, it is difficult to provide accurate solution. The major problem lies in the collection and mining of data. Rise in telemedicine, the doctors giving diagnosis in different channels through different companies makes it harder for the doctor to update the patients' records which in turn results in no data at the end and AI ML cannot provide a solution. The solution could be to come up with a new way to record and update the patients' and doctors' records for both in-person and virtual visits. For example, in the European Union, stringent data protection regulation act has been enforced so that the organization must not use and store data for their personal purpose; if found guilty of breaching patients' confidentiality, they have to pay a fine of 4% of companies' annual turnover.

- **Improving cybersecurity:** Security and privacy protection are certainly very important issues of IoT applications, particular healthcare IoT. This is because healthcare IoT tends to use location, personal and context information of users in order to provide its services [24]. As discussed, earlier protection of data is most important for the users to get confidence in smart healthcare digitalization process. The study conducted by IBM found that HealthCare organization is associated with high possibilities of data breach, which is three times more than in any other domain. Accurate authentication deficiency and excessive user permission are other main reasons which lead to the data breach in smart healthcare sector. More software technology is coming together in smart healthcare, such as adaptation of Internet of Medical Things that will be more likely to cause software attacks. There must be a cybersecurity team behind the product working continuously for the removal of bug threats from the third-party hackers. There is not only data breach but there are also bugs in the updated software for removing the bugs There must also be a technical team working for the removal of bugs and update the product before and after the launch.
- **Digital user experience:** The design of the product like a connected IoT monitor device, mobile or web application must be developed in a way so that its user interface and experience are user-friendly because the age range of people using the product can be anywhere between 3 and 100. The UI and UX team must take into consideration and developer user-friendly product.
- **Operator interface:** This interface allows network operators to register to the SHS in order to manage current and historical information from environmental sensors, set rules and alarm notifications [1]. An inconvenient-designed healthcare device might make the patient to remove the device and limit the data which is able to be collected. The user interface should be as convenient and intuitive as possible. Even people who are not familiar with the software should be able to use the complete functionality, e.g., new user data, constraints of different sorts and history access [25]. If the software of the healthcare device is difficult to use, it will also result in the medical professional not to prescribe the device to the other patients. It does not matter how strong the technology or the development of the product is, it all comes down to the user interface and the user experience; therefore, this is the most important thing to take into consideration in developing a smart healthcare device.
- **Quality assurance testing in healthcare:** It is important to ensure that the software is capable to deliver the required task and service to the user.

1.9   FUTURE RESEARCH IN SMART HEALTHCARE

The major challenges include interoperability of interconnected devices in the cloud, cybersecurity preventing attacks, collection of more medical patient-related data and efficient management of all the devices connected to the cloud [3, 13–18, 20–22, 26–28].

The other challenges include usage of ideas to reduce the cost for developing and management of the device. The approach of the future healthcare must be patient-centric healthcare approach which means that the healthcare is there to support the patient not only in the diagnosis and treatment aspect but also the other aspects as discussed in the problems with access to healthcare. The new development in health-care should be of immediate diagnosis of diseases based on the everyday difficulties faced by the patients so as to stop the spread at initial stage. The future research also includes the risk prediction and the prevention of any new virus. The main paths for future research revolve around

- challenges about engaging patients or citizens in designing e-health services,
- the necessity to develop purely disciplinary research and reach a common taxonomy,
- patient empowerment,
- the impact of digitalization on healthcare practices and the relationship between patients and healthcare professionals, and
- insufficient strategic and policy reflection about the impact of digitalization [29].

In near future, researchers can work towards improvement of healthcare as its rev-olution 4.0, which will be useful and convenient to the society 5.0 (refer Figure 1.2).

Hence, in this chapter, the authors discuss about the CPSs and its usages. The authors explain about the importance of CPS and medical CPSs. The authors describe in detail about the types of attackers and attacks in the medical CPSs. The authors also speak about the issues and challenges of medical CPSs in the future. They first introduce the technologies emerged due to COVID, such as processes in AI, cloud computing, Big Data, blockchain and IoT. They discuss about the appli-cation of artificial intelligence, Internet of Things and Internet of Medical Things development primarily in the COVID-19 eras.

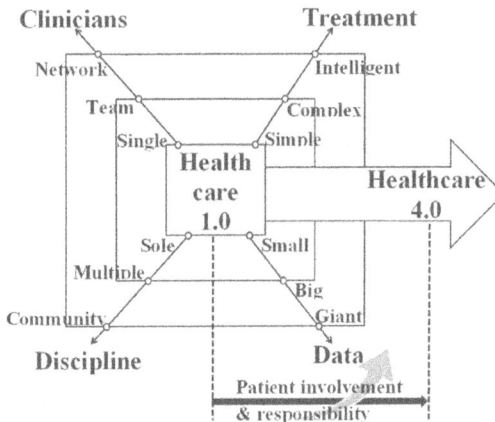

FIGURE 1.2   Healthcare 1.0 to healthcare 4.0.

1.10 CONCLUSION

Smart healthcare has to be well maintained by both the users in the smart environment and the developers working in the backend who develop, upgrade and update the products. Without further research, the challenges discussed previously about the smart healthcare will not be welcomed by the users using smart healthcare in telemedicine. In this chapter, we have discussed the challenges faced by the users in smart healthcare and also the solutions to few challenges or the approach or the way the problem can be resolved. By focusing on the challenges and developing hassle-free smart healthcare, the vision of smooth functioning of medical facilities can become a reality.

REFERENCES

1. L. Catarinucci et al. "An IoT-Aware Architecture for Smart Healthcare Systems." *IEEE Internet of Things Journal*, vol. 2, no. 6, pp. 515–526, December 2015. https://doi.org/10.1109/JIOT.2015.2417684
2. H. Zhu et al. "Smart Healthcare in the ERA of Internet-of-Things." *IEEE Consumer Electronics Magazine*, vol. 8, no. 5, pp. 26–30, September 1, 2019. https://doi.org/10.1109/MCE.2019.2923929
3. M.M. Nair, A.K. Tyagi and R. Goyal. Medical Cyber Physical Systems and Its Issues. International Conference on Recent Trends in Advanced Computing 2019, ICRTAC, 2019.
4. A. Kankanhalli, J. Hahn and S. Tan et al. "Big Data and Analytics in Healthcare: Introduction to the Special Section." *Information Systems Frontiers*, vol. 18, pp. 233–235, 2016. https://doi.org/10.1007/s10796-016-9641-2
5. C. Kaul, A. Kaul and S. Verma. "Comparative Study on Healthcare Prediction Systems Using Big Data." 2015 International Conference on Innovations in Information, Embedded and Communication Systems (ICIIECS), pp. 1–7, 2015. https://doi.org/10.1109/ICIIECS.2015.7193095
6. S. Dash, S.K. Shakyawar and M. Sharma et al. "Big Data in Healthcare: Management, Analysis and Future Prospects." *Journal of Big Data*, vol. 6, p. 54, 2019. https://doi.org/10.1186/s40537-019-0217-0
7. A. Alabdulatif, I. Khalil, X. Yi and M. Guizani. "Secure Edge of Things for Smart Healthcare Surveillance Framework." *IEEE Access*, vol. 7, pp. 31010–31021, 2019. https://doi.org/10.1109/ACCESS.2019.2899323
8. A. Solanas, F. Casino, E. Batista and R. Rallo. "Trends and Challenges in Smart Healthcare Research: A Journey from Data to Wisdom." 2017 IEEE 3rd International Forum on Research and Technologies for Society and Industry (RTSI), pp. 1–6, 2017. https://doi.org/10.1109/RTSI.2017.8065986
9. M.M. Islam, A. Rahaman and M.R. Islam. "Development of Smart Healthcare Monitoring System in IoT Environment." *SN Computer Science*, vol. 1, p. 185, 2020. https://doi.org/10.1007/s42979-020-00195-y
10. M. Nasr, M.M. Islam, S. Shehata, F. Karray and Y. Quintana. "Smart Healthcare in the Age of AI: Recent Advances, Challenges, and Future Prospects." *IEEE Access*, vol. 9, pp. 145248–145270, 2021. https://doi.org/10.1109/ACCESS.2021.3118960
11. S.P. Bhavnani, J. Narula and P.P. Sengupta. "Mobile Technology and the Digitization of Healthcare." *European Heart Journal*, vol. 37, no. 18, pp. 1428–1438, December 2016.
12. M. Ojha and K. Mathur. "Proposed Application of Big Data Analytics in Healthcare at Maharaja Yeshwantrao Hospital." 2016 3rd MEC International Conference on Big Data and Smart City (ICBDSC), pp. 1–7, 2016. https://doi.org/10.1109/ICBDSC.2016.7460340

13. G.H. Sai, K. Tripathi and A.K. Tyagi. "Internet of Things-Based e-Health Care: Key Challenges and Recommended Solutions for Future." In P.K. Singh, S.T. Wierzchoń, S. Tanwar, J.J.P.C. Rodrigues and M. Ganzha (eds), *Proceedings of Third International Conference on Computing, Communications, and Cyber-Security.* Lecture Notes in Networks and Systems, vol. 421. Singapore: Springer, 2023. https://doi.org/10.1007/978-981-19-1142-2_37

14. A.K. Tyagi, A. SU, G. Aghila and N. Sreenath. "AARIN: Affordable, Accurate, Reliable and Innovative Mechanism to Protect a Medical Cyber-Physical System Using Blockchain Technology." *IJIN*, vol. 2, pp. 175–183, October 2021.

15. S. Kute, A.V. Shreyas Madhav, A.K. Tyagi, A. Deshmukh. "Authentication Framework for Healthcare Devices Through Internet of Things and Machine Learning." In V. Suma, X. Fernando K.L. Du and H. Wang (eds), *Evolutionary Computing and Mobile Sustainable Networks.* Lecture Notes on Data Engineering and Communications Technologies, vol. 116. Singapore: Springer, 2022. https://doi.org/10.1007/978-981-16-9605-3_27

16. S. Kute, A.K. Tyagi, R. Sahoo and S. Malik. "Building a Smart Healthcare System Using Internet of Things and Machine Learning." In R. Fernandez and T.F. Fernandez (eds), *Big Data Management in Sensing: Applications in AI and IoT.* River Publishers, pp. 159–178, 2021.

17. S. Kute, A.K. Tyagi and M.M. Nair. "Research Issues and Future Research Directions Toward Smart Healthcare Using Internet of Things and Machine Learning." In R. Fernandez and T.F. Fernandez (eds), *Big Data Management in Sensing: Applications in AI and IoT.* River Publishers, pp. 179–200, 2021.

18. S. Kumari, P. Muthulakshmi and D. Agarwal. Deployment of Machine Learning Based Internet of Things Networks for Tele-Medical and Remote Healthcare. In V. Suma, X. Fernando K.L. Du and H. Wang (eds), *Evolutionary Computing and Mobile Sustainable Networks.* Lecture Notes on Data Engineering and Communications Technologies, vol. 116. Singapore: Springer, 2022. https://doi.org/10.1007/978-981-16-9605-3_21

19. S.B. Cáceres. "Electronic Health Records: Beyond the Digitization of Medical Files." *Clinics (Sao Paulo)*, vol. 68, no. 8, pp. 1077–1078, 2013. https://doi.org/10.6061/clinics/2013(08)02. PMID: 24037000; PMCID: PMC3752637.

20. A.A. Siyal, A.Z. Junejo, M. Zawish, K. Ahmed, A. Khalil and G. Soursou. "Applications of Blockchain Technology in Medicine and Healthcare: Challenges and Future Perspectives." *Cryptography*, vol. 3, no. 1, p. 3, December 2019.

21. A.M. Krishna and A.K. Tyagi. "Internet of Things Based e-Healthcare System: An Useful Review on Critical Issues and Challenges." *International Journal of Advanced Science and Technology*, vol. 29, no. 3, pp. 3223–3237, December 2020. 3223 ISSN: 2005-4238 IJAST, 2019 SERSC.

22. A.K. Tyagi, R. G and A. SU. Role of Emerging Technologies in COVID 19: Analyses, Predictions, and Future Countermeasures (December 16, 2020). Available at SSRN: https://ssrn.com/abstract=3749782 or http://dx.doi.org/10.2139/ssrn.3749782

23. M.H. van Velthoven, C. Cordon and G. Challagalla. "Digitization of Healthcare Organizations: The Digital Health Landscape and Information Theory." *International Journal of Medical Informatics*, vol. 124, pp. 49–57, 2019. ISSN 1386 5056.

24. D. He, R. Ye, S. Chan, M. Guizani and Y. Xu. "Privacy in the Internet of Things for Smart Healthcare." *IEEE Communications Magazine*, vol. 56, no. 4, pp. 38–44, April 2018. https://doi.org/10.1109/MCOM.2018.1700809

25. A. Kochanke. "Digitization in the Healthcare Industry: The Cloud Scheduler." *XRDS*, vol. 26, no. 3, pp. 34–37, Spring 2020. https://doi.org/10.1145/3383382

26. V. Jayaprakash and A.K. Tyagi. "Security Optimization of Resource-Constrained Internet of Healthcare Things (IoHT) Devices Using Asymmetric Cryptography for Blockchain Network." In D. Giri, J.K. Mandal, K. Sakurai and D. De (eds), *Proceedings*

of International Conference on Network Security and Blockchain Technology. ICNSBT 2021. Lecture Notes in Networks and Systems, vol. 481. Singapore: Springer, 2022. https://doi.org/10.1007/978-981-19-3182-6_18

27. M.M. Nair, A.K. Tyagi and N. Sreenath. "The Future with Industry 4.0 at the Core of Society 5.0: Open Issues, Future Opportunities and Challenges." 2021 International Conference on Computer Communication and Informatics (ICCCI), pp. 1–7, 2021. https://doi.org/10.1109/ICCCI50826.2021.9402498

28. A.K. Tyagi, T.F. Fernandez, S. Mishra and S. Kumari. "Intelligent Automation Systems at the Core of Industry 4.0." In A. Abraham, V. Piuri, N. Gandhi, P. Siarry, A. Kaklauskas, A. Madureira (eds), *Intelligent Systems Design and Applications*. ISDA 2020. Advances in Intelligent Systems and Computing, vol. 1351. Cham: Springer, 2021. https://doi.org/10.1007/978-3-030-71187-0_1

29. V. Mabillard and J. Mattijs. "Digitization and Co-Production of Healthcare: Toward a Research Agenda." Working Papers CEB 21-021, ULB – Universite Libre de Bruxelles, 2022.

2 AI and IoT for Smart Healthcare

Background and Preliminaries

Prabhjot Kaur, Sharad Chauhan,
Meenu Gupta, and Ashish Kumar

CONTENTS

2.1   Introduction 23
2.2   Related Work 24
2.3   Different Applications of 5G and 6G in Healthcare.....................................27
    2.3.1   Continuous Monitoring Using 5G 27
    2.3.2   User Identity Verification in the 5G MEC Network 27
    2.3.3   Smart Diabetes 5G..27
    2.3.4   Robotic Telesurgery Using Tactile Internet 27
    2.3.5   6G for Healthcare 28
2.4   Different 6G Technologies under Healthcare...28
    2.4.1   Internet of Everything...28
    2.4.2   Edge Intelligence 29
    2.4.3   Artificial Intelligence..29
2.5   Holographic Communication for Healthcare 30
2.6   VR and AR Under Healthcare..30
2.7   Artificial Intelligence in Healthcare..31
    2.7.1   Types of Diseases Focused by AI..32
    2.7.2   Machine Learning for Diagnosis of Healthcare Diseases.................33
    2.7.3   Deep Learning for Diagnosis of Healthcare Diseases......................34
2.8   Internet of Medical Things (IoMT)..35
    2.8.1   Intelligent Wearable Devices (IWD) 35
    2.8.2   Blood Sample Reader 36
2.9   Challenges in Healthcare..36
2.10 Conclusion 37
References...37

2.1   INTRODUCTION

The prevention of diseases has become a crucial aspect of healthcare due to the population's aging and the rise in chronic patients. Regular exercise, good nutrition, and recurring preventive controls not only promote prevention as a strategy to maintain

DOI: 10.1201/9781003321668-2

a healthier environment but also as a way to avoid serious conditions from getting worse. To meet patient requests, the future health sector will need to address the rise in chronic conditions and the lack of available therapies. Emerging technologies can be used in behavioral systems and protective policies to recognize probable health concerns early on and make it possible to schedule the necessary actions, including concurrently monitoring treatments and creating new assessments [1]. The global market for smart health is anticipated to increase at an average annual growth rate of 16.2% between 2020 and 2027, which was reaching 143.6 billion in 2019. To quickly enter health records and connect people, resources, and organizations, platforms for health systems that make use of wearable appliances, the Internet of Things (IoT), and mobile Internet are referred to as "smart healthcare." The actors involved in intelligent medical treatment are broad and include doctors, personnel, hospitals, and research organizations. It includes a flexible framework with numerous dimensions, such as the detection and prevention of disease, evaluation and assessment, management of healthcare, patient choice, and medical research [2].

The astonishing and empowering qualities of 6G communication technology have drawn the attention of many academics [3]. These qualities have been demonstrated via impressive breakthrough advancement in most fields, and they are expected to become apparent starting in 2030. Additionally, numerous scientific and technical methods as well as important contributions have been made by researchers worldwide regarding 6G.. In delicate and priceless healthcare circumstances, Artificial Intelligence (AI) and 6G are playing a vital role in fairly allocating resources. Unlike applications powered by 5G for smart healthcare, 6G is the real facilitator of AI. The primary indicators for diagnosis in healthcare with high bandwidth and minimal delay are "Virtual/Augmented Reality (VR and AR)."

The inability of "5G-driven VR/AR" in healthcare to enable a real-time platform for end users is one of its limits for multimedia transmission. It is crucial to use the right parameters while validating the "Fuzzy-based sustainable, Interoperable, and Reliable Algorithm (FISRA)" in e-healthcare systems [4]. With its high frequency, low latency, improved connectivity, and great stability, 6G are one of the newest, most potent, and smartest technologies available.

2.2   RELATED WORK

Mucchi et al. have discussed the importance of 6G technology in healthcare in the future. As a future aspect, 6G will be seen as the replacement for 5G technology. Our existing systems in healthcare are not sustainable in the future due to the rapid increase in population all over the world. Authors have proposed about wireless health perspective that could be followed by everyone in a proper way in their life that will be a vital and new way for the community. 6G technology provides the feasibility for wireless health by cooperating with the Internet considering the human body to be the part of the Internet. These smart wearable devices are used for recovering information related to health in daily life [1].

Abdullatif et al. have discussed the issue of the increase in chronic diseases in the last few years due to which causes of death also increases. So, the authors proposed that a smart healthcare system is required to improve the services provided in medical sciences. For managing proper services, reducing cost, and improving scalability, some intelligent healthcare is required instead of one-to-one interaction with patients. The authors have discussed reinforcement learning which provides support to an intelligent healthcare system. In their research work, they have discussed various challenges in healthcare and how they provide benefits by using reinforcement learning. They have also proposed emerging techniques used in these areas [2].

Khan et al. have proposed Internet of Everything (IoE) enabled intelligent services that are the future of wireless services. Fifth Generation (5G) technologies support the IoE services but for complex services; it didn't complete all requirements. So, for that, we required 6G to enable advanced technologies. In their research work, author have proposed some advanced technologies based on 6G like machine-learning (ML) techniques, networking, and computing technologies. They have also proposed some open areas for research in the future based on 6G technologies like AI-based adaptive transceivers, smart harvesting systems, smart business models, security models based on decentralization, blockchain-based smart business models, etc. [3].

Padhi et al. have discussed the issues existing in healthcare systems because of unbalance distribution of medical resources in rural areas. They have proposed cognitive data intelligence that can be used in monitoring the health status of people. They have also proposed one approach based on the Tactile Internet, cognitive intelligence, and IoT and termed as 6GCIoHE. This approach provides high performance in the field of healthcare in real time so that patients get better treatment. This will provide a theoretical framework in the field of cognitive healthcare by using cognitive intelligence capability [4].

Janjua et al. have suggested that diseases created by natural disasters affected people and society. Authors showed in their study that deaths and illness have increased in pandemic situations due to the non-availability of proper resources. But if proper action is taken within a particular time then we can stop this situation. In the current COVID-19 scenario, a proper system always is a factor in saving lives in this pandemic scenario. Wireless communication using 6G will be the basic need for such a system for developing a healthcare system. It is always a requirement that proper treatment will be provided to all patients physically or remotely. For that, healthcare systems require proper equipment and latest technologies. In their research work, authors have discussed healthcare communication challenges with proper solutions [5].

Sheth et al. have discussed in their research work that up to 2030, all development in 6G will be completed and adopted for communication. Various organizations are working on the problems and challenges of 6G. 6G technologies provide ultra-high and ultra-low latency which are useful for different applications that are not feasible with 4G or 5G technologies. The 5G technologies have some security and privacy problems and it is not suitable for some applications. In such a scenario, AI plays an important role by providing feasible solutions for these problems. In this research work, authors have proposed 6G technology based on AI technology which is suitable for future applications. For avoiding security and privacy issues, AI technology is incorporated with different applications [6].

Sodhro et al. have proposed AI-enabled healthcare applications that are efficient as well as cost-effective. AI-enabled 6G technologies provide an e-healthcare system that is efficient for almost every human being. They have proposed a cyber-physical system (CPS) by using it we can facilitate the healthcare system by connecting personal devices through the Internet. Cloud computing will be used for extracting and monitoring data from sensors and uploading them to the cloud. Due to the different types of data extracted from sensors, there is always the requirement for a smart, interoperable, and reliable healthcare system framework. In this research work, authors have suggested one model for getting ECG data to examine the health of the patients. They have also proposed a fuzzy-based algorithm that is smart enough to decide a case of providing priority to patients based on their conditions. Authors have proposed a cloud-based model for connecting healthcare with mobile. The given research work is better with previous approaches on different parameters like reliability, interoperability, and accuracy in the perspective of medical health [7].

Alshehri et al. have proposed future technologies related to the healthcare system which include AI, IoT, the Internet of Medical Things (IoMT), and 6G wireless technologies. They have suggested smart healthcare will be a requirement of the future and produce revenue in coming years. Authors have conducted a survey in their research work based on IoT and IoMT technologies in the healthcare system. This research work shows some challenges in the current scenario and provides some future directions in the field of smart healthcare system [8].

Nasr et al. have suggested that due to the increase in chronic diseases there is always a requirement for a better healthcare system. Smart healthcare system based on AI and ML is the more popular and better system for managing health issues in hospitals, nursing homes, and medical institutions. The authors have focused on this smart healthcare system with the help of wearable and smart devices for monitoring health-related issues. They have also suggested social robots for helping and assisting the living environment. The authors also highlighted software architecture for creating and integrating smart healthcare systems with the help of AI and analytic tools. This proposed system has discussed the smart healthcare framework, the functionality of the model, calculating performance and comparative analysis, and limitations of the smart healthcare system [9].

Jiang et al. have discussed that due to the development of AI technology, there is a change in healthcare data and analytic techniques. Authors in their research work have discussed the current scenario of AI and its future in smart healthcare system. AI techniques to help manage structured and unstructured data. They have discussed various AI techniques used in healthcare systems like neural networks, deep learning, and support vector machines for managing structured data. They have also focused on various areas in medical science like cancer detection, neurology, etc. where these AI techniques provide benefits. These techniques are also beneficial in the detection, diagnosis, and providing treatment in the medical field [10].

Secinaro et al. have proposed their reviews as the contribution of AI techniques in the healthcare system. They have discussed various applications of AI in the healthcare system. By the use of these AI techniques, it is better for managing health services, patient data, clinical decision-making, and diagnosis of diseases. It provides benefits in predicting the diseases and treatment of patients for these diseases.

It provides quality analysis, and knowledge-based management of data which also helps researchers in the field of healthcare [11].

Doupe et al. have discussed the role of ML in the healthcare system. ML is used to predict cost and quality in the healthcare system. Authors have developed an algorithm for predicting the outcome and included different steps in their works like data collection, learning parameters, and evaluation in this algorithm. In their research work, they have applied three approaches: first is the decision tree method for identifying different risks for an outcome. Second is a deep-learning method for identifying different patterns and third is ensemble methods for improving the prediction of improvements. These ML approaches will be helpful in different research problems [12].

2.3 DIFFERENT APPLICATIONS OF 5G AND 6G IN HEALTHCARE

2.3.1 CONTINUOUS MONITORING USING 5G

The requirement for ongoing patient monitoring is real. A system for diagnosing patients and warning them is built with the use of AI. The system demonstrated the shortcomings of 4G technology and the need for 5G technology using architecture simulations of 4G and 5G technologies. A case study on heart diseases demonstrated the validity of the efficient tool as a health surveillance tool.

2.3.2 USER IDENTITY VERIFICATION IN THE 5G MEC NETWORK

Because IoT data is so large and takes so long to analyze, mobile edge computing (MEC) uses a cellular base station to deliver data to the cloud. The validity of users' importance must be taken into consideration while assigning wireless resources to manage the data transference as well as processing preference on a cell network specifically designed for medical products [10]. Consider the case where the user's priorities are not verified. Then, a user having less necessity can allot more wireless assets to him, leaving low-importance users with insufficient wireless resources.

2.3.3 SMART DIABETES 5G

It is crucial to advance diabetes treatment and a prevention strategy since diabetes has an impact on both general health and the economy. The current problems with diabetes detection include an absence of a system for information interchange, the absence of ongoing advice to prevent and treat diabetes, and a lack of tailored analysis of vast volumes of information from numerous origins [11]. And for that reason, this diabetic treatment incorporates techniques such as smart fabrics and a 5G mobile network.

2.3.4 ROBOTIC TELESURGERY USING TACTILE INTERNET

The cognitive system, which is based on a 5G network and AI, includes physical and emotional stimuli. For wireless Internet connection to the tactile Internet, the

5G wireless network might make an appropriate reference system. In contrast to the conventional surgical concept, the telesurgery robot is a groundbreaking surgical technique that is employed in nominally protruding treatments all over the world.

2.3.5   6G FOR HEALTHCARE

Better patient condition tracking, the creation of automated healthcare warnings, and immediate as well as pertinent meeting with healthcare professionals are made possible by the merging of AI-powered algorithms with 6G. All of this helps to reduce hospital stays, mortality, and morbidity rates, as well as overall medical expenses. All modes of transmission – off-body, in-body, and on-body – are included in the body layer. Real-time data can be sent to edge devices and the cloud through off-body communications [13]. Particles or nanostructures which serve as biological transmission systems serve as the body's sensors [12]. The human body's biological cells have sparked a noble uprising known as the internet of bio-nano things (IoBNT), which enables inner-body monitoring and handling. The appropriate steps are then wirelessly activated after the nurse or the doctor receives the therapeutic data. Since it will enable IoBNT and IoNT connections, 6G technology is significant in this regard. Each human sense is used in the human bond approach to collect and send data. A human being's "thoughts" or experiences could soon be sent to another person. We can consider 6G as a "material" automation that provides an attractive experience for the users by utilizing the data stored by the sensors of emotions. It is feasible to provide enhanced services including patient monitoring, diagnosis, help, and treatment. VLC stands for visible light communication, a kind of visual wireless tool [14]. Light rays are used by VLC to deliver data. It is capable of gathering data from the body, facilitate extended user transmission, and take advantage of the architecture which could offer a network for improved communication.

2.4   DIFFERENT 6G TECHNOLOGIES UNDER HEALTHCARE

To fulfill the commitment, 6G communication techniques need accompanying technologies. 6G communication technology must be integrated with AI; it is an AI-driven tool. Additionally, 6G would allow the IoE to add different cloud services and help advance several industries. Also, 6G technology requires edge technology to offer cloud services to intelligent devices. So, numerous technologies make up 6G communication technology.

2.4.1   INTERNET OF EVERYTHING

Capturing, communicating, caching, thinking, computing, and controlling in 6G. Capturing involves high-level sensing. Holographic communication in healthcare is impossible without it. The recorded information is transformed into automated data, kept in a local cache, and sent instantly to distant places. Digital data may occasionally be further transformed into signals and sent to additional hardware for processing [15]. However, before computing, cognition aids in the preparation of workable conclusions based on input. They are wise decisions that aid in simplifying the computation. To regulate the actions conducted by smart devices for healthcare, computed data are sent to such devices.

2.4.2 EDGE INTELLIGENCE

Cloud computing will be used by 6G to store large data, process, and analyze [5]. Intelligent devices produce data that is sent to the cloud for storage, but this uses up transmission bandwidth. The exponential expansion of data has pushed technology nearer to information origin today. The edge technology is what this is. According to 6G's claims [16], it has a large ability to deliver slick services to billions of intelligent gadgets. The smooth and high-speed Internet services that 6G will offer to intelligent devices, which are essential for healthcare, will be provided through edge technology. In its edge nodes, edge technology continuously gathers, computes, and analyses health data [10]. The nodes were situated nearer to smart healthcare equipment. In a transmission, data of the user are transmitted to the edge devices. The end devices also calculate the healthcare information. Edge nodes then examine the data to most appropriate action to take. For instance, the edge node will analyze user health information it receives from smart healthcare tools to examine any type of deficiency in the user. The end nodes get continuous transmissions of healthcare information. The edge node keeps track of the medical data [17].

AI is utilized to detect patterns in the massive amount of health-related data that edge nodes receive and calculate such patterns for study. Using AI, edge nodes might create a picture, data, and edge analytics for videos. Giga sight is decentralized hybrid cloud architecture for video edge analytics. However, significant computing power is needed for AI methods. At the moment, running AI algorithms demands a lot of computational resources and power, both of which are restricted to edge nodes. To execute, they rely on the cloud. However, one of the network nodes in 6G will be the edge node. To give healthcare systems intelligence services, all nodes in the 6G network would be capable of AI.

2.4.3 ARTIFICIAL INTELLIGENCE

A completely AI-driven communication network will be 6G [5]. Using 6G, every component of network transmission would be smarter, enabling it to make decisions on its own when necessary. With 6G, the entire planet will be covered, which includes air, space, as well as the ocean. This is only possible by "intelligent AI" being created from the various communication components. AI algorithm implementation results in great performance and accuracy in communication networks. Healthcare powered by AI enhances clinical diagnostics and decision-making [18]. AI is needed in the healthcare industry to do jobs instantly. Data preprocessing is not necessary for deep learning (DL). Instantaneous data could be used as input because it does the computation using original health data. Additionally, in computing a significant number of network characteristics, it exhibits great accuracy. In a similar vein, other AI system currently being investigated on healthcare data is deep reinforcement learning (DRL).

Reinforcement learning involves the structure first formulating some judgments before seeing the outcomes. Based on observation, the decision is once more computed to produce the optimal result. DRL combines the advantages of deep neural networks and reinforcement learning methods [19]. DRL provides good performance within a short calculation time as a result. Federated AI will also share its information with other intelligent devices, improving healthcare. AI algorithms have performed well. Algorithms for AI demand pricey infrastructure. Proactive caching is another area where AI is recommended. All AI algorithms are quite computationally intensive. The heavy computation task requires more time and energy. However, 6G is unable to offer such comfort. The AI algorithms which would be employed in 6G will have issues. For instance, the neural networks have many layers. To improve the performance of 6G, which increases the efficiency of healthcare, research is being done to improve AI procedures having reduced calculation period and reduced power utilization.

2.5 HOLOGRAPHIC COMMUNICATION FOR HEALTHCARE

A hologram is a tangible representation of an interference pattern that creates a three-dimensional (3D) light field with dispersion. The created picture retains the actual object's depth, aberration, as well as other characteristics. Holographical transmission makes a hologram of the object by using cameras at various angles. It will utilize the integrated and improved core services of URLLC and eMBB. To deliver great service quality and stream high-definition videos, significant data rates are necessary. Furthermore, real-time speech and quick control responses demand very low latency. Holographic communication will represent a significant advance in healthcare. Additionally, 6G can deliver this service. 6G holographic communication will promote human interaction. In some emerging circumstances, the doctors must wait for the diagnosis from the professional doctor(s). However, holographic communication allows the patient's expert doctor(s) to be diagnosed while traveling. Moreover, she can oversee the doctors at an initial health intervention. In several cases, patients must visit several doctors before receiving a proper diagnosis, or the hospital may not offer the necessary treatment. The patient might need to travel to different cities or countries. It imposes both physical as well as monetary hardship on the sufferer in such circumstances. Additionally, it is exceedingly difficult for patients to travel when they are ill. However, doctors can diagnose patients remotely thanks to holographic communication. The only place the patient can go for treatment is the hospital. The use of holographic communication will also enable skilled medical professionals to give care across remote regions while still residing in suburbs or cities [20]. The 6G holographical transmission will aid in the global connectedness of healthcare, much like the 6G global coverage.

2.6 VR AND AR UNDER HEALTHCARE

The use of augmented reality (AR) makes actual objects appear more virtual. Additionally, it combines a variety of sensory faculties, including auditory, visual, somatosensory, and haptic. Along with real-time interaction, augmented reality also

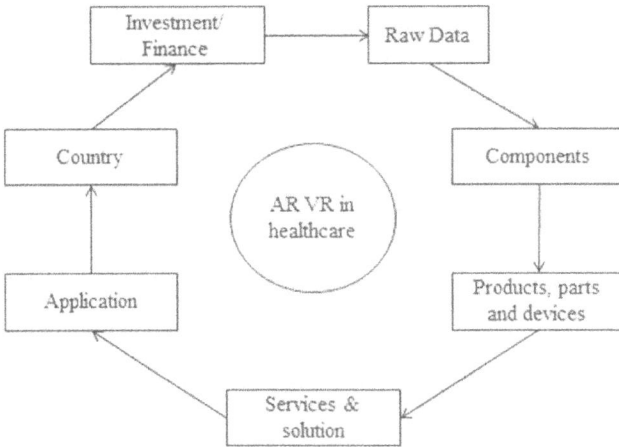

FIGURE 2.1   AR and VR in healthcare.

accurately renders 3D pictures of both virtual and actual items. The display of a created or digital world where nothing is genuinely real is referred to as virtual reality (VR). The primary service for AR and VR will be the combined and enhanced URLLC and eMBB. High-data rates are required for broadcasting high-definition videos as well as for providing high-quality service. Furthermore, good Internet speed is necessary for concurrent speech as well as quick controlled responses. The maximum data bandwidth of 1 Tbps and user experience of more than 10 Gbps with more than 0.1 ms of latency required by AR and VR can be provided by MBBLL [2]. Both AR and VR are at development stage at the moment as shown in Figure 2.1. 6G may, however, provide fresh opportunities for its application in the health sector. Without making any incisions, AR will make it possible to see into a patient's body. Doctors can also change the depth of the area of the body in question.

For improved visibility, the specified body part might also be made larger. The use of 6G will allow clinicians to view patients remotely. For improved diagnosis, holographic communication and augmented reality can be integrated. Doctors can practice medical operations in virtual reality without using actual patients. When doing risky, complex operations or surgeries, it will be highly beneficial [21]. These will all be intelligent gadgets having 6G Internet access. As was said before, for remote healthcare study or diagnostics, a smooth, as well as high-resolution presentation, can be generated using 6G.

2.7   ARTIFICIAL INTELLIGENCE IN HEALTHCARE

Recently, AI technologies have had a significant impact on the healthcare industry, sparking a lively debate on whether AI doctors would eventually take the place of human doctors. Soon, AI can help doctors make better clinical decisions or perhaps take the place of human judgment in some functional areas of healthcare, but we do not believe that human doctors will be replaced by machines (e.g., radiology).

New successful implementations of AI in healthcare are now achievable, due to the quick advancement of Big Data analytical methodologies and the expanding accessibility of healthcare data [4]. In the medical literature, there has been a lot of discussion over the advantages of AI. AI can utilize complex procedures to "learn" traits out of a variety of healthcare data and then use the learned information to enhance medical practice. It can also have auto-correcting as well as learning capabilities to enhance the accuracy as per user response. By providing real-time clinical knowledge from journals, textbooks, and medical practices to assist with optimal patient concerns, an AI system can assist doctors. Additionally, a system powered by AI can help reduce the inevitable diagnostic and therapeutic errors that happen with human medical care. There are two main categories of AI devices. The first category includes ML techniques that examine structured data, such as imaging, genomic, and EP data shown in Figure 2.2. The ML methods applied in healthcare applications aim to categorize patient traits or forecast the possibility that a disease would reveal itself [5]. The second category consists of natural language processing (NLP) methods that add to and improve organized medical data by extracting data from unstructured sources like clinical notes and medical journals. The goal of NLP techniques is to transform unstructured text into structured data that can be read by machines and analyzed using ML methods.

2.7.1 TYPES OF DISEASES FOCUSED BY AI

Although there is a rising volume of studies on AI in the health sector, these three disease categories, cardiovascular disorders, cancer as well as nervous system illnesses – remain its main emphasis.

1. **Cancer**: A double-blinded validation research showed IBM Watson for oncology could be a reliable AI model for supporting cancer detection. Also identified skin cancer subgroups by analyzing clinical photos.
2. **Neurology**: Bouton et al. created an AI system to help quadriplegic patients regain control over their movements. Additionally, testing was done on an

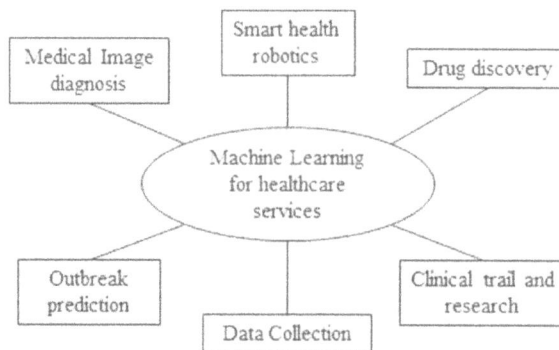

FIGURE 2.2 Machine learning for healthcare services.

off-line man–machine interaction that manages upper-limb prosthesis by timing the release of vertebral sensory neurons.

3. **Cardiology**: In [6] talked about the possible use of an AI system to detect heart problems through cardiac images. The Arterys Cardio DL program, which uses AI to automatically generate customizable ventricular separation based on traditional cardiovascular MRI scans recently received FDA approval to go on sale in the US.

It is not entirely surprising that attention has been focused on these three disorders. Early diagnosis is essential in preventing the deterioration of a patient's health status because all three diseases are major causes of death [6]. Additionally, by enhancing the analytical techniques on genetics, imaging, EP, or EMR, which is the core of the AI model, timely diagnoses may be possible.

2.7.2 MACHINE LEARNING FOR DIAGNOSIS OF HEALTHCARE DISEASES

ML generates data analysis techniques to derive characteristics from the data. ML algorithms use patient "traits" as well as occasionally interesting clinical results as input. Basic characteristics of a patient, like gender, age, and illness history, are frequently combined with disease-specific characteristics like gene expressions, diagnostic imaging, EP tests, medication, clinical symptoms, physical examination results, and many more. Along with characteristic data, the medical study mainly gathers patient health results. These include quantitative illness levels, patient survival rates, and disease markers [1]. ML algorithms can be categorized into two main groups: supervised learning and unsupervised learning, depending on whether the results are included. Although directed learning is ideal for analytical modeling by creating few correlations between the patient's characteristics (used as input) and the desired outcome, unsupervised learning is well recognized for feature extraction (as output). Lately, semi-supervised learning was presented as a combination of directed as well as and undirected study that is appropriate in situations where the result for certain subjects is unknown [22].

Clustering and principal component analysis (PCA) are both popular techniques for unsupervised learning. Without using the outcome data, clustering assembles participants with comparable qualities into clusters. Clustering methods generate cluster labels for the patients by enhancing and limiting the resemblance of the patients between and throughout groups. Three popular clustering algorithms are hierarchical clustering, Gaussian mixture clustering, and K-means clustering. When a variable is examined across a variety of parameters, like the number of genes in genome-wide association research, PCA is mostly used for dimension reduction [7]. The finest results are typically linked with the inputs which are most closely related to the results and are determined through a training procedure in supervised learning, which takes into account the individuals' qualities as well as their outcomes. Typically, the outcome compositions change based on the required results. Some instances of results are the possibility of having a particular clinical event, the expected magnitude of a disease, or the projected duration of lifespan [23].

Relevant methods include support vector machines (SVM), decision trees, naive Bayes, logistic regression, closest neighbor, discriminant analysis, random forests, and neural networks. The fact that determining the prototype specification is a curving optimization technique with a global optimum solution is a significant characteristic of SVM. Additionally, a variety of convex optimization methods now in use are easily adaptable for SVM implementation. SVM has thus been widely applied in medical research.

Decision trees, which resemble flowcharts and are common aids for medical decision-making, direct readers toward categorizing based on the low or high risk of a result. Using a decision tree, the study's sampled population is divided into successively small subsets, each of which has a different probability of the desired outcome. A good decision tree will divide the sampled population into groups whose probability of the result varies widely between groups but not much within groups [8]. A decision tree's advantage is its capacity to take into account nonlinear correlations among various factors that define subgroups in a data-driven manner. ML techniques based on decision trees may be most useful to healthcare system scientists whenever a research problem examines the variations of the threat of result among subpopulations or while taking into account numerous (and possibly multidimensional) complicated impacts on the risk of clinical outcomes that might be challenging to anticipate via conventional logistic regression [24].

Random forests and gradient boosting machines (GBM) are the two most used techniques for preventing overfitting in trees (RF). GBMs aggregate a variety of trees, each being built to reweight portions of the data, wherein mistakes caused by the initial tree help the following iteration's learning of a more ideal tree (called a boosting strategy). While RF also generates many decision trees, it aggregates a forest of several trees, in which each tree has individually trained to a randomized bootstrap-resampled version of the data (a procedure known as bagging), with a randomly selected portion of parameters chosen for suitable branch determination [5].

2.7.3 DEEP LEARNING FOR DIAGNOSIS OF HEALTHCARE DISEASES

Even though "deep learning" has increased in usage in Web and marketing literature, it belongs to a well-established and fundamentally old-style ML technique: the creation of neural networks. In a neural network, the outputs of one set of data manipulations feed the parameters to the subsequent sequence of manipulations. In the network, each transformer (or neuron) gets a calibrated input combination that reflects a calibrated value of the observable values (for the first layer of neurons) or from a previous layer of neurons (for the second and subsequent layers of neurons), and thereafter produces a result relying on a nonlinear transformation function called the activation function [9]. With the advancement of neural network design, it is now possible to train these models "end to end" using backpropagation or by simultaneously teaching every linked component. It is common to refer to the aforementioned network class as a multilayer perceptron. Different data types are used in multilayer perceptron estimator modifications. Convolutional neural networks, which make use of spatial dependencies among picture pixels, can be used in the investigation of images. Convolutional neural networks are employed in healthcare research for ophthalmology or radiology applications.

2.8   INTERNET OF MEDICAL THINGS (IoMT)

The "Intelligent Internet of Medical Things" (IIoMT) will develop and fulfill a variety of functions for the welfare of humanity in the 6G communication paradigm. AI-powered IIoMTs are smart machines that make decisions on their own and utilize communication protocols to do so. Along with IIoMT, IoE will also develop, allowing medical devices to connect to the Internet. MRI and CT scans are two examples. The scanner will scan the objects and use 6G technology to relay the data to distant areas. A pathologist can examine this data immediately. Almost all healthcare devices could be capable of Internet access, allowing for quick conclusion-making [25]. Therefore, the limitations of time, place, and money will be overcome via IIoMT as shown in Figure 2.3. Another illustration is the ease with which distant doctors may treat cancer patients. It takes time right now to determine if a cancer patient has benign or aggressive cancer. However, soon, 6G communication technologies will enable real-time cancer detection. Additionally, specialist hospitals are not necessary for doctors or patients [26].

It costs money and time. As a result, remote physicians will work with local physicians to treat cancer patients. The death rate for cancer patients who are diagnosed early can be almost eliminated. But these sensors must be created. This situation applies to numerous illnesses in addition to cancer. Consider cardiovascular therapies.

2.8.1   INTELLIGENT WEARABLE DEVICES (IWD)

Internet-connected intelligent wearable devices (IWD) send physical and intellectual information to testing as well as observation facilities. The heartbeat, blood tests, blood pressure, body weight, health issues, and nutrition will all be monitored by this technology. We'll get the test results back to you right away. Additionally, IWD gains knowledge from a person's personal body history and counsels them

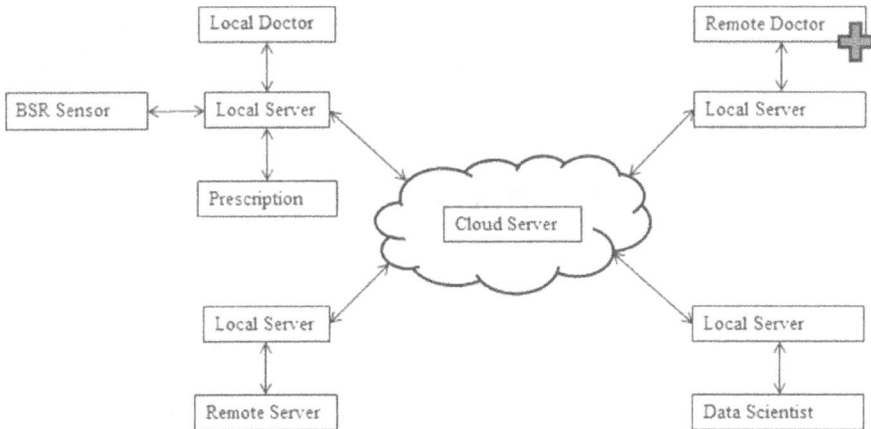

FIGURE 2.3   Healthcare system.

on their next course of action, such as suggesting a stroll or a run. IWD will keep a record of each individual's habits, diet, and health history. IWD can, therefore, recommend foods to eat in case of any inadequacies [16]. If minor physical issues like deficiencies are discovered, the number of visits to the hospital will reduce. Thus, it will lower hospital expenses and free up the hospital to concentrate on more complicated problems. Additionally, a blood sample will be read by IWD and transmitted for pathological results. As a result, IWD may be used to detect cancer in its early stages. IWD can, therefore, enhance health conditions and lengthen human life. Additionally, it is essential in services for the elderly because these services call for intensive care. IWD in the future will include several functionalities in a single device. One gadget will contain all of the functions. Such devices will cost a lot when they are first released, but as time goes on, the price will drop and more people will be able to purchase them.

2.8.2 BLOOD SAMPLE READER

The human body depends on blood, and most ailments can be identified by blood tests. For a traditional blood sample, a human being must be injected with a needle. However, there is a lot of research being done on devices for drawing blood without using needles. For example, Lipani et al. [27] developed a new needle-free way for diabetes sufferers to monitor their blood glucose levels. The sophisticated wearable blood sample reader (BSR) sensors would be without needles. The health sector will undergo a modification thanks to BSR sensors. All the specifications of blood like RBC, WBC, etc. can be correctly examined. The 6G Internet will continue to be accessible to this BSR sensor. Periodically, automatically, or with the patient's consent, a specimen of blood would be delivered to a testing facility for analysis.

As a result, checking blood samples won't require any personal intervention. This gadget will be essential for monitoring and providing intensive care for the elderly. Furthermore, BSR sensors might quickly put an end to the COVID-19 pandemic. The number of patients has surpassed millions, and nations are running low on medical supplies. The medical personnel becomes infected when blood is drawn using a needle [28]. Instantaneous spread monitoring of the COVID-19 virus can be done easily by the BSR sensor. Thus, it can be of great assistance in times of epidemics as well as pandemics. BSR sensors can, therefore, become a healthcare tool that is most in demand in the future.

2.9 CHALLENGES IN HEALTHCARE

The development of e-health makes it possible to gather, process, and analyze vast amounts of data from several devices and locations (such as hospitals, clinics) to deliver effective healthcare services. The development of edge nodes (such as cellphones) with integrated sensors, cameras, high-performance processing, and storage resources allows each patient or user to produce vast amounts of data whenever and wherever they choose. The patients can produce, gather, and share irregularly huge volumes of real-time data on their functioning and the environment around them [29]. Thus, I-Health systems become a heterogeneous and extremely dynamic environment due to the anomalies in producing and collecting medical data as well as the dynamism of the networks [30]. Furthermore, such dynamics are too complicated to be represented by static conventional optimization or simple stochastic assumptions. Experience-based learning is often required in such a highly mobile workplace.

2.10 CONCLUSION

ML algorithms can be helpful for researchers in health services that want to enhance the prediction of a healthcare outcome and have access to huge datasets for training and developing an estimation algorithm. ML techniques can provide generalizable data-driven estimators when choosing between a large number of covariates and when the result of concern might be influenced by intricate dynamic relationships and interaction effects. Intellectual healthcare should enhance the standard of living. The components of intelligent healthcare specifically include IWD, IIoMT, HIH, and H2H. AI combination, superior mobile connection, and assistance from cloud computing as well as edge computing are requirements for any IIoMT. BSR sensors are essential to IIoMT. IWD will be a ground-breaking medical device that comes with various sensors, including BSR. Numerous diseases will be automatically diagnosed with its assistance, and a person's health will be significantly improved. Additionally, there will be no need to visit the hospital for regular checkups like blood pressure, sugar levels, and blood work. Also, to check for any abnormalities, information related to personal health is sent to the health-monitoring center by IWD regularly. While IoBNT, in-body, and on-body communication, which is essential for the medical sector and could be time-saving as well as affordable for the government and end users, can be used for real-time patient monitoring with 6G technologies, there are drawbacks. As was already mentioned, these issues may be ethical, technological, or privacy-related and will need to be resolved to usher in a new era of cutting-edge technology that can suit industrialized countries.

REFERENCES

1. L. Mucchi et al. "How 6G technology can change the future wireless healthcare," *2nd 6G Wirel. Summit 2020 Gain Edge 6G Era, 6G SUMMIT 2020*, 2020, doi: 10.1109/6GSUMMIT49458.2020.9083916.
2. A.A. Abdellatif, N. Mhaisen, Z. Chkirbene, A. Mohamed, A. Erbad, and M. Guizani. "Reinforcement Learning for Intelligent Healthcare Systems: A Comprehensive Survey," pp. 1–31, 2021 [Online]. Available: http://arxiv.org/abs/2108.04087.
3. L.U. Khan, I. Yaqoob, M. Imran, Z. Han, and C.S. Hong. "6G wireless systems: A vision, architectural elements, and future directions." *IEEE Access*, vol. 8, pp. 147029–147044, 2020. doi: 10.1109/ACCESS.2020.3015289.
4. P.K. Padhi and F. Charrua-Santos, "6G enabled tactile internet and cognitive internet of healthcare everything: Towards a theoretical framework." *Appl. Syst. Innov.*, vol. 4, no. 3, pp. 1–29, 2021. doi: 10.3390/asi4030066.
5. M.B. Janjua, A. E. Duranay, and H. Arslan. "Role of wireless communication in healthcare system to cater disaster situations under 6G vision." *Front. Commun. Networks*, vol. 1, pp. 1–10, December 2020. doi: 10.3389/frcmn.2020.610879.

6. K. Sheth, K. Patel, H. Shah, S. Tanwar, R. Gupta, and N. Kumar. "A taxonomy of AI techniques for 6G communication networks." *Comput. Commun.*, vol. 161, pp. 279–303, 2020. doi: 10.1016/j.comcom.2020.07.035.

7. A.H. Sodhro and N. Zahid. "Ai-enabled framework for fog computing driven e-health-care applications." *Sensors*, vol. 21, no. 23, 2021. doi: 10.3390/s21238039.

8. F. Alshehri and G. Muhammad. "A comprehensive survey of the internet of things (IoT) and AI-based smart healthcare." *IEEE Access*, vol. 9, pp. 3660–3678, 2021. doi: 10.1109/ACCESS.2020.3047960.

9. M. Nasr, M.M. Islam, S. Shehata, F. Karray, and Y. Quintana. "Smart healthcare in the age of AI: Recent advances, challenges, and future prospects." *IEEE Access*, vol. 9, pp. 145248–145270, 2021. doi: 10.1109/ACCESS.2021.3118960.

10. F. Jiang et al. "Artificial intelligence in healthcare: Past, present and future." *Stroke Vasc. Neurol.*, vol. 2, no. 4, pp. 230–243, December 2017. doi: 10.1136/svn-2017-000101.

11. S. Secinaro, D. Calandra, A. Secinaro, V. Muthurangu, and P. Biancone. "The role of artificial intelligence in healthcare: A structured literature review." *BMC Med. Inform. Decis. Mak.*, vol. 21, no. 1, pp. 1–23, 2021. doi: 10.1186/s12911-021-01488-9.

12. P. Doupe, J. Faghmous, and S. Basu. "Machine learning for health services research-ers." *Value Heal.*, vol. 22, no. 7, pp. 808–815, 2019. doi: 10.1016/j.jval.2019.02.012.

13. E.N.K. Sharad and I.K. Aulakh. "Evaluation and implementation of cluster head selection in WSN using Contiki/Cooja simulator." *J. Stat. Manag. Syst.*, vol. 23, no. 2, pp. 407–418, 2020. doi: 10.1080/09720510.2020.1736324.

14. R. Caruana and A. Niculescu-Mizil. "An empirical comparison of supervised learn-ing algorithms." *ICML 2006 – Proc. 23rd Int. Conf. Mach. Learn.*, vol. 2006, pp. 161–168, 2006.

15. R. Caruana, N. Karampatziakis, and A. Yessenalina. "An empirical evaluation of supervised learning in high dimensions." *roc. 25th Int. Conf. Mach. Learn.*, pp. 96–103, 2008. doi: 10.1145/1390156.1390169.

16. M. Servetnyk and R. Servetnyk. "Emerging applications, technologies, and services in wireless communications: 5G to 6G evolution." *J. Sci. Pap. "Social Dev. Secur.*, vol. 11, no. 2, April 2021. doi: 10.33445/sds.2021.11.2.1.

17. P.K. Paul, B. karn, and R Rajesh. "Cloud computing & its deployment model: A short review." *Int. J. Appl. Eng.*, pp. 29–36, 2015, doi: 10.5958/2322-0465.2015.00005.2.

18. I.S.M. Ali Tunc and E. Gures. "A survey on IoT smart healthcare: Emerging technolo-gies, applications, challenges, and future trends." *Inf. Theory (Cs.IT); Netw. Internet Archit.*, 2021. doi: https://doi.org/10.48550/arXiv.2109.02042.

19. M.M. Kamruzzaman, I. Alrashdi, and A. Alqazzaz. "New opportunities, chal-lenges, and applications of edge-AI for connected healthcare in internet of medi-cal things for smart cities." *J. Healthc. Eng.*, vol. 22, pp. 1–14, February 2022. doi: 10.1155/2022/2950699.

20. S.M.M.S. Akbar, Z. Hussain, and Q. Z. Sheng. "6G survey on challenges, requirements, applications, key enabling technologies, use cases, AI integration issues and security aspects." *Netw. Internet Archit.*, 2022. doi: https://arxiv.org/abs/2206.00868.

21. S. Nayak and R. Patgiri. "6G communication: A vision on the potential applications." *Lect. Notes Electr. Eng.*, vol. 869, pp. 203–218, 2022. doi: 10.1007/978-981-19-0019-8_16.

22. K. Pahwa and S. Chauhan. "Big Data and Machine Learning in Healthcare: Tools Challenges." *Proc. – 2021 3rd Int. Conf. Adv. Comput. Commun. Control Networking, ICAC3N 2021*, pp. 326–330, 2021. doi: 10.1109/ICAC3N53548.2021.9725714.

23. S. Chauhan, S. Singh Kang, and Deepshikha. "Cluster based techniques leach and modified LEACH using optimized technique EHO in WSN." *Int. J. Innov. Technol. Explor. Eng.*, vol. 8, no. 9 Special Issue, pp. 363–372, 2019. doi: 10.35940/ijitee.I1058.0789S19.

24. S. Chauhan, R. Arora, and N. Arora. "Researcher Issues and Future Directions in Healthcare Using IoT and Machine Learning." In *Smart Healthcare Monitoring Using IoT With 5G*, Ist. edition, G.C.M. Gupta and V.H.C. de Albuquerque (eds). Boca Raton, London, New York: CRC Press, Taylor and Francis Group, pp. 177–196, 2021.

25. T.B. Ahammed, R. Patgiri, and S. Nayak. "A vision on the artificial intelligence for 6G communication." *ICT Express*, May 2022. doi: 10.1016/j.icte.2022.05.005.

26. S.A.A. Hakeem, H.H. Hussein, and H. Kim. "Vision and research directions of 6G technologies and applications." *J. King Saud Univ. - Comput. Inf. Sci.*, vol. 34, no. 6, pp. 2419–2442, June 2022. doi: 10.1016/j.jksuci.2022.03.019.

27. G. Gui, M. Liu, F. Tang, N. Kato and F. Adachi. "6G: Opening new horizons for integration of comfort, security, and intelligence." *IEEE Wirel. Commun.*, vol. 27, no. 5, pp. 126–132, 2020. doi: 10.1109/MWC.001.1900516.

28. S. Chen, Y.-C. Liang, S. Sun, S. Kang, W. Cheng, and M. Peng. "Vision, requirements, and technology trend of 6G: How to tackle the challenges of system coverage, capacity, user data-rate and movement speed." *IEEE Wirel. Commun.*, vol. 27, no. 2, pp. 218–228, April 2020. doi: 10.1109/MWC.001.1900333.

29. M. Katz, P. Pirinen, and H. Posti. "Towards 6G: Getting ready for the next decade." *Proc. Int. Symp. Wirel. Commun. Syst.*, vol. 27, pp. 714–718, August 2019. doi: 10.1109/ISWCS.2019.8877155.

30. K.B. Letaief, W. Chen, Y. Shi, J. Zhang, and Y.J.A. Zhang. "The roadmap to 6G: AI empowered wireless networks." *IEEE Commun. Mag.*, vol. 57, no. 8, pp. 84–90, 2019. doi: 10.1109/MCOM.2019.1900271.

3 Security and Privacy Issues in Smart Healthcare Using Machine-Learning Perspectives

*Ashish Kumar, Neha Gupta, Paarth Bhasin,
Sharad Chauhan, and Imane Bachri*

CONTENTS

3.1   Introduction 41
3.2   Related Works 43
3.3   Malicious Healthcare Hacks and Machine Learning 43
    3.3.1   Malicious Attacks in the Healthcare Industry 43
    3.3.2   Machine-Learning Algorithms in Healthcare 45
    3.3.3   Healthcare Hackers versus Machine Learning 46
3.4   Smart Healthcare Industry and Cybersecurity 47
    3.4.1   Robotics-Based Healthcare Industry 48
    3.4.2   Smart Healthcare System versus Cybersecurity 49
3.5   Challenges and Future of Machine Learning in Healthcare Cybersecurity 51
3.6   Impact of 6G 51
    3.6.1   5G and Its Limitations 51
    3.6.2   6G and Its Distinct Advantages 52
    3.6.3   Challenges and Trends in 6G for Future 52
3.7   Data Security 53
3.8   Difficulty in Inclusive Approach 53
3.9   Technical Requirements 53
3.10 Conclusion 53
References 53

3.1   INTRODUCTION

The healthcare industry is growing to address the increasing patients' demand and requirement. Nowadays, healthcare industry focuses on providing smart healthcare solutions to make patient self-dependent. Smart healthcare includes access to patient medical history anytime, anywhere. Machine leaning facilitates all these benefits in healthcare domain by addressing all the industrial challenges and modifying work-flow process of people information digitization [1]. This digitization has increased the volume of online data and, hence, healthcare domain has become prone to cyber-attacks.

Healthcare systems utilize Internet to ensure the anytime access of digitized data. Hence, the threat of cyber-attacks and security breaches is increasing daily. Hackers try to steal the healthcare data and can cause financial loss to the industry [2]. The information related to people is in danger, so it is necessary to protect data from unauthorized access. Hackers can breach into the system, infect the network and access critical information using malware or ransomware [3]. Hackers can monetize the attack and demand ransom from the people or organization. Security and privacy of the data is essential in the healthcare industry. There is a need for cybersecurity in healthcare industries to protect the patient's vital information from unauthorized access. In addition, antivirus software should be implemented for network security. Software should be updated constantly to protect network from newer threats. Also, machine-learning algorithms can be used for cybersecurity of data and to defend against the hackers.

Machine learning is one of the prevalent technologies for cybersecurity. Machine learning can defend a system from cyber-attacks. With the help of a suitable algorithm, one can read hackers' behaviours; it can also help to improve network and antivirus software [4]. Machine-learning algorithms, such as logistic regression, KNN, and Naive Bayes has applications in cybersecurity for health-care information. Machine learning can automate the healthcare processes and provide intensive treatment to the patient. Machine-learning algorithms can be trained on healthcare data and can diagnose chronic diseases such as cancer, benign tumours at an early stage. Self-learning networks can be used in health-care for analyzing the clinical findings such as X-ray, CT-scans, and MRI for diagnosis of disease. Also, machine learning has made the task of administrative staff easier and convenient.

In the era of COVID-19, technologies are helping the government in many fields. They can gather information about COVID-19 virus, easily monitor the patient's health, store patient's information, and track the Covid patient eas-ily. In India, corona patients are easily located with the Aarogya Setu app, and necessary medical aid can be provided for the treatment. Also, for Covid vac-cination, technologies assist the organization in a fast and quick gathering of the related information. Despite these advantages, various disadvantages are also associated with this technology. The model's accuracy is paramount in smart healthcare as minor errors may lead to severe consequences. Therefore, in this chapter, we will cover the use of machine learning, smart healthcare, and application of robots in healthcare industries, cybersecurity, and malicious attacks in healthcare.

It is the most common form of AI (artificial intelligence), which allows machines to first learn from the data and develop a pattern that helps in specific tasks. It con-sists of various sets of algorithms to perform the task.

3.2 RELATED WORKS

In the healthcare industry, machine learning has proposed prediction models for the early diagnosis of diseases. These models enhance the success rate of the treatment. In addition, healthcare organization can manage their data by using suitable machine-learning algorithms. Also, machine learning defends against cyber-attacks in the healthcare domain. In smart healthcare, AI-based robots work in cleaning, delivery, and assisting in surgery. However, robot-based surgery could be dangerous as a minor error can lead to a patient's death.

We have studied various machine-learning algorithms and their application in the healthcare industry. The details of the substantial work are summarized, and highlights are tabulated in Table 3.1.

3.3 MALICIOUS HEALTHCARE HACKS AND MACHINE LEARNING

With the advancement in the healthcare industry, cybersecurity is one of the foremost concerns. Hackers are regularly trying to breach the system and gain control of the potential information of the patient or the medical staff. Also, the credit card/debit card information that is stored online to make payment for the treatment is at risk. All this attracts the threat of cyber-attack in healthcare industries [9]. Attackers can steal all the financial information of patients and employees. In addition, they can disturb the treatment process by changing the data as all the information related to treatment is stored in the online database [10].

Machine learning is one of the most popular technologies providing solutions to cater cyber-attacks [8]. It processes the data and finds a pattern to enable decision-making. In the healthcare industry, machine learning can diagnose the early detection of diseases. Many organizations are using AI-based robots to provide advancement in the medical field [15]. The following section will detail the application of machine-learning algorithms to detect various malicious attacks in healthcare.

3.3.1 MALICIOUS ATTACKS IN THE HEALTHCARE INDUSTRY

Primarily, the attacker gains control of all the information to demand ransom. They can also use the debit card/credit card number to steal the money from the bank account [11]. In addition, attackers can manipulate the treatment history and impact the treatment process. Critical cyber-attacks have been reported in the healthcare industry, and the details are as follows:

- Once the attacker gains access to the network, they can easily encrypt files until the organization pays a specific ransom demanded by the hacker [9, 10].
- After gathering all the information, they can sell it to the other organization to know all the strategies of running the business.
- Hackers can use health insurance-related data and claim insurance [10].

TABLE 3.1

Details of Potential Work in the Domain of Healthcare Industry

Authors	Methods	Summary
Bhardwaj et al. [1].	Machine learning	They have explained about the use of machine learning in the healthcare field.
M. Chen et al. [2].	Stochastic Gradient Descent, CNN.	Used hospital dataset from city such as Wuhan (China) and predicted the risk of diseases.
Torres et al. [3].	Naive Bayes, SVM	Reviewed and summarized the various machine-learning algorithm. Application of machine-learning techniques for cybersecurity is also discussed.
Majumder et al. [4].	Artificial intelligence	Benefits of smart healthcare were highlighted and the cybersecurity using AI.
Bhatnagar et al. [5].	Machine learning, Naive Bayes, Decision trees.	Role of robotic process automation in pharmaceutical industries has been described, the impact of Ayurveda in Indian pharmaceutical sectors has also been described.
Fraley et al. [6].	Machine learning, TensorFlow	With the help of machine learning and TensorFlow, they have experimented to evaluate how machine learning could be leveraged for security event management.
Safavi et al. [7].	Blockchain technology	They have discussed the various possible threats in the smart healthcare system and proposed some solutions, they have summarized the various papers.
Newaz et al. [8].	Artificial Neural Network (ANN), Decision Tree (DT), Random Forest (RF), and K-Nearest Neighbours (KNN)	Model is prepared using different machine-learning algorithms. Action management module which notifies the healthcare professional in the event of any malicious activity in the smart healthcare system. And their accuracy has compared to each other.
Y. Xin et al. [9].	Machine learning, deep learning, SVM, KNN, Decision Tree.	Reviewed various machine learning and deep learning method for network security.
Zeadally et al. [10].	Artificial intelligence, Machine learning, KNN, SVM, etc.	Discussed cyber threats and proposed some solution based on AI. They have discussed various machine-learning algorithm in their work.
Liu et al. [11].	Machine learning, SVM, etc.	Authors have proposed various machine learning-based models to deal against security threat.
Wiens et al. [12].	Machine learning.	Use of machine learning in the healthcare industry has been discussed with the challenges of machine learning in the healthcare field.
Patel et al. [13].	IOT (internet of things), Big Data.	Types of robots and their application in the medical field has been described in the paper. Also, challenges of using robot in the medical field have also been described.
Yoon et al. [14].	Artificial intelligence	Summarized the success of robots in healthcare industries.
Chowdhury et al. [15].	Machine learning, SVM, random forest, Naive Bayes, Decision Tree.	Prepared a model using various machine-learning approaches for malware detection.

- After knowing the pay methods of patients in hospitals, they can use debit or credit card numbers and hack the bank account [11].
- They can manipulate treatment details as each patient's treatment details are mentioned in the database. In medical situation, change of medicine or treatment can lead to a patient's death.
- They can use mobile numbers to hack mobile and utilize the information for unethical activities.
- After gaining all the information, hackers can blackmail doctors into doing erroneous work.

There are various such attacks in healthcare industries nowadays, so it is essential to protect our data. Machine-learning algorithms provide the solution to prevent these attacks, and the details are as follows.

3.3.2 MACHINE-LEARNING ALGORITHMS IN HEALTHCARE

Machine-learning algorithms have changed the traditional diagnosis and treatment procedure in healthcare. Machine learning-based systems help in the early diagnosis of death-leading diseases like cancer and malignant tumours. Machine-learning techniques can be broadly classified as supervised learning and unsupervised learning.

- *Supervised learning* is a type of machine-learning algorithm in which models are trained using labelled data. Supervised techniques can be used for classification and regression. Examples of supervised learning are logistic regression [2], SVM [3], and linear regression, etc.
- *Unsupervised learning* is a type of machine-learning algorithm in which pattern is detected using unlabelled input data. It predicts the pattern of data on its own. It does not need any supervision from outside. Unsupervised techniques can be used for clustering and association.

Examples of unsupervised learning are hierarchical clustering, K-Means [8], etc. With the help of a suitable algorithm, we can train our machine and get desired results. Various machine-learning algorithms applied in healthcare are:

- **Logistic regression** is one of the popular supervised machine-learning algorithms. It is a classification algorithm used to predict the probability of the desired variable. Using this algorithm, the likelihood of the occurrence of a disease can be predicted [2]. Logistic regression can be used to identify malicious botnet traffic to prevent the cyber-attack [16].
- **Naive Bayes** is one of the most accessible supervised learning classification algorithms that can quickly predict diseases. This algorithm can also be used to prevent healthcare data from attackers [3].
- **K-Nearest Neighbour (KNN)** can be used for classification and regression [8]. In [17], the authors utilized KNN on healthcare data and provided the breast cancer detection model.

- **Support vector machine (SVM)** is a supervised learning type that analyses data for regression and classification. SVM can be used to detect cyber-attacks and malware [3, 11].

In sum, these algorithms help to improve the accuracy of medical treatment. The mortality rate can be reduced substantially by these advances in healthcare. In addition, healthcare useful information can also be prevented from attackers by applying these techniques in the cybersecurity model.

Figure 3.1 illustrates the basic methodology for implementing a suitable machine-learning algorithm in python. At the start of any machine-learning project, we need to import all the appropriate libraries which can be used during the making of the model. Python libraries such as pandas, matplotlib, pyplot are used for basic implementation. The evolution of the model is necessary to know the accuracy and errors. For error calculation, MSE (mean square error), RMSE (root mean square error), and MAE (mean absolute error) can be used. The next section will detail about the challenges faced by machine-learning algorithms to deal with healthcare hackers.

3.3.3   HEALTHCARE HACKERS VERSUS MACHINE LEARNING

Hackers steal the potential information from the organization for their own benefits. Terrorist organizations try to hack the research to find the biological weapon. Many hackers are just doing it for ransom or to sell the data. Cyber-attacks may be internal or external. Passwords can be leaked by the internal worker for money [9] or one can

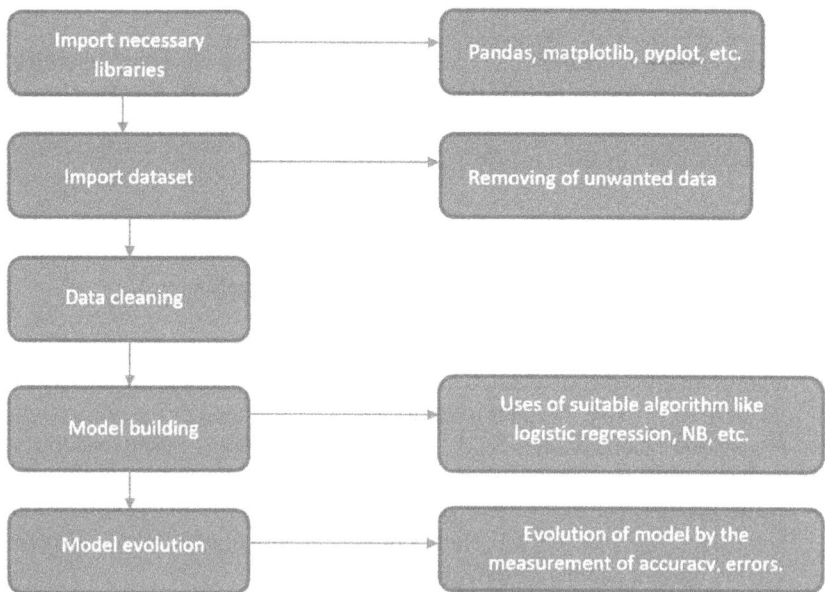

FIGURE 3.1   Step-by-step procedure for implementing the machine-learning algorithms in python.

help the hacker in system breaching. All these problems can be solved using machine learning.

Machine learning is a type of AI in which machine first find the pattern in the data given and then gives the desired output. A suitable algorithm and proper process are necessary for a better, accurate model in machine learning [14]. With the help of machine-learning algorithms, we can know the hacker's behaviour. We can understand their pattern of hacking and use this knowledge to defend our system against hacker. A threat detection system can be proposed using machine-learning techniques such as Naive Bayes, SVM, and others. Algorithms like fuzzy logic and neural network have been successfully used for malware detection [15].

Attacks like phishing are a type of crime in which hackers gain all users' information by fraud websites [18]. With the help of machine-learning approaches, one can find out the authorship of phishing attacks [6, 19]. Machine learning can be used to protect the network and modify antivirus software which helps to defend against cyber-attacks.

3.4 SMART HEALTHCARE INDUSTRY AND CYBERSECURITY

WHO (World Health Organization) defines smart healthcare as information and communication technology applications in healthcare, including disease control and monitoring, education, and research. The roles of technologies in healthcare are growing, with all industries taking help from technologies to ease their work. Healthcare industries make use of machine learning to manage their data. Nowadays, most healthcare data are uploaded on the server, which hackers can hack. Many hospitals started to get help from AI-based robots to have more successful surgeries [20]. They benefit from the latest technologies in the treatment to enhance the success rate. With machine learning, doctors can predict diseases at an early stage. In the COVID-19 pandemic, technologies are helping the government store all the information about death, recovery, and infected people. It is also helping in the vaccine drive, and government can gather all the information related to vaccination very fast.

With the growing technologies, the risk of cybercrime is also increasing. Now, hackers have many ways to break into the system [19]. Privacy and security are essential as all the information related to patients is stored in the database. Once the hacker gains control of the system, they can use the information for illegal work. They can take all information related to research and sell it to another organization. The various terrorist organization are also trying to hack the research-based industry to gain research-related information. Various news has come which claim that in the time of COVID-19 pandemic, one country tries to steal the information related to Covid vaccine from other countries.

In this era of social media, hackers can easily gain information about any people and organization. Social media companies are always trying to secure the information related to users, but vulnerability in technologies leads to cyber-attacks. In [21], the authors discussed various vulnerabilities in existing technologies and emerging cyber-attacks and different methods to overcome this challenge.

Cybersecurity is critical to defending against such attacks to protect people's privacy and security [22]. Many organizations use antivirus software to protect their system from hacker's viruses, as after breaching into the computer, they install the virus in the system. Organizations are using machine learning to know the behaviour of hackers [23, 24]. By knowing their pattern, one can defend their system from hackers. Many healthcare industries are taking the help of machine learning and deep learning to make their server better, so they can be protected against cybercrime.

Various precautions should also be taken to avoid cyber-attacks. One should use a strong password in their system. We should change our passwords regularly. Don't share passwords or email id with an unknown person. People should be aware of cyber-attacks and cybersecurity. We should avoid spam emails. We should not open any malicious link which can lead our phone or computer to a cyber-attack. Secure all necessary files with a strong password. The organization should use trusted software to avoid any cyber-attack.

3.4.1 ROBOTICS-BASED HEALTHCARE INDUSTRY

Many healthcare industries worldwide are taking the help of robots in the medical field [12]. First, the robots are trained according to human behaviour, and then they follow the same actions [4]. The use of robots not only decreases human effort but also improves efficiency. It saves time and money for the organization. It can work day and night continuously like a machine, so industries started to shift from human workers to robots [14]. The robot can be used in various fields like cleaning, delivery, treatment, etc. [13].

Various types of robots can be used in healthcare industries. The details are as follows:

- **Service robot:** This type of robot can help in cleaning, delivery, and stock control. Robots make human work easy and accurate. Healthcare industries are taking the help of robots for cleaning purposes as they save a lot of time and money. The use of robot is growing in the delivery area. Also, it can be used for the delivery of medicines in the healthcare industry. Many pharmaceutical manufacturing industries are also taking the help of robots in the working area, which reduces workers' workload. The uses of robots in packaging are shown in Figure 3.2.

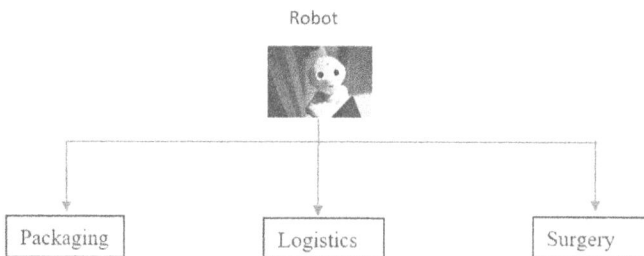

FIGURE 3.2   Role of robots in various industries.

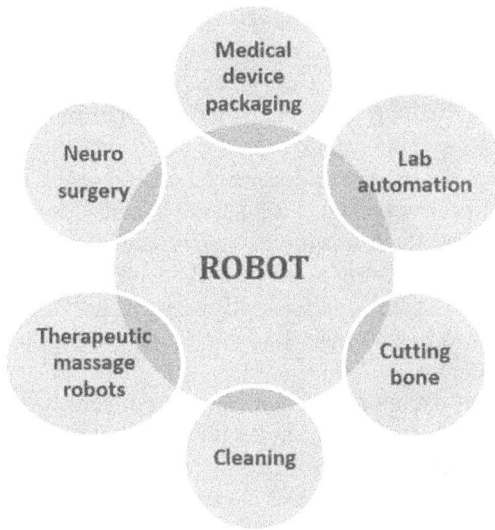

FIGURE 3.3 Application of robots in the medical field.

Surgical robot: This type of robot can help in treatments. It can help in stern and severe surgeries. Robots can provide better treatment according to instructions provided to them. It can easily do complicated surgery effectively and accurately. The robot doing surgery has been shown in Figure 3.3.

In [25], authors described the uses of healthcare robots for older people at home, various problems that older people face at home, and how robots can be used to overcome the difficulties. Robots can be used for home assistance. There is a need for assistance to senior people who can talk to them, do their general work, and do nursing work.

In Figure 3.3, various uses of robots in the medical field are described. Robots can be used in severe neurosurgery. The usage of robots in typical surgeries increases the success rate of treatments and reduces the risk of errors. In addition, robots can be used in medical device packaging. They can be used for lab automation purposes. The robots can also be used for therapeutic massage and the treatment of bones. Nevertheless, robots can be used to clean areas where humans can have the risk of infections.

Despite these advantages of robots in healthcare industries, there are certain disadvantages also. A robot is a machine and can't be fully trusted. Any technical issues can occur at any time and may risk the patient's life. There is the requirement of cybersecurity in case of hacking the robot. Hackers can control the robot's activity remotely and make it do unethical and harmful jobs. One major problem is that the jobs of people are at risk. With the use of robots, the need for human worker decreases. In developing countries like India, it will be a significant challenge.

3.4.2 SMART HEALTHCARE SYSTEM VERSUS CYBERSECURITY

Smart healthcare system uses modern technologies, but with growing technologies, the need for cybersecurity is also increasing. Many organizations nowadays started to use the latest technology for better, easy, and efficient work [12]. There are various applications of machine learning in smart healthcare to ensure cybersecurity [10]. It also helps in malware detection [15]. Machine learning-based systems can help the organization in developing their industries and managing internal data. These systems can store patient's information and the treatment details too.

Cybersecurity is essential because organizations are using wireless technology, the internet, and servers to store data [26]. All the information is stored on the server and hackers can hack all the info with the help of machine learning. Organizations can update their server with better performance. Security of the network is also very much necessary as the hacker can hack all the network. Organizations are using various technologies to defend their system from cyber-attacks. The organization can keep backup data also.

Healthcare systems use modern technology-based medical equipment for treatment, so if the hacker breaks into the system, they can change the system's instructions. Here also the need of cybersecurity is necessary. We can improve our network to defend against the attacker. Medical devices' security and periodic equipment inspection are also essential [27]. Some smart healthcare techniques are discussed next, which can help in healthcare industries and also help to protect the system from cyber-attacks [28].

- The disease prediction model forecasts the risk of diseases in the patient's body. M. Chen *et al.* [2] proposed a model based on convolutional neural network-based multimodal disease risk prediction (CNN-MDRP) and observed an accuracy of 94.8%.
- The malware detection model locates malicious activity related to cyber-attacks. Newaj *et al.* [8] discussed machine learning algorithm-based models and achieved 91% accuracy.
- The disease diagnosis model classifies the existence and non-existence of a particular disease. Mansour *et al.* [29] discussed the method (CSO-CLSTM model) for disease diagnosis with an accuracy of 96.16% for heart disease diagnosis and 97.26% for the diagnosis of diabetes.

The use of robots is also increasing in healthcare industries, and it leads to an organization towards security risk. Hackers can gain control of the robot, and the robot could do any criminal activity. So, by using better technologies in robots, we can defend the robots against cybercrime. Various use of cybersecurity is there in the hospitals [30, 31]. The details of the various ways by which the system can be defended are as follows.

- By improving the password into a strong password, changing the password from time to time can defend us against internal cyber-attacks.
- Improving our server network can defend us against external cyber-attacks.
- Using suitable IT technologies, one can detect malicious emails, software, websites, messages, and external links.
- By improving the wireless communication system, cyberattacks can be defended.

- Updating the technologies with the latest technology can also help us to defend against cybercrime.
- By using antivirus software, malicious hacks can be detected.
- Workers' education can also help to stop cyber-attacks. All the workers working inside the hospital should be aware of cybersecurity risks.
- Patient education is also helping to defend against cyber-attack. Patients should learn how to use all smart systems and new technologies and be aware of cybersecurity risks.

3.5 CHALLENGES AND FUTURE OF MACHINE LEARNING IN HEALTHCARE CYBERSECURITY

There are various challenges of machine learning in healthcare cybersecurity. The need for cybersecurity is growing with the increasing use of modern wireless, internet technologies and the growing use of smart healthcare tools in healthcare industries [32, 33]. The healthcare industry has all the responsibility to secure patients' privacy as all the personal data is stored in their database. We have to improve the technology and accuracy of our model so they can work correctly and accurately. When we use AI-based robots, accuracy of the robot is in question [34, 35]. Even a small bit of error in surgery time can lead to a patient's death. Hence, we have to improve the implementation technology of robots to enhance efficiency and accuracy. In machine learning, one should measure the accuracy using various algorithms and apply the best algorithms based on accuracy [36, 37].

Technology is changing with time, and we should also adjust accordingly. Many possibilities are there for the future in machine learning. The main challenge in machine learning is that the accuracy is affected if one can't appropriately apply algorithms. There is a requirement for a medical robot that can work accurately and ease the difficulties in the surgery field. We can make a system using machine learning to read the behaviour of diseases and increase the mortality rate.

3.6 IMPACT OF 6G

In India, 5G is recently launched in few metro cities. Before discussing the benefits of 6G in healthcare industry, it is essential to analyze 5G and its limitations.

3.6.1 5G AND ITS LIMITATIONS

With the incoming of 5G technology, the world is able to experience its benefits and is making use of its high-data transfer speeds which can go up to a few gigabytes per second. 5G has helped by improving the latency, data transfer rate, and reliability of internet connectivity. It also has had multiple applications in the healthcare industry [38].

However, it has its own shortcomings which have a huge impact on the healthcare industry. With medical organizations storing patients' private data on databases to improve data access for the medical workers, 5G technology increases the risks of hacking. Moreover, the speed of 5G is insufficient to match the pace of innovation of medical technologies.

3.6.2 6G AND ITS DISTINCT ADVANTAGES

The high speed of 5G is outperformed by the upcoming 6G technologies. With speed clocking to a few terabytes per second expands the possible applications of the internet services even further. 6G promises to offer applications in healthcare such as internet of bio-nano things (IoBNT), intelligent nanoscale inner body communications, in-body, on-body, off-body communications, visible light communication (VLC), holographic connectivity, ubiquitous connectivity, and many more [39]. By integrating AI-powered algorithms to 6G, we can more accurately track the patients' condition and develop automated healthcare alerts and relevant real-time interactions with all healthcare providers [39]. This not just helps the patients in places where human resources may be expensive but also helps in scaling of the services thereby giving the ability to reach a large number of patients. Applications of 6G are illustrated in Figure 3.4.

3.6.3 CHALLENGES AND TRENDS IN 6G FOR FUTURE

6G technology is still in its initial phases of research and has managed to have multiple applications in the healthcare industry. However, going ahead, the challenges in the implementation of the technology is yet to be discovered. Specifically, 6G will offer challenges in the following areas:

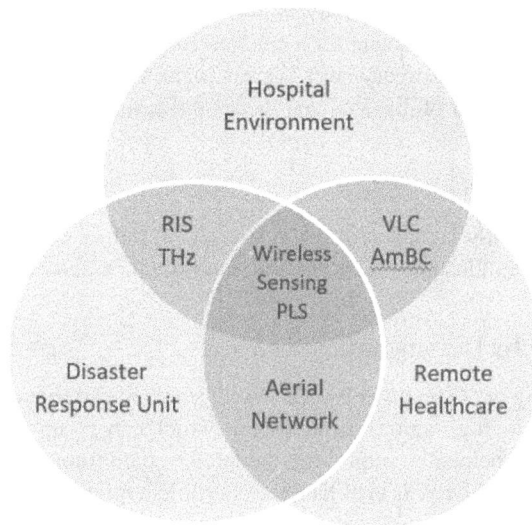

FIGURE 3.4 Applications of 6G.

3.7   DATA SECURITY

Considering the scale and reach of 6G applications, one of the greatest challenges will be faced in the areas of privacy and data security. Multiple authentication systems and complex cryptography would perhaps be required to counter this.

3.8   DIFFICULTY IN INCLUSIVE APPROACH

Keeping in mind India's diversity, especially in case of healthcare, healthcare literacy, and access to healthcare processes, the 6G environment will offer considerable barriers to be removed to reach out to the masses to achieve inclusive benefits.

3.9   TECHNICAL REQUIREMENTS

For 6G to succeed, we will need to have seamless communication network requirements so that combining and correlating data with real-time monitoring is possible so as to have real cost and time-effective benefits for both government agencies as well as the general masses.

3.10   CONCLUSION

In this chapter, we have discussed the potential cybersecurity risks in the healthcare industry. Machine learning-based cybersecurity algorithms ensure the integrity and confidentiality of the user's data to reduce cyber-attack risk. Use of smart technologies in healthcare is making it susceptible to cyber-attacks. Various cyber-attacks that can be a potential risk to the user's data and the need for cybersecurity in the healthcare industry have been highlighted in detail. Merits of machine-learning technologies that can defend medical process from cybercrime have been discussed at length. Robotics-based healthcare industries, the uses of robots in the medical field, and the risk of using these modern technologies in healthcare have been reviewed. Implementation of smart healthcare industry has been highlighted to address the real-time problems of users. Uses of technologies in the healthcare industry, cyber-attack, risk of cybercrime, the need of cybersecurity, information about machine learning in the field of healthcare, and use of machine-learning algorithms in cybersecurity have been discussed. The various challenges and future of machine learning in healthcare cybersecurity and 6G technology in machine learning have also been described to identify further research.

REFERENCES

1. Bhardwaj, R., Nambiar, A. R., & Dutta, D. (2017). "A Study of Machine Learning in Healthcare." 2017 IEEE 41st Annual Computer Software and Applications Conference (COMPSAC), pp. 236–241. doi:10.1109/COMPSAC.2017.164
2. Chen, M., Hao, Y., Hwang, K., Wang, L., & Wang, L. (2017). "Disease prediction by machine learning over big data from healthcare communities." *IEEE Access*, 5, 8869–8879. doi:10.1109/ACCESS.2017.2694446

3. Martinez Torres, J., Iglesias Comesana, C., & Gracia-Nieto, P. J. (2019). "Review: Machine learning techniques applied to cybersecurity." *International Journal of Machine Learning and Cybernetics*, 10, 2823–2836.
4. Majumder, A. K. M. J. A., & Veilleux, C. B. (May 11, 2021). *Smart Health and Cybersecurity in the Era of Artificial Intelligence* [Online First], IntechOpen. doi:10.5772/intechopen.97196
5. Bhatnagar, N. (2019). "Role of robotic process automation in pharmaceutical industries." In: Hassanien, A., Azar, A., Gaber, T., Bhatnagar, R., F. Tolba, M. (eds), *The International Conference on Advanced Machine Learning Technologies and Applications (AMLTA2019)*. AMLTA 2019. Advances in Intelligent Systems and Computing, vol 921. Cham: Springer. https://doi.org/10.1007/978-3-030-14118-9_50
6. Fraley, J. B., & Cannady, J. (2017). "The promise of machine learning in cybersecurity." *SoutheastCon*, 2017, 1–6. doi:10.1109/SECON.2017.7925283
7. Safavi, S., Meer, A. M., Keneth Joel Melanie, E., & Shukur, Z. (2018). "Cyber Vulnerabilities on Smart Healthcare, Review and Solutions." 2018 Cyber Resilience Conference (CRC). doi:10.1109/cr.2018.8626826
8. Newaz, A. I., Sikder, A. K., Rahman, M. A., & Uluagac, A. S. (2019). "Health Guard: A Machine Learning-Based Security Framework for Smart Healthcare Systems." 2019 Sixth International Conference on Social Networks Analysis, Management and Security (SNAMS), pp. 389–396. doi:10.1109/SNAMS.2019.8931716
9. Xin, Y. *et al.* (2018). "Machine learning and deep learning methods for cybersecurity." *IEEE Access*, 6, 35365–35381. doi:10.1109/ACCESS.2018.2836950
10. Zeadally, S., Adi, E., Baig, Z., & Khan, I. A. (2020). "Harnessing artificial intelligence capabilities to improve cybersecurity." *IEEE Access*, 8, 23817–23837. doi:10.1109/ACCESS.2020.2968045
11. Liu, Q., Li, P., Zhao, W., Cai, W., Yu, S., & Leung, V. C. M. (2018). "A survey on security threats and defensive techniques of machine learning: A data-driven view." *IEEE Access*, 6, 12103–12117. doi:10.1109/ACCESS.2018.2805680
12. Wiens, J., & Shenoy, E. S. (January 1, 2018). "Machine learning for healthcare: On the verge of a major shift in healthcare epidemiology." *Clinical Infectious Diseases*, 66, (1), 149–153. doi:https://doi.org/10.1093/cid/cix731
13. Patel, A. R., Patel, R. S., Singh, N. M., & Kazi, F. S. (2017). "Vitality of Robotics in Healthcare Industry: An Internet of Things (IoT) Perspective." In: Bhatt C., Dey N., Ashour A. (eds), *Internet of Things and Big Data Technologies for Next Generation Healthcare*. Studies in Big Data, vol 23. Cham: Springer. https://doi.org/10.1007/978-3-319-49736-5_5
14. Yoon, S. N., & Lee, D. (2018). "Artificial intelligence and robots in healthcare: What are the success factors for technology-based service encounters?" *International Journal of Healthcare Management*, 1–8. doi:10.1080/20479700.2018.1498220
15. Chowdhury, M., Jahan, S., Islam, R., & Gao, J. (2018). "Malware detection for healthcare data security." *Security and Privacy in Communication Networks*, 407–416. doi:10.1007/978-3-030-01704-0_22
16. Bapat, R. *et al.* (2018). "Identifying Malicious Botnet Traffic Using Logistic Regression." 2018 Systems and Information Engineering Design Symposium (SIEDS), pp. 266–271. doi:10.1109/SIEDS.2018.8374749
17. Al-Hadidi, M. R., Alarabeyyat, A., & Alhanahnah, M. (2016). "Breast Cancer Detection Using K-Nearest Neighbor Machine Learning Algorithm." 2016 9th International Conference on Developments in eSystems Engineering (DeSE), pp. 35–39. doi:10.1109/DeSE.2016.8.

18. Pandey, A., Gill, N., Sai Prasad Nadendla, K., & Thaseen, I. S. (2019). "Identification of phishing attack in websites using random forest-SVM hybrid model." *Intelligent Systems Design and Applications*, 120–128. doi:10.1007/978-3-030-16660-1_12

19. Martínez Torres, J., Iglesias Comesaña, C., & García-Nieto, P. J. (2019). "Review: Machine learning techniques applied to cybersecurity." *International Journal of Machine Learning and Cybernetics*. doi:10.1007/s13042-018-00906-1

20. Kolpashchikov, D., Gerget, O., & Meshcheryakov, R. (2022). Robotics in healthcare. Handbook of Artificial Intelligence in Healthcare: Vol 2: Practicalities and Prospects, 281–306.

21. Jang-Jaccard, J., & Nepal, S. (2014). "A survey of emerging threats in cybersecurity." *Journal of Computer and System Sciences*, 80(5), 973–993. doi:10.1016/j.jcss.2014.02.005

22. Coventry, L., & Branley, D. (2018). "Cybersecurity in healthcare: A narrative review of trends, threats and ways forward." *Maturitas*, 113, 48–52. doi:10.1016/j.maturitas.2018.04.0

23. Ahmad, M. A., Eckert, C., & Teredesai, A. (2018). Interpretable Machine Learning in Healthcare, in Proceedings of the 2018 ACM International Conference on Bioinformatics, Computational Biology, and Health Informatics (BCB '18), ACM, NY, USA, 559–560. https://doi.org/10.1145/3233547.3233667

24. Qayyum, A., Qadir, J., Bilal, M., & Al-Fuqaha, A. (2021). "Secure and robust machine learning for healthcare: A survey." *IEEE Reviews in Biomedical Engineering*, 14, 156–180. doi:10.1109/RBME.2020.3013489

25. Robinson, H., MacDonald, B., & Broadbent, E. (2014). "The role of healthcare robots for older people at home: A review." *International Journal of Social Robotics*, 6, 575–591. doi:https://doi.org/10.1007/s12369-014-0242-2

26. Ali, K. A., & Alyounis, S. (2021). "Cybersecurity in Healthcare Industry." 2021 International Conference on Information Technology (ICIT), pp. 695–701. doi:1110.09/ICIT52682.2021.9491669

27. Fu, K., & Blum, J. (2013). "Controlling for cybersecurity risks of medical device software." *Communications of the ACM*, 56(10), 35. doi:10.1145/2508701

28. Mansour, R. F., Amraoui, A. E., Nouaouri, I., Diaz, V. G., Gupta, D., & Kumar, S. (2021). "Artificial intelligence and internet of things enabled disease diagnosis model for smart healthcare systems." *IEEE Access*, 9, 45137–45146. doi:10.1109/access.2021.3066365

29. Jalali, M., & Kaiser, J. (2018). "Cybersecurity in hospitals: A systematic, organizational perspective." *Journal of Medical Internet Research*, 20(5), e10059. URL: https://www.jmir.org/2018/5/e10059

30. Conaty-Buck, S. (2017). "Cybersecurity and healthcare records." *American Nurse Today*, 12(9), 62–64.

31. Tian, S., Yang, W., Grange, J. M. L., Wang, P., Huang, W., & Ye, Z. (2019). "Smart healthcare: Making medical care more intelligent." *Global Health Journal*. doi:10.1016/j.glohj.2019.07.001

32. Ayala, L. (2016). *Cybersecurity for Hospitals and Healthcare Facilities*. Apress. doi:10.1007/978-1-4842-2155-6

33. Riek, L. D. (2017). "Healthcare robotics." *Communications of the ACM*, 60(11), 68–78. doi:10.1145/3127874

34. Luh, F., & Yen, Y. (2020). "Cybersecurity in science and medicine: Threats and challenges." *Trends in Biotechnology*. doi:10.1016/j.tibtech.2020.02.010

35. Janjua, M. B., Duranay, A. E., & Arslan, H. (2020). "Role of wireless communication in healthcare system to cater disaster situations under 6G vision." *Frontiers in Communications and Networks*, 1, 610879.

36. Kumar, A., & Jain, R. (2021). "Behavioral Prediction of Cancer Using Machine Learning." In Cancer Prediction for Industrial IoT 4.0: A Machine Learning Perspective, pp. 91–105. Chapman and Hall/CRC Press.
37. Kumar, A., & Ahluwalia, R. (2021). "Breast Cancer Detection Using Machine Learning and Its Classification." In Cancer Prediction for Industrial IoT 4.0: A Machine Learning Perspective, pp. 65–78. Chapman and Hall/CRC.
38. Al-Jawad, F., Alessa, R., Alhammad, S., Ali, B., Alqanbar, M., & Rahman, A. (2022). "Applications of 5G and 6G in Smart Health Services." *International Journal of Computer Science and Network Security*, 22, 173–182. doi:10.22937/IJCSNS.2022.22.3.23
39. Saeed, U., Shah, S. A., Khan, M. Z., Alotaibi, A. A., Althobaiti, T., Ramzan, N., & Abbasi, Q. H. (2022). "Intelligent reflecting surface-based non-LOS human activity recognition for next-generation 6G-enabled healthcare system." *Sensors*, 22(19), 7175.

4 A Framework for Virtual Reality in Healthcare
Insight for Disaster Preparation

Tina Dudeja, Akanksha Dhamija, Tanisha Madan,
Richa Sharma, Narina Thakur, and Zarqua Neyaz

CONTENTS

4.1 Introduction 57
4.2 Literature Survey 61
4.3 Proposed Methodology 62
    4.3.1 Development Procedure of Simulator Backend and Frontend 63
    4.3.2 Pediatric Triage 66
4.4 Conclusion 66
References 67

4.1 INTRODUCTION

Technologies such as AR/VR in education and gaming have already built their foundations. This review reflects on the application of this technology in emergency preparedness. Disaster is a phenomenon that cannot be expected and that causes harm, illness, and death. It takes place naturally, and each person has to cope with it and its after-effects. The concept here is to create a virtual 3D world to support the first learners in the training process with minimum costs and giving them real impressions of the situation. The ratio of deaths during a disaster will reduce considerably using these tools and the first responders or crisis relief forces will operate faster and more effectively. According to a study conducted by Texas University, about 45% of those qualified in AR/VR applications have 30% quicker real-life activities [1]. With rising smartphone proliferation and the popularity of artificial intelligence, tremendous R&D has been undertaken in order to explore more cost-friendly and efficient sensor technology and graphic-processing units [2], which have contributed to the development of inexpensive, augmented, and enhanced reality applications. These advances have allowed scientists in various fields to create managed virtual environments to communicate with digitally generated stimuli [3]. Decision-makers in environmental sciences and emergency management will use augmented and increased reality technologies to replicate different environmental situations to ensure that the situation is practical and safe [4–5]. The focus of this chapter is on creating a virtual environment that combines technologies – augmented reality and virtual reality – that

DOI: 10.1201/9781003321668-4

is more economical and respondents receive an atmosphere similar to situations and training in cases of calamity or emergency [1].

This work intends to add to the body of knowledge on training for disaster risk reduction. Investigations are conducted into the usage of virtual environments for training. Unfortunately, not many nations are completely prepared to face such catastrophes, and as a result, the urban poor are the group most at risk. Disasters are not always caused by environmental risks. They only become a problem when residents of the impacted areas can no longer endure or manage their impacts. By educating community members in the chosen region about the risks posed by typhoons and floods, the national warning systems in place for these hazards, and the precautions they may take to ensure their own and their families' well-being, we hope to empower them. Apart from this, we need a system which helps the above-mentioned communities with proper training using AR/VR technology.

The main feature of next-generation medical facilities is the incorporation of innovation in healthcare. Healthcare innovation must be viewed as a human-centred process that makes use of complex, advanced, distributed medical services and processes. When operating a VR surgical simulation system, one can imitate the realism of the actual procedure and lower the incidence of errors during the actual operation in the future. VR surgical simulation systems provide trainee or inexperienced surgeons with surgical training [6–7]. Actively promoting the well-being of citizens is one of the goals of the healthcare system. In this context, it is crucial to define advanced ICT solutions for preventive care, health status monitoring, and health and wellness education using data from environmental, wearable, and even in-body sensors. It makes it possible to build a network of continuously updated patient clinical data, assisting medical practitioners in making decisions [8]. By taking several factors into account, 6G technology can alter wireless healthcare in the future (technological, ethical and regulatory, sociological, etc.). 6G is viewed as a complete and pervasive connectivity fabric that enables the collection of many/all the required data from individuals (healthy and not), ranging from the activation of on-demand health check-ups to how much water a person has consumed daily (using sensors on the bottle, for example) to how many calories they have consumed daily (using sensors on/into the body) [9]. A growing number of patients impacted by disasters and a shortfall of medical resources to meet patients' needs for care will be an issue of the future healthcare system. Since future health services will depend on ICT, adoption is essential. The ability to measure some health indicators in real time, assess the patient's overall condition, and automatically share the clinical data collected from triage cards among all members of the care team are all essential for the customised management of the patient's health. These factors should be prioritised when managing the health of patients who have experienced a disaster. Distribution of triage cards for medical emergencies via wireless 6G technology is the vision of our research.

Triage cards are basically used in both healthcare industry and non-healthcare industry. In non-healthcare industry, they may be used for priority of project, publication and in healthcare industry, it may be used to distinguish among critical patients and non-critical patients. In our research paper, we have covered its usage in healthcare industry. They may be used at the time of war, disaster, and in situation when ambulances are less in number and there are more number of patients. In that case, triage cards are used to distinguish between patients. Coloured tape or marker pen may be used to mark the patient [10]. Triage cards generally consist of:

1. Patients identification
2. Progress of patient
3. Record of casualty

It may be used to identify the priority if the patients need immediate medical treatment. Triage cards are classified into:

Immediate: Those who need immediate medical treatment as they are critical but can survive.

Observation: Those who are stable and out of danger but still require immediate medical treatment. These patients are taken to hospital because they have better recovery rate than immediate patients.

Wait: Less Injured. These patients need medical attention but after patients in the immediate and observation category.

Expectant: The person has died or may be beyond the help of a doctor therefore cannot be cured.

Dismiss: These patients have no injury or with minor injuries that do not require any medical attention.

These five classes are coloured with different colours for differentiation. All information will be stored in the database so that it can be used in future. Automated triage system takes around 6 minutes to access the result as proposed in the paper [11]. Automated triage system is computerised triage system that gives more specific and accurate results than simple triage system which needs more resources.

The fusion of AR and VR technologies aim to create interfaces that have fewer screen time and more connections with humanity. The picture of tragedy in his paper was seen in the real world by Leebmann et al. [12]. Images of people concealed in rubble, destruction simulations, and interventions were imposed using structures of increased reality (ARS). ARS system architecture includes positioning, photogrammetry, inertia, and GPS differential navigation. The main goal of the paper is to decrease the number of deaths caused by a lack of planning for disasters by incorporating technology such as AR/VR into the industry, which has risen in recent years. Disaster impacts not only people's lives but also the environment, environmental growth, etc. A significant factor in avoiding the detrimental effects of catastrophe preparation of people and first responders needs to be considered on primary basis [12]. Figure 4.1 explains the movement of data from the centre hub to the sub-hubs.

Individuals with special skills, including firefighters and specialist rescue teams, may be involved in research and rescue operations. To check that these people require special clothes and breathing devices to protect them from environmental threats, they can enter the emergency area before participating. Once the victims have been

Communications center

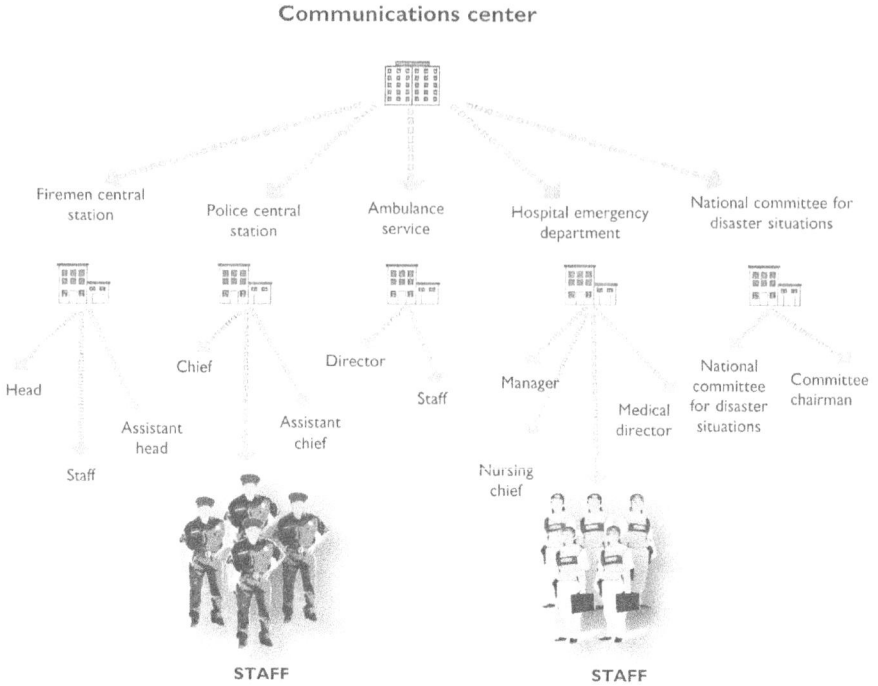

FIGURE 4.1   Movement of information.

identified by search and rescue teams, they must be brought to an assessment point of risk-free victims (field triage). The patients get first-aid according to their condition after this initial triage [13].

Many successful and practically implemented models have been deployed using VR interfacing and are facilitating humans with their functionalities. Few following models recognized are:

1. Gujarat Institute of Disaster and Management has created two models using VR interface which are used to create awareness among school students. The first model is an earthquake simulator which is an android application. The stimulator stimulates an environment of earthquakes in the school. The second model is a fire stimulator that stimulates the scenario of a fire in the classroom. This model is also an android application.
2. The University of Florida has created a web-based virtual reality game "burn centre" which will train and help healthcare workers and people with understanding the situation and injuries. The trainers or contributors can even earn credits from the game.
3. Indian Railway Institute of Disaster Management has created a train accident application using VR interface and is even training the railway officers for the situations that occur during railway accidents.

The theoretical work of the model is essentially defined. The second section explains the research done in the form of literature survey, with parts explaining the working of the model. The third section explains the proposed methodology in the field. The chapter ends with a conclusion in the last section.

4.2 LITERATURE SURVEY

This section examines the latest work in the field of AR/VR technology and 6G technology in healthcare employed by various writers in their literature-based study.

P. Jorge [14] proposed end-to-end analysis of performance delay and evaluated the criteria of reliability in 6G offered via VR framework services which is a challenging technology. The construction of end-to-end delay by application of supermartingale envelopes for reliable VR prediction for specified service profile. The proposed results have been compared to simulation results following ana-lytical predictions using theory of Markov queue. K. Omori [15] implements the procedure for control of infection in the affected area by utilising the VR groups which comprise the favoured response to consecutive learning method. It proves as a beneficial tool which provides each group with a similar circular content. After training, it uses the objective structured clinical examination. J. Bazyar [16] provides the range of the triage tags and the principles definite for every system including detailed circumstances of the area, the assortment of the disasters and emergencies, along with services and resources. It will test its model accuracy in instance of situations for actually injured victims. Since there will be a deficiency of accurate triage systems in clinics, countries need to have a triage system to effectively cast-off during disasters and emergencies. J.M. Franc [17] proposed a methodology called METASTART as it is a meta-analysis which recommends the START (simple triage and rapid treatment) method which does not provide enough accuracy to aid as a consistent disaster triage device. Though the accuracy of START method resembles disaster triage, progress of a further accurate triage technique should be immediately pursued.

Ronald B. et al. [18] focuses on applicability of triage systems for medical emer-gencies through a computational model depending upon the usage of the model. It may be using a wireless communication medium or an IoT-based chip capable of prioritising patients urgently in need. Most of the recent systems have been using START technology. The author proposed to develop a portable monitoring device to keep track of the health of patients through triage colour indications and storing all the information in a cloud-based repository for data acquisition. It also dealt with analysing the symptoms of the patients and dynamically acting upon them. Jokela et al [19] examined the dependability of a pro RFID and cell phone technology in two simulated mass casualty incidents. mTriage software is used on cell phones provided to rescue personnel at the disaster scene for RFID reading/writing. Tags linked to victims' "zipper collars" and Logica Merlot Office Media Mobile software on laptops and tablets officers stationed at the evacuation and treatment facility. The automated triage system, developed by the study in, is an automated triage system. The system is made up of triage decision-making algorithms, graphical user interfaces (GUIs) created with Microsoft Visual Studio, and biological modules. Through sensors built within the e-Health Kit V2.0, this system gathers the patient's vital signs, syndrome, and primary symptoms, processing the information using an Arduino Uno. Through serial communication, this platform communicates and transmits the data acquired to the GUI (created for Windows) for display[20]. A system that is tuned to assist the most damaged persons in emergency circumstances (IBSC) comprising of Near Field Communication wristbands given to the sufferers, a web service, and a mobile app (issued to medical staff and assistants). The smartphone app is intended to give medical professionals the victims' geolocation as well as a guide that suggests the best path to take care of them depending on the seriousness of their diseases and using a triage approach. The Travelling Salesman Problem is used as the foundation for routing resolution, and it is solved by utilising a k-partition method to divide the vast number of victims into several groups.

B. Lima [21] introduces a strategy for hospital emergency rooms to prioritise patients provided it comprises two primary parts: a smart priority suggestion and patient-monitoring system and an innovative hospital emergency smart band (HESB) (SPRPC). A. Follmann [22] proposes the time and calibre of triage which were compared using a triage algorithm created with augmented reality and telemedicine support. An Android software created especially for use with Smart Glasses adds information in terms of augmented reality using two separate techniques: by visualising a triage algorithm in data glasses and by making a telemedical link with a senior emergency physician using the embedded camera.

4.3 PROPOSED METHODOLOGY

The software is designed in such a way that it uses AR and VR interfaces in order to create a real-life atmosphere. The interfaces are created using various applications such as unity, echo AR, and Adobe XD. These interfaces are further linked with different stimuli(s) so that the person getting the training feels like they are actually in the situation and can work accordingly. The model will be trained in various situations such as earthquakes, fire emergencies, tsunami, and landslides.

1. The trainees will also get information about the triage tag which is one of the most important tags for the safety of individuals that have suffered or are injured at that moment. The triage tags are used to indicate how badly the person is injured and how soon he/she needs to be taken for medication. These tags are used to tell the doctors or other medical helpers who should be taken first for the treatment, who can wait, and who is dead. To learn about these tags is very important for the first responders in order to help every individual correctly.

2. After training by the stimulator, the trainees will be given an assessment that they must resolve. Their understanding and how their mind behaved during the situations would be represented as a result of the assessment, as shown in Figure 4.2.

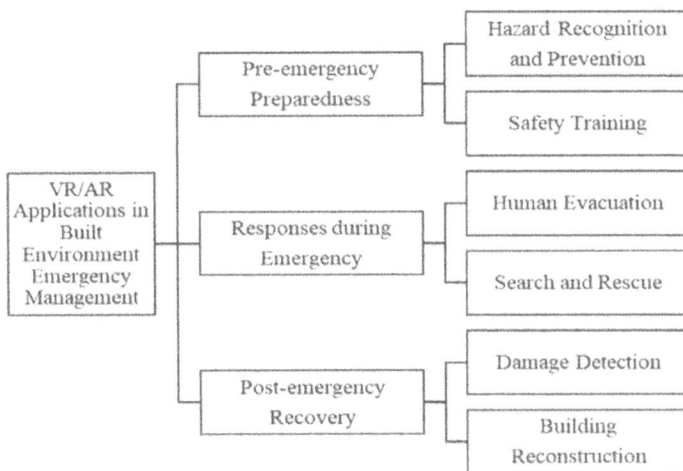

FIGURE 4.2 Key learning of the stimulator.

4.3.1 Development Procedure of Simulator Backend and Frontend

1. Firstly, the frames for specific situations will be designed using designing softwares.
   These frames will be converted to 3D form using unity and echo AR and then joined together to create scenes.
2. Frontend and Backend of the software will be designed and developed using JavaScript, AdobeXd, HTML, and CSS.
3. After the compilation of the software, testing will be done. Bugs will be removed if any and then final testing will be done.
4. The software will work easily on devices such as smartphones or using VR headsets. It will be eco-friendly and will cost around 3,000–4,000 rupees. The sensors used will give vibrations, water sprinkles which will feel like happening in reality.

The model will be used together with online videos and presentations. This will enhance the understanding of trainees. The learners can learn and perform at their pace. In addition, VR applications also provide interactive services such as voice communication. The trainees will be tested with the help of triage tags and a series of tests will be taken. They will be marked upon how they handle each type of victims and how they use tags to help the staff and victims, as shown in Figure 4.3.

Triage is a mechanism that enables care and transport goals to be established in order to save the most lives. It is carried out during the rescue process and uses priority treatment standards for patients, which differentiate between those who need urgent stability and carriage and those who can wait. Triage also requires patients to be identified for emergency surgery through a more comprehensive examination. The primary

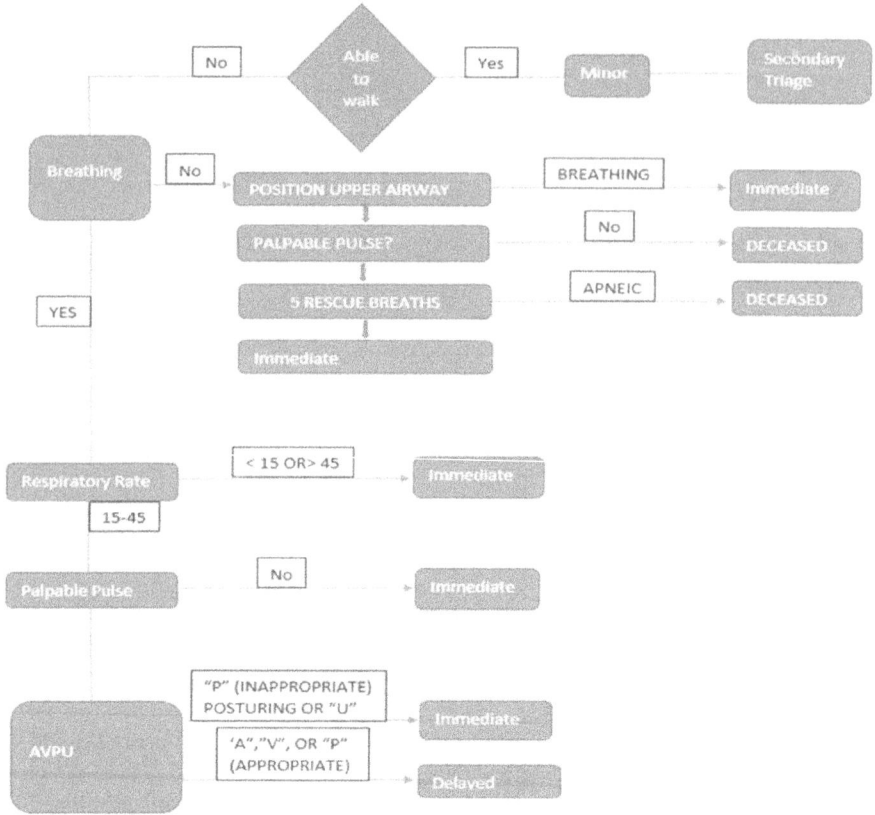

FIGURE 4.3 Paediatric triage working.

triage within an MCI is a fast assessment such that any victim can be assessed in a small space of time and care goals can be decided, as shown in Figure 4.4.

When patients are taken to the collecting site, the triage team must evaluate each individual victim immediately and refrain from delivering care other than haemorrhage management and short airway repositioning. Specific algorithms like the START were used to simplify this method using a colour-coding scheme (simple triage and rapid treatment). The START triage assesses respiration, pulse/perfusion and mental state. Before initial surgical intervention, all patients are treated first. During this assessment, any victim will receive an indicator of the degree of medical emergency with a particular colour-coded sticker, tape, or marker.

Decisions are taken solely on the basis of the state of the survivor. Patients are graded orange, yellow (moderately or as a matter of urgency), red (seriously or emergent), and patients who are gradually wounded (deceased) will be marked black. Three stages for field triage are carried out:

Triage on the ground: It classifies casualties in order to distinguish those who would be transported to the specialised emergency station straight away.

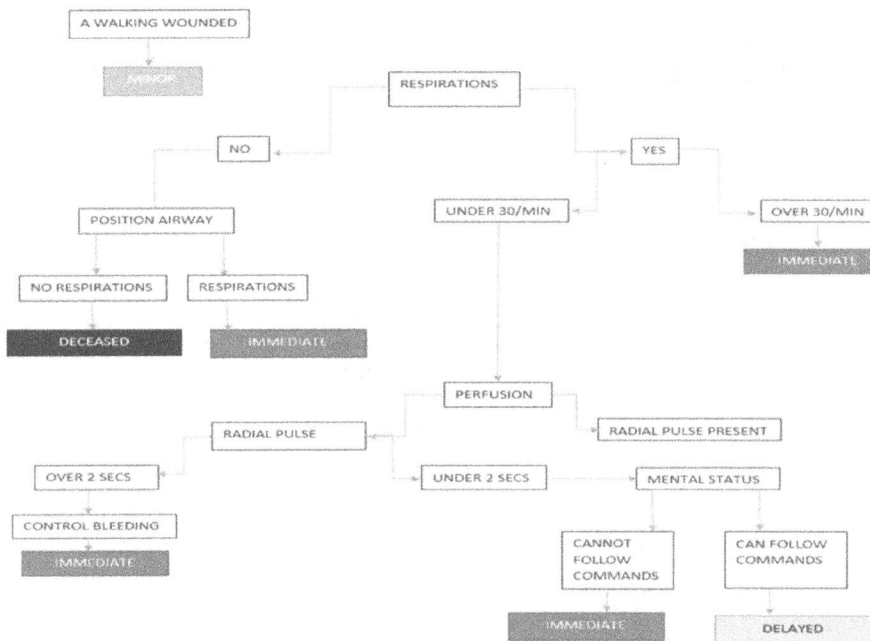

FIGURE 4.4 Working of triage tag.

On-site triage: It normally takes place by first-aid services or medical emergency technicians. If the technicians lack extensive triage expertise, they propose classifying the patients into categories "yellow" and "red." It is further classified into classification and evacuation triage cards which are described in Tables 4.1 and 4.2.

Triage for medical care: It establishes the level of care required. This type of triage should be done by an emergency physician, anaesthesiologist, or surgeon.

TABLE 4.1
Classification of Medical Triage

Colour	Specifications
Red	Settling is expected immediately.
Yellow	Medication that is delayed could be suitable.
Green	These victims may or may not have to be treated. This group covers ambulatory people and people with minor divisions and minor injuries or flames.
Black	Deceased

TABLE 4.2
Evacuation Triage

Colour	Specifications
Red	These victims have the highest priority for transport, ideally with a specialist crew to a tertiary hospital as surgery or organ maintenance or ICU services are required.
Yellow	The second-highest priority for transportation is these patients, including those who are currently healthy but who can pay or need an emergency operation.
Green	If possible, after being reviewed and trusted, these victims should be released on site. Those with minor injuries can, where available, be treated or forwarded to primary care.
Black	Transportation to the morgue.

4.3.2 PEDIATRIC TRIAGE

An updated triage algorithm based on physiological parameters applied to the standard set of pediatric principles is the JumpStart triage scheme. This system understands, unlike the adult triage system, that an apneic infant will continue to provide a degree of infusion until an irreversible heart loss secondary to anoxia occurs. These children will live with continued or resurrected respiratory activity that is not detected by the application of the START system, which does not require a palpation of pulses in patients whose apnea occurs after opening the airway.

4.4 CONCLUSION

Planning is vital in order to mitigate threats and hazards in case of a catastrophe. It should go from the family unit to the local society and its multiple bodies on separate levels. Both communities should create their own municipal crisis or emergency plan. The state and national strategy for this local emergency plan must be appropriately planned. Disaster preparations should include the specific needs of the residents affected and the possible movement of certain people who may pose threats to public health. The fundamental elements of the emergency plan are the following: scenario analysis, assumptions, priorities, targets, site organisation, tasks and duties, preparation, and the collection of relevant information. The strategy requires a practical evaluation, intensive preparation, and alignment of existing resources. A logistics scheme including the post office, specialised emergency office, evacuation and transportation, hospital treatment should be instituted for a reaction to mass casualties. This structure should be organised and ready-to-organise patient treatment for any component market.

This chapter presented a model or software to help and train the first respondents during a disaster. Training for disaster preparedness is essential for people living in areas prone to natural calamities. This software will not only help the first respondents but also the local people to understand the situation so that they can at least help their family and close ones till the help reaches them. The software will train and will inform people about the things, techniques they can use. The software is cost-effective, eco-friendly, and easily accessible. The simulator is used to train and teach first responders the techniques that can be used to save as many lives as possible lives during a calamity.

REFERENCES

1. Hsu, E., Li, Y., Bayram, J., Levinson, D., Yang, S. and Monahan, C. "State of virtual reality based disaster preparedness and response training." *PLoS currents,* vol. 5, 2013.
2. Deng, Z., Yu, Y., Yuan, X., Wan, N. and Yang, L. "Situation and development tendency of indoor positioning." *China Commun.*, vol. 10, no. 3, pp. 42–45, 2013.
3. Anthes, C., García-Hernández, R. J., Wiedemann, M. and Kranzlmüller, D. "State of the art of virtual reality technology." In 2016 IEEE Aerospace Conference, March 2016, pp. 1–19.
4. Freina, L. and Ott, M. "A literature review on immersive virtual reality in education: State of the art and perspectives." In *The International Scientific Conference eLearning and Software for Education*, April 2015, vol. 1, p. 133. "
5. Mucchi, L., Jayousi, S., Caputo, S., Paoletti, E., Zoppi, P., Geli, S. and Dioniso, P. "How 6G technology can change the future wireless healthcare." In 2020 2nd 6G Wireless Summit (6G SUMMIT), March 2020, pp. 1–6. IEEE.
6. Dascal, J., Reid, M., IsHak, W. W., Spiegel, B., Recacho, J., Rosen, B. and Danovitch, I. "Virtual reality and medical inpatients: A systematic review of randomized, controlled trials." *Innov. Clin. Neurosci.*, vol. 14, no. 1–2, p. 14, 2017.
7. https://www.disabled-world.com/calculators-charts/triage.php
8. Chong, H. A. and Gan, K. B. "Development of automated triage system for emergency medical service." In 2016 International Conference on Advances in Electrical, Electronic and Systems Engineering (ICAEES), November 2016, pp. 642–645. IEEE.
9. Leebmann, J., "An augmented reality system for earthquake disaster response." *International Archives of the Photogrammetry, Remote Sensing and Spatial Information*, vol. 34, 2004.
10. Zhou, Z., Chang, J. S. K., Pan, J., and Whittinghill, D. "Alternate reality game for emergency response training: A review of research." *Journal of Interactive Learning Research*, vol. 27, no. 1, pp. 77–95, 2016.
11. Ahuja, R. B. and Bhattacharya, S. "ABC of burns: Burns in the developing world and burn disasters." *BMJ*, vol. 329, no. 7463, pp. 447, 2004, https://doi.org/10.1136/bmj.329.7463.447. PMid: 15321905 PMCid: PMC514214.
12. Available: https://indianrailways.gov.in/railwayboard/uploads/directorate/safety/pdf/2019/DM%20PLan-2019.pdf. [Accessed: 19 January 2021].
13. Mitsuhara, H., Shishibori, M., Kawai, J. and Iguchi, K. "Game-based evacuation drills using simple augmented reality." In 2016 IEEE 16th International Conference on Advanced Learning Technologies (ICALT), July 2016, pp. 133–137. IEEE.
14. Gomez-Ponce, J., Abbasi, N. A., Willner, A. E., Zhang, C. J. and Molisch, A. F. "Directionally resolved measurement and modeling of THz band propagation channels." *IEEE Open J. Antennas Propag.*, vol. 3, pp. 663–686, 2022.
15. Omori, K. et al. "Virtual reality as a learning tool for improving infection control procedures," *Am. J. Infect. Control*, 2022, ISSN 0196-6553, https://doi.org/10.1016/j.ajic.2022.05.023.
16. Bazyar, J., Farrokhi, M. and Khankeh, H. "Triage systems in mass casualty incidents and disasters: A review study with a worldwide approach." *Open Access Maced J. Med. Sci.*, vol. 7, no. 3, pp. 482–494, February 12, 2019. https://doi.org/10.3889/oamjms.2019.119. PMID: 30834023; PMCID: PMC6390156

17. Franc, J. M., Kirkland, S. W., Wisnesky, U. D., Campbell, S. and Rowe, B. H. "MetaSTART: A systematic review and meta-analysis of the diagnostic accuracy of the simple triage and rapid treatment (START) algorithm for disaster triage." *Prehosp. Disaster Med.*, vol. 37, no. 1, pp. 106–116, February 2022. https://doi.org/10.1017/S1049023X2100131X. Epub 2021 Dec 17. PMID: 34915954.

18. Roland, B. and Christian, H. N. "The last decade of symptom oriented research in emergency medicine: Triage, work-up, and disposition." *Swiss Med. Wkly.*, vol. 149, no. 41–42, pp. 2–9, 2019. https://doi.org/10.4414/smw.2019.20141.

19. Jokela, J. et al. "Increased situation awareness in major incidents' radio frequency identification (RFID) technique: A promising tool." *Prehosp. Disaster Med.*, vol. 27, no. 1, pp. 81–87, 2012. https://doi.org/10.1017/S1049 023X1 20002 95.

20. Rivero-García, A., Santos-González, I., Hernández-Goya, C. and Caballero-Gil, P. "IBSC system for victims management in emergency scenarios." In IoTBDS 2017 – Proceedings of the 2nd International Conference on Internet of Things, Big Data and Security, 2017, no. IoTBDS, pp. 276–283. https://doi.org/10.5220/0006298702760283.

21. Lima, B. and Faria, J.P. "Towards real-time patient prioritization in hospital emergency services." 2018. https://doi.org/10.1109/HealthCom.2018.8531089.

22. Follmann, A., Ohligs, M., Hochhausen, N., Beckers, S. K., Rossaint, R. and Czaplik, M. "Technical support by smart glasses during a mass casualty incident: A randomized controlled simulation trial on technically assisted triage and telemedical app use in disaster medicine." *J. Med. Internet Res.*, vol. 21, no. 1, pp. 1–10, 2019. https://doi.org/10.2196/11939.

5 Mobile Healthcare Applications

Critical Privacy and Security Issues, Challenges, and Solutions

Sunita Kumari, Arush Sachdeva,
Anant Bansal, and Deepanshu Pal

CONTENTS

5.1 Introduction 70
    5.1.1 Contributions 72
    5.1.2 Organization of the Chapter 72
5.2 Background..72
    5.2.1 Mobile Healthcare Applications...72
    5.2.2 Privacy Policy..74
    5.2.3 6G 74
5.3 Related Work 75
5.4 Threat and Vulnerability Analysis 83
    5.4.1 Threat Modeling 84
        5.4.1.1 Threat Agents...84
    5.4.2 Attack Surface and Vulnerabilities.......................................84
5.5 Testing Methods..87
    5.5.1 Static Analysis 87
    5.5.2 Dynamic Analysis 88
    5.5.3 Web Server Connection 89
    5.5.4 Privacy Policy Inspection 89
5.6 Case Study 89
    5.6.1 App Selection and Preparation 89
    5.6.2 Test Environment, Database, and Other Tools 90
    5.6.3 Results of Testing..90
5.7 Reviewed Methodology 90
    5.7.1 Review Planning..90
        5.7.1.1 Research Objective 90
        5.7.1.2 Research Questions..91
        5.7.1.3 Research Criteria 92
    5.7.2 Literature Research..92
        5.7.2.1 Exploring Database..92

DOI: 10.1201/9781003321668-5

69

        5.7.2.2   Analyzing Existing Surveys...92
        5.7.2.3   Finding Gaps...93
    5.7.3   Conducting Review...94
        5.7.3.1   Creating Taxonomy..94
        5.7.3.2   Finding Solutions 96
5.8 Evaluation 96
    5.8.1   Evaluation Objectives 96
    5.8.2   Evaluation Methods 96
        5.8.2.1   Data Collections..96
        5.8.2.2   Security and Privacy Challenges 103
        5.8.2.3   mHealth Cloud Storage... 108
        5.8.2.4   Privacy and Security Issues in Digi Health
                  Application of 6G.. 108
        5.8.2.5   Mobile Devices Security Measures 109
        5.8.2.6   HealthCare Applications Infrastructure 110
5.9 Discussion... 110
    5.9.1   Legal Discussion.. 110
    5.9.2   Dark Web – An Inspiration for Data Thefts.................................... 110
    5.9.3   Roles of Institutions in Regulating Privacy and Healthcare-
            Related Issues 112
5.10 Results.. 112
    5.10.1 Manual Analysis.. 112
        5.10.1.1 Static Code Analysis.. 114
        5.10.1.2 Dynamic Code Analysis 114
5.11 Conclusion and Future Work 117
Acknowledgment 118
References..118

5.1 INTRODUCTION

The use of mobile phones has transformed radically over the years. Now the usage of mobile phones does not terminate on just phone calls and SMS. Nowadays, mobile phones are mini-computers that can help us with everything from healthcare to video calls and gaming to banking, making our lives easier. Advantages and disadvantages are two sides of a coin. The multifarious use of phones brings certain limitations as well.

There is a growing awareness that recognizes the potential of mobile healthcare applications to contribute to the betterment and well-being of society. With the passing years, there has been a shift in the mode of medications taken by the people. Especially in the time of Covid, people avoided visiting hospitals and mobile healthcare emerged to be a golden option for them. The features provided by mobile healthcare apps have made users forget the face-to-face consultation with doctors. The attributes of these apps like real-time monitoring, 24/7 doctor support, low fees charged by doctors, and diet plans have made it an even more efficient way of medication and this feature of healthcare applications attracts many users toward it.

Although healthcare applications appear to be a commendable choice for medical facilities but at the same time, there is a noticeable growth in privacy issues faced by users. There is a growing concern about the information shared with the mHealth applications which may lead to malicious hacking, DoS, DDoS attacks, device hijacking, unauthorized access, disclosure of personal health information, data ownership disputes, and privacy violations.

According to Indian IT regulations, applications developed by Registered Medical Practitioners (RMPs) must completely comply with the Indian Medical Council (Professional Conduct, Etiquette and Ethics) Regulations, 2002, as well as the relevant provisions of the IT Act, data protection and privacy laws, or any applicable rules announced from time to time for safeguarding patient privacy and confidentiality and regulating the management and transmission of such personal information. This will be legally binding, and it must be followed. Prior to listing any RMP on its online platform, technology platforms must do due diligence. Every RMP featured on the site must have his or her name, qualification, and registration number, as well as contact information. Patients cannot be counselled by technology platforms based on artificial intelligence/machine learning, nor can they be prescribed drugs. Only an RMP has the authority to counsel or prescribe, and must engage directly with the patient in this regard. While current technologies like artificial intelligence, the Internet of Things, advanced data science-based decision support systems, and others may aid and support an RMP in patient evaluation, diagnosis, or treatment, the ultimate prescription or counselling must be delivered directly by the RMP. If a specific technology platform is determined to be in breach, BoG, and MCI may designate the platform as blacklisted, and no RMP may utilize it to deliver telemedicine [1]. One of the well-known data collectors discovered that 80% of all Covid monitoring apps leak data and that roughly 70% of apps have at least one high-level security risk after analyzing healthcare apps [2].

The edited book chapter can be summarized in the following points:

- Users of mobile healthcare applications although they have numerous advantages over direct consultation with doctors but this brings serious security and privacy issues [3].
- It has been well analyzed that those features and permissions have been present in healthcare applications and the risks they pose for the users.
- Experience shared by the users has also been analyzed and it is found that mined data can be sold easily on the dark web.
- Solutions for users as well as developers have been discussed regarding this problem. Legal obligations that can be imposed by required authorities are also discussed in this chapter.

Three basic necessary regulations for data protection as per

- Comprehensive privacy policies – The applications should provide privacy policies such that data breaches can be controlled in every manner leading to the completeness of privacy policies.

- Uniformity of data collection – The data collected by the application should not be more than what is declared in their respective privacy policies [4].
- Security of data transmission – The data transmitted to the server of the apps for improving their services must not be forwarded to any third party and it should be ensured that no external element has access to the data before, after, and during transmission.

5.1.1 CONTRIBUTIONS

- In this chapter, the following research contributions are discussed: Analysis of mobile healthcare applications using different software to identify the data which is being forwarded to third-party servers.
- Analysis of permissions, features, and privacy policies of healthcare applications to identify challenges faced by these applications to comply with privacy laws of India and to analyze the risk posed by users of these applications.
- Analysis of Personal Health Information (PHI) which is being traded on the other side of the web [5].
- Description and analysis of notions and reviews of the users toward healthcare applications.
- Discussions of privacy laws as per the Indian Penal Code to protect mHealthCare applications users of India.
- Elucidation of different organizations related to healthcare and security as well as their duties and responsibilities toward the nation.
- Proposal of a novel framework to enhance the privacy and security of mobile healthcare application users.

5.1.2 ORGANIZATION OF THE CHAPTER

The rest of the chapter is organized as follows. The next section discusses the background, the second section explains threats and vulnerability, the third section describes testing methods, the fourth section discusses about the case study, the fifth section studies a reviewed methodology, the sixth section explains evaluation, the seventh section includes discussion, and the eighth section elaborates on results. and the last section summarizes the conclusion and future work [5].

The following Figure 5.1 summarizes the chapter in the form of a diagram.

5.2   BACKGROUND

This section is written to make the reader understand the topic and its importance. It provides the prerequisites for the chapter and summarizes the currently known literature on the topic.

5.2.1 MOBILE HEALTHCARE APPLICATIONS

Also known as mHealthCare applications, these are some new-generation applications that are used to easily connect the physician and the patient. In times of COVID, it was impossible for people to visit a doctor for normal ailments due to the

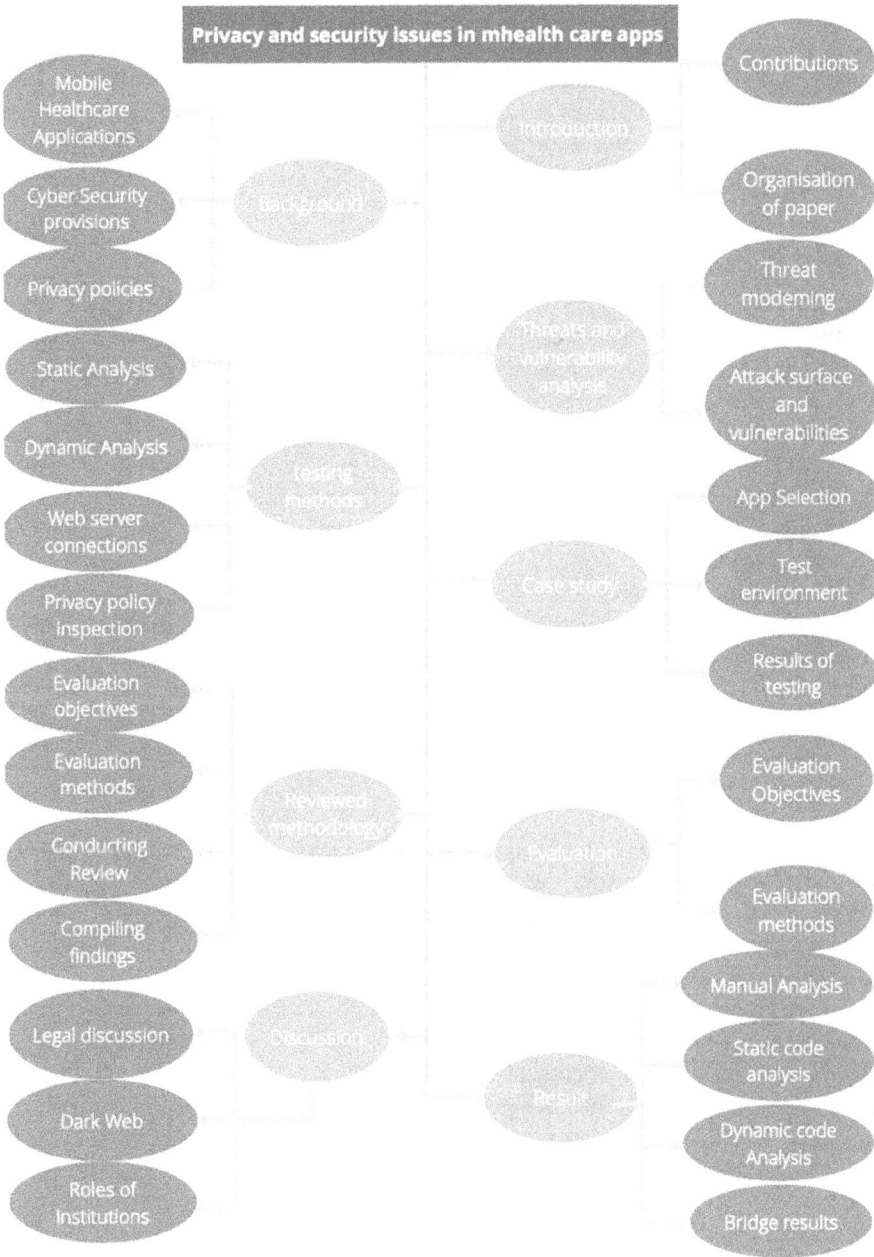

Privacy and security issues in mhealth care apps

Mobile Healthcare Applications

Cyber Security provisions

Privacy policies

Static Analysis

Dynamic Analysis

Web server connections

Privacy policy inspection

Evaluation objectives

Evaluation methods

Conducting Review

Compiling findings

Legal discussion

Dark Web

Roles of Institutions

Background

Testing methods

Reviewed methodology

Discussion

Introduction

Threats and vulnerability analysis

Case study

Evaluation

Result

Contributions

Organisation of paper

Threat modeming

Attack surface and vulnerabilities

App Selection

Test environment

Results of testing

Evaluation Objectives

Evaluation methods

Manual Analysis

Static code analysis

Dynamic code Analysis

Bridge results

FIGURE 5.1 Article roadmap.

outbreak of the virus. In such emergency conditions, healthcare applications became a lifesaver. They are featured such that they could provide instant consultation to the ill. Due to the presence of real-time monitoring of heartbeat, steps, pulse, etc., they have made themselves more proficient and user-friendly. Their extensive use has led to a revolution in the medical science industry. Along with this, these applications also present a serious cyber security threat to their users. To download these applications, one must approach Play Store or App Store followed by which they can download the required app by searching it. After the installation of the app, some general information is asked during the process of registration after which the user will be able to use the app.

5.2.2 PRIVACY POLICY

Applications often require personal data to be operated and this generated the need for the formation of a complete and easily understandable privacy policy for the applications. A privacy policy is a legal document displayed on software that describes the usage of data of app users by the application. The privacy policy is proposed, approved, and uploaded on platforms like Google Play Store, App Store, Windows Store, etc. to inform the users about the amount of personal data collected, the reason for the collection of data, and the way of using the personal data collected [6].

In most healthcare applications, user data is collected and provided to third-party servers. It is clearly mentioned in the privacy policy of such applications but due to the negligence of users, sometimes it becomes a trap for them. These policies are ambiguous and difficult to understand leading to legal complications in case a user registers a complaint against the app developer. It is also noted that some vital information related to user data privacy is written in such a manner that it becomes difficult for a user to analyze the cyber risk he/she faces after accepting such policies.

5.2.3 6G

Mobile cellular networks are required to achieve both coverage and capacity for their subscribers. 1G network was introduced in the 1980s to deliver voice exchange services from one place to another. It used the technology of analog signals. But due to less transmission efficiency, excessive cost, low availability, and hard handovers, 2G was introduced. 2G technology was based on digital modulation techniques and it is used to deliver both voice and SMS. Although 2G tried to ensure the encryption of data using the Subscriber Identity Module (SIM), it was facing certain issues like end-to-end encryption, authentication, etc. which led to an increase in the illegal use of such devices. Then 3G emerged in the 2000s and provided high internet speed. It was able to support services like web browsing, TV streaming, etc. 3G improved its security services using Authentication and Key Agreement (AKA) as well as two-way authentication. Unfortunately, 3G networks were also vulnerable to threats associated with internet protocol such as unauthorized access to data, threats to integrity, denial of services, etc. With every innovative technology, there came new challenges to be faced and humans kept on developing recent technologies. Similarly, 4G came around 2009–2010, and these networks provided better spectrum efficiency and reduced latency which in turn was helpful in achieving the needs of digital video broadcasting, high-definition television, and video chats. 4G networks were used as IP backbone networks, wireless core networks, wireless access networks, smart mobile terminals, etc. The foremost shortcoming was that it was even more vulnerable to security and privacy threats as users interact even more closely while using this technology. We are standing in a world where 5G has recently been introduced in some parts of the world to ensure faster speeds, more complete systems, more secure architectures, and an increased number of connections. Security and privacy issues in 5G can be divided into three tiers of architecture – access networks, backhaul networks, and core networks. Privacy protection methods have been advanced using machine-learning algorithms. To address signaling overloads, key agreement protocols and lightweight authentication are used to support communications for an enormous number of devices. Along with this, devices can be grouped together using AKA protocols. After the recent development of 5G, 6G looks like the next logical step. It is expected to offer more than five times more reliability and bandwidth as compared to 5G. 6G is anticipated to meet the requirements for future generations where self-driving cars, remote 3D teleportation, and metaverse is a reality. While 5G has already lowered the latency to less than 10 milliseconds, 6G has the capability to further lower it down to the order of nanoseconds, which makes real-time automation possible.

6G takes advantage of sub-millimeter waves to deliver not just high-speed internet but also lower latencies and higher reliability. 6G is envisioned as energy-efficient, high-range, extensive, and cost-effective with enhanced security. 6G can be used to introduce modern technologies like multiple accesses, waveform design, channel coding schemes, network slicing, numerous antenna technologies, and cloud edge computing.

5.3 RELATED WORK

We have analyzed around 15 papers and their contributions and challenges are discussed in the related work section. Following is a table incorporating the gist of those research papers:

Ref. No	Authors	Paper	Contribution	Challenges
[7]	Leonardo Horn Iwaya, Aakash Ahmad, and M. Ali Babar	Security and Privacy for mHealth and uHealth Systems: A Systematic Mapping Study	The study carefully finds, classifies, compares, and analyses the state-of-the-art in m/uHealth system security and privacy. To characterize the types, frequency, and demographics of published research, synthesize and categorize research topics, recurrent issues, significant solutions, and their reported assessments, a systematic Mapping Study was done on 365 qualitatively selected studies.	Specific control families (e.g., focusing entirely on individual involvement), types of applications, or technology should be the subject of literature studies. For over-represented regions, literature reviews or mapping studies can be done since they can be narrowed down and further analyzed (e.g., if feasible, at a control level instead of a family level).

(Continued)

Ref. No	Authors	Paper	Contribution	Challenges
[8]	Ming Fan, Le Yu, Sen Chen, Hao Zhou, Xiapu Luo, Shuyue Li, Yang Liu, Jun Liu, Ting Liu	An Empirical Evaluation of GDPR Compliance Violations in Android mHealth Apps	Mobile health apps are used as a peephole in this article to investigate the current state of GDPR compliance in Android apps. HPDROID is a proposed automated system that identifies the data practices indicated in the app privacy policy and the data-relevant behaviors in the app code, bridging the semantic gap between the general principles of GDPR and app implementations. Then, using HPDROID, three types of GDPR compliance problems are identified, including an insufficient privacy policy, inconsistency in data gathering, and data transfer security. An empirical review of 796 mHealth applications is conducted to meet the objectives.	Because the study of system-provided encryption algorithms is dependent upon, the paper's methodology will fail if the self-implemented encryption function is used.
[9]	Melissa J. Harvey, Michael G. Harvey	Privacy and Security Issues for Mobile Health Platforms	The security engineering process is explained in this article, and it may help healthcare companies establish an architecture-level security plan that complies with privacy and security regulations and industry efforts. The article highlights the many security architecture scenarios in which the protection strategy will be applied and to underlines the need of integrating security across these contexts. Industry and government security best practices are presented in the third section of the study, which may help healthcare companies create security architectures that satisfy their particular privacy and security needs.	The challenges include designing a legal and regulatory-compliant architecture-level protection plan for minimizing threats and vulnerabilities. These needs are best handled at the architecture and design phase of the security engineering process when vulnerabilities are introduced and may be fixed for a lower cost. To instill user trust in the system, robust security safeguards should be implemented into the system. To enable access to health data repositories and to provide eHealth information and services to all populations, cost-effective cloud technologies

Ref. No	Authors	Paper	Contribution	Challenges
				should be used. To increase the quality of health information obtained from health data repositories and to enable sophisticated mobile health apps that employ streaming analytics, Big Data analytics should be introduced into the system.
[10]	Konstantin Knorr, David Aspinall	Security Testing for Android mHealth Apps	In this research, a testing strategy for Android mHealth apps is given, which is based on threat analysis and takes into account attack scenarios and vulnerabilities unique to the domain. To show the concept, it was applied to apps for treating hypertension and diabetes, and numerous severe flaws were discovered in the most popular apps.	The article recommends digging deeper into the app's purpose and the data acquired. While the paper focused on simple numerical data harvests and direct data leakages, a more sophisticated examination may look into how detailed data can leak indirectly (for example, through summaries).
[11]	Miloslava Plachkinova, Steven Andrés, Samir Chatterjee	A Taxonomy of mHealth Apps – Security and Privacy Concerns	The research provides a taxonomy for mHealth apps that includes the most important security and privacy features. The taxonomy was put to the test using 38 of the most popular Android and iOS health apps. According to the findings, having a single method for categorizing mHealth apps in terms of security and privacy is necessary and advantageous. This study adds to the literature since it builds on previous work and offers information to a still-unexplored topic like mobile healthcare.	More study is needed to look at the dimensions of the taxonomy, which may be divided down into numerous subcategories or by performing user studies.
[12]	Rajindra Adhikari, Deborah Richards and Karen Scott	Security and Privacy Issues Related to the Use of Mobile Health Apps	The goal of this study is to look into the strengths and weaknesses of data privacy and security in some of the most popular mHealth apps. This project entails conducting a systematic literature review	The purpose of this article is to examine app security mechanisms and encryption approaches.

(*Continued*)

Ref. No	Authors	Paper	Contribution	Challenges
			and a comparative analysis of the 20 most popular mHealth apps in order to identify a set of risk and safety features that can help consumers choose mHealth apps and provide guidelines for the development of mHealth apps with appropriate security and privacy features.	
[13]	Achilleas Papageorgiou, Michael Strigkos, Eugenia Politou, Efthimios Alepis, Agusti Solanas, and Constantinos Patsakis	Security and Privacy Analysis of Mobile Health Applications: The Alarming State of Practice	In this article, we look at some of the most popular freeware mobile health apps in terms of security and privacy. Selected mobile health applications were subjected to static and dynamic analysis, as well as specialized testing of their features. The paper's distinctive characteristics include long-term evaluations of the life cycle of the examined applications and our general data protection regulation compliance auditing approach. The findings of the research show that the majority of the examined applications do not follow well-known practices and principles, including legal constraints imposed by current data protection rules, putting millions of users' privacy at risk.	During the implementation phase, technical issues such as tracking and deleting user-disseminated data to third parties, as well as establishing and developing internal procedures that meet GDPR auditing and data protection regulations, will be encountered.
[14]	Leysan Nurgalieva, David O'callaghan, and Gavin Doherty	Security and Privacy of mHealth Applications: A Scoping Review	Using a scoping review technique, this study explores the latest research on the security and privacy of mHealth apps. It examines suggested data security and privacy evaluation approaches and frameworks for mHealth apps, as well as research-based design suggestions. This work compiles recent studies on the subject to aid researchers, app	Some of the limitations are related to the generalizability of the findings, which might be attributable to specific healthcare settings and issue areas, patient groups studied, or app categories examined. Another drawback is the potential for consistent weighting in mHealth evaluations.

Ref. No	Authors	Paper	Contribution	Challenges
			designers, end-users, and healthcare professionals in the development, evaluation, recommendation, and adoption of mobile health applications.	Furthermore, assumptions and judgments are made based on the information provided, which may be limited. Other methodological flaws mentioned were a lack of stakeholder participation, which might lead to the omission of essential evaluation criteria and views. Another major constraint is the results not being full and the need to update and modify them.
[15]	Stacy Mitchell, Scott Ridley, Christy Tharenos, Upkar Varshney, Ron Vetter, Ulku Yaylacicegi	Investigating Privacy and Security Challenges of mHealth Applications	The present level of data security in mobile apps is evaluated in this study by doing a physical forensics investigation of many popular mHealth apps. The article describes the types of personal data that can be revealed both before and after applications are deleted and/or protected on a mobile device.	The paper would like to focus on the following: (a) the creation of a white paper that can be submitted to various government agencies at the local, state, and federal levels, including the FDA, which is interested in guidelines for mobile health applications; (b) the submission of recommendations to device and equipment manufacturers and mobile application developers to improve their offerings; and (c) the creation of patient education material that addresses a variety of topics.
[16]	Muzammil Hussain, Ahmed Al-Haiqi, A.A. Zaidan, B.B. Zaidan, Kiah M., Salman Iqbal, S. Iqbal, Mohamed Abdulnabi	A Security Framework for MHealth Apps on the Android Platform	The major goal of this study is to present a cohesive, practical, and effective framework for improving the security of medical data linked with Android mHealth applications while also protecting the privacy of their users. The proposed framework delivers the necessary protection through a collection of security	The goal of this study is to look into and analyze the security and privacy concerns that mHealth applications face, and then propose a security framework to safeguard that class of apps. Although other types of smartphone applications (such as financial, educational, and

(Continued)

Ref. No	Authors	Paper	Contribution	Challenges
			checks and policies that safeguard mHealth apps against both classic and newly discovered vulnerabilities. The framework is divided into two layers: a Security Module Layer (SML), which implements the security-check modules, and a System Interface Layer (SIL), which connects SML to the Android OS. Through SIL, SML enforces security and privacy regulations at many layers of the Android platform. To demonstrate its practicality and evaluate its performance, the proposed framework is tested by a prototypic implementation on genuine Android smartphones. The framework's efficacy and efficiency are assessed. Effectiveness is measured by comparing the framework's performance against a set of assaults, while efficiency is measured by comparing the performance overhead in terms of energy consumption, memory, and CPU utilization to that of a stock version of Android.	communication apps) were not expressly included in the study and assessment, there is no reason why the proposed method cannot be applied to them. This solution was also developed entirely on the Android platform, with no other mobile platforms being explored for the framework's deployment. In principle, porting the solution to other platforms is possible, but owing to the close interaction between the framework's architecture and the internals of the Android operating system, the magnitude of modifications may be large in practice. Nonetheless, because Android is by far the most extensively used smartphone platform, using it to construct the target framework seems like a fair choice. The fast advancement of technology in the realm of smartphone computing has also hampered this study.
[17]	Shimaa A. Abdel Hakeem, Hanan H. Hussein and HyungWon Kim	Security Requirements and Challenges of 6G Technologies and Applications	This article delves into the critical issues and challenges that 6G networks face in terms of security, privacy, and trust. Furthermore, the typical technologies, as well as the security problems associated with each technology, are explained. This article discusses the 6G security architecture and how it differs from the 5G security architecture. The security risks and challenges of the 6G	The security and privacy threats associated with 6G technology are significant. The amount of power required by 6G is a significant issue, and 6G cells must be designed from small to minuscule to meet the novel technological needs, which necessitates the development of complex hardware and designs. Furthermore, to maintain the privacy of

Ref. No	Authors	Paper	Contribution	Challenges
			physical layer are also discussed. In addition, the AI/ML layers are examined, as well as the recommended security solution for each layer. The article discusses the growth of security in legacy mobile networks, as well as their security issues and the most important 6G application services and their security needs. Finally, this study covers the dependability of 6G networks as well as potential remedies.	federated learners, secure data transfers are essential, and scalability of the requisite computing, communication, and storage resources is a difficulty for AI/ML.
[18]	Yang Lu	Journal of Industrial Integration and Management	This research examines the underlying concepts of 6G security, explores key technologies linked to 6G security, and discusses a variety of 6G security concerns. This study will be useful to anybody interested in the security challenges around 6G.	In the 6G era, the number of IoT devices will approach 80 billion, and many of these devices will pose new security issues. IEEE 802.15.4, 6LoWPAN, CoAP, and other significant IoT communication protocols are now in use. The communication security of these protocols is based on encryption methods such as elliptic curve encryption (ECC). These protocols will no longer be secure with the introduction of quantum computing and the growth in the capability of next-generation computing systems.
[19]	Ceara Treacy, Fergal McCaffery, Anita Finnegan	Mobile Health & Medical Apps: Possible Impediments to Healthcare Adoption	This study looks into two mHealth sub-topics: mobile health apps (MHAs) and mobile medical apps (MMAs), which have grown in popularity as smartphones and tablets have become more common. The study covers difficulties that are preventing MMAs from developing and innovating, as well as the	There are still concerns about applications that are MMAs but have not gone through the regulatory procedure. It is up to the developers to interpret the requirements, and given the complexity and time constraints, many developers pitch their applications as having a

(Continued)

Ref. No	Authors	Paper	Contribution	Challenges
			medical field's embrace of MMAs. The regulatory context is discussed, as well as challenges such as communication and ambiguity about the regulatory status of MMAs, time and expense, safety concerns, and security and privacy concerns.	health and wellness focus. MHAs and MMAs are unlikely to have a significant influence on healthcare unless regulatory agencies assume responsibility for ensuring their safety. MHAs will always be perceived as a novelty without the certainty of safety. Similarly, use of applications in the arena of significant health conditions will be difficult to emerge unless consumers can be certain that their data is safe and their privacy is protected. If apps are to be completely adopted by medical doctors and consumers, further care must be given to the integrity, usability, and safety of the applications.
[20]	Dongjing He, Muhammad Naveed, Carl A. Gunter, Klara Nahrstedt	Security Concerns in Android mHealth Apps	This study offers a series of three analyses of Google Play mHealth applications that reveal that mHealth apps employ insecure internet connectivity and third-party servers in large numbers. Under HIPAA, both behaviors would be deemed problematic, implying that the growing usage of mHealth applications might lead to the less secure treatment of health data unless mHealth suppliers change how they share and retain data.	**Upgrade to the latest Android version** Android is continually changing its behavior in order to avoid new attacks. For example, since Jelly Bean (Android 4.1), an app may only gather and see log messages that originate from itself, reducing the risk of logging information leaking. A malicious program can grant itself the READ LOGS permission on a rooted device (i.e., a device that enables any app to run with administrator permissions on Android) by performing the "'pm grant" command. This implies that keeping sensitiveinformation in system logs is still risky for an app. According to data collected by the

Ref. No	Authors	Paper	Contribution	Challenges
				Android platform in March 2014, about 40% of all Android smartphones are running the Jelly Bean version. Because there are so many Android users and so many mHealth applications, it is profitable for hostile actors to look for ways to extract sensitive personal healthcare data from mHealth apps.
				Agreements between users Many applications have been reported to urge users to reveal their private health information by giving a privacy policy that has been agreed upon by the users. In the survey, the majority of applications make privacy rules available to users either via an URL link within the app or when the app is initially opened. Users have little control or awareness over how health data is stored and sent, so applications should at the very least encrypt all data in transit and at rest. Understanding the privacy policies of mHealth applications, we feel, will be an intriguing future study area. Users should be aware of the terms under which they accepted to use the app and how their data will be handled.

5.4   THREAT AND VULNERABILITY ANALYSIS

While using any application, its users need to analyze whether they are facing cyber threats or not. In this software world, it is less likely that any application is sending data to any third-party server. Even if data is being sent to a third-party server, it increases the responsibility of the third party to respect the privacy of the personal data of a user. In the section on threat and vulnerability analysis, it will be discussed what threats a user may face, what information is of more importance to an external attacker, and what types of attacks a user may face.

5.4.1 Threat Modeling

The major threats to the privacy of medical data as stated by [3] are as follows:

- Interfering and damaging medical data (integrity issue) [10]
- Loss of data (accessibility issue)
- The unofficial revelation of data (confidentiality issue)

Now we need to analyze what information is more valuable for trackers and third parties. We need to assign the value of the information to the user as per the needs of external agents.

5.4.1.1 Threat Agents

A threat agent [10] or threat actor is any entity that brings harm or compromises the security of an organization. It can be any person, group, or organization. But the terms "hacker" and "threat agent" cannot be used interchangeably as hackers intentionally damage security using specialized tools and exploits, but threat agents on the other hand might be unintentional and need not have technical knowledge. We can say that hackers are a subset of threat agents. Threat agents can be broadly classified into:

1. APT groups
   APT Groups are nation-state stealth actors constantly engaged in espionage, IP stealing, or political manipulation. Since they are highly skilled and use custom malware or zero-day vulnerability, they are difficult to discover and remain undetected for extended periods.
2. Insider threats
   They are the people working inside the organization. They can be a serious threat as they enjoy privileged access. Insider threats are not always intentional but are also due to employee negligence or error.
3. Lone wolves
   These types of people hack for fun. They are also called script kiddies as they are not skilled enough to design their tools. They use tools made by other hackers. These are usually younger people who hack just because they can.

5.4.2 Attack Surface and Vulnerabilities

Organizations, irrespective of their size, face the risk of cyber-attacks [10]. This is because data collected by these organizations like credit/debit cards, name, age, phone number, and other sensitive information is of significant use to these attackers. This data can be easily sold on the dark web. Cyber-attacks are done for financial incentives, but in some instances, they are also done for fame. These iniquitous people deploy distinct types of attacks on the host machine like malware, phishing, MiTM, DoS, and SQL Injection. Once these machines are compromised, the required data can be easily extracted. To ease their job, these hackers exploit various vulnerabilities present in the application. Vulnerabilities are of two types – client side and server side. Some of the common vulnerabilities faced are directory traversal, integer overflow errors, hardcoded access key, out-of-bounds write errors, OS Command Injection, and previously freed memory.

The major types of cyber-attackers are:

1. Recreational hackers
   These are the types of hackers that hack for fame or to impress someone. They usually have limited resources and use existing exploits.
2. Cybercriminals
   These are people or groups of people that hack the application solely to steal the company's sensitive data. They usually hack into other people's computers to launch attacks to safeguard their identities. They are the most notorious and active type of hackers. They are the major threat to an app's security.
3. Hacktivists
   Unlike the previous two types, these types of hackers do not hack for money, data, or fame, they hack to show their resentment toward the government. They are usually organizations that see themselves fighting for justice.
4. State-sponsored attackers
   These are the types of attackers that are state-funded. They are hired by the government to identify and exploit national infrastructure vulnerabilities, exploit systems, and gather intelligence. They are highly skilled and have plenty of resources.

Attacks that can be performed are of the following types:

1. Malware
   Malware is any software or piece of code that is harmful to the system. It is usually inserted into the system using social engineering (a method that leverages human error to gain confidential information or remote access). "Malware" is quite a broad term that is inclusive of adware, worms, trojans, bots, ransomware, etc. Attackers can also use the infected system to perpetrate their hostile intentions like forming a botnet which is a network of infected systems.
2. Man-in-the-middle attacks
   It is the type of attack in which the attacker positions between the user and the application, thus eavesdropping on the communication, and deceiving the user and the application that normal conversation is going on. It is typically done to steal login credentials, financial information like credit/debit card numbers, and sensitive personal information. This information can be used for impersonation, illicit password changes, and many other malicious activities.

3. Denial of service

   Denial of service (DoS) attack is an attack that slows down or crashes the server. It is fulfilled by overloading the server with traffic or exploiting an existing vulnerability that makes the server unstable and causes it to crash. A more advanced form of this attack called distributed denial of service (DDoS) attack is perpetuated when multiple infected systems orchestrate a synchronized denial of service onto a single target. Since the attack is being carried out from multiple systems, it makes it difficult to track the attacker.

4. SQL injection

   SQL injection attack is a type of attack in which sensitive personal information can be extracted from the database by inserting or injecting a SQL Query via the input data from the client to the application. In some scenarios, this can escalate to compromise the server, perform a denial-of-service attack, or even leave a backdoor into the system.

5. Zero-day exploit

   A zero-day exploit as its name suggests is an attack launched by the hacker the day he/she learned about the vulnerability and the developer has "zero days" to fix it. The perpetrator takes advantage of this and launches malware before the developer has an opportunity to fix it.

6. Cross-site scripting

   Cross-site scripting is a method in which the attacker masquerades as a trusted website and sends a malicious script to the browser. Since the script came from a trusted source, the browser executes this script. As the script deceives the browser by conveying that it came from a trusted source. Thus, the script can access any session tokens, cookies, or other sensitive data used with that site, or even rewrite the HTML.

7. IoT attacks

   In these types of attacks, the whole IoT network is compromised. This can comprise of devices, networks, data, and users. The attack surface for these types of attacks can be devices, communication channels, and applications/software. Once inside the network, attackers can steal important sensitive data or shut down the network.

Attackers exploit many vulnerabilities in applications. However, naming and explaining every vulnerability is not feasible, therefore, some of the common vulnerabilities exploited are explained next:

1. Directory traversal

   It is a vulnerability in which the perpetrator randomly reads the files on the server which is running an application. These files could contain credentials for backend systems, operating system files, application codes, etc. In some scenarios, the attacker might be able to modify these files, thus changing the application behavior.

2. Integer overflow error

   It arises during the execution when the program tries to store a value greater than the value that the allocated memory location can store leading to a wrap-up (the value is wrapped to a small negative value). If this condition is left unhandled, then the result can be used to manage to loop, allocate memory, and several other scathing consequences.

3. Hardcoded access key
   Hardcoded access keys are plain text passwords, SSH keys, DevOps secrets, encryption-decryption keys, etc. which are embedded in the code. Manufacturers often hardcode passwords to facilitate deployments at scale. Passwords are usually hardcoded into software applications, BIOS, and other firmware across computers, mobiles, servers, IoT devices, DevOps Tools, and routers. The attackers leverage this vulnerability to hijack the firmware of devices, systems, and software.

4. Out-of-bounds write errors
   It occurs when the program attempts to write past or beyond the allocated buffer. It usually occurs when a pointer is incremented or decremented and it goes outside of the valid memory buffer and results in the corruption of sensitive information or a system crash.

5. OS command injection
   OS command injection allows the attacker to execute commands on the operating system. This arises when the web application sends unvalidated system commands to be executed. Because of the scant input validation, the perpetrator can inject their commands to be executed on the shell level which is introduced to operating system by cookies, forms, or HTTP headers.

5.5 TESTING METHODS

Testing methods are important to address mobile healthcare applications' security, privacy, and safety. These tests are required to ensure encryption of the application, and safety checking inputs for valid ranges which helps to ensure that vulnerabilities like SQL injection, DoS, cross-site scripting, and MiTM are unfeasible. The authors in paper [10] describe the methods to check the overall security of an application that can be divided into four parts, namely:

5.5.1 STATIC ANALYSIS

It is a way to scrutinize the code before it is compiled and run. It helps us to find out coding issues such as programming errors, coding standard violations, undefined values, and syntax errors. A similar analysis is done for healthcare applications to examine security threats to the user due to coding errors. It is based on the information found on the APK file, including manifested and compiled code [21].

- Proper SSL usage – A faulty report of SSL implementation from Mallodroid [22] shows potential for MITM attack, lack of encryption, or missing integrity protection, which could allow a threat of data leak.
- Debug flag – Debug flag is a flag that can be raised in a code to check the current values of a code. A tool Drozer [23] can help in debugging the Android app and check any case of data leak by using debug flag.

- Content providers – The content provider class allows the app to share data with another app with its action control structure. This structure should be carefully drafted and implemented to restrict any data leak; this vulnerability can be tested using Drozer [23].
- Use of encryption – Encryption ensures the prevention of data even on data leaks. The proper implementation of encryption can be tested by using standard cryptographic functions generated by APK tool [19]. If data is revealed as a result, the data would be considered highly vulnerable.
- Poor use of certificate parameters – [24] The current standard certification parameter is X.509 parameters of this certification can be CN (Common Name), OU (organization unit), O (Organization), L (Location), S (State) and C (country name). Poor use of certification can be tested using OpenSSL [21].
- Code quality – A poorly written code can cause multiple bugs, and several standard bugs can be found using Find bugs [25], the number of bugs found determines the quality of the code.
- Malware and privacy scanners – Advertisement and tracker cookies can cause serious threats as they can collect some sensitive data. They can be detected by using the Add-ons detector [26].
- Add-ons – Viruses and malware along with privacy trackers can be found using McAfee Security [27], Avast [28], etc.

5.5.2 DYNAMIC ANALYSIS

It is a process of testing, analyzing, and evaluating an application while it is being used. It improves memory issues, decreases crashes during execution, and corrects bugs. Hence, it is used to test running [21] applications for potentially exploitable vulnerabilities the cause of which is too complex to be discovered by static analysis. The foremost advantage of static analysis is that it examines all execution paths and variable values and not just those used during execution.

- Input check
  Checking if an app is accepting input out of normal range, whether it is popping any warning or not, is it accepting any invalid input, for example, name in the column of age.
- Data security
  Checking if the app is saving any unencrypted data either on disk or server, it can be done using Droidwall [29] and Wireshark [5].
- Data cleaning
  Testing if the app has an in-built feature to delete data after the completion of processes.
- Privacy policy
  The privacy policy is a policy that defines users' agreement on the usage of personal data. This test checks whether the app has a privacy policy or not.
- Permissions check
  Checking the number of permissions the app is taking and how many of those are relevant to the features provided by the app.

- Backup and logs
  Checking whether the app makes any unencrypted backup of data or locates any on the server. This can be done using adb [30].

5.5.3 WEB SERVER CONNECTION

Some healthcare applications interface data with a dedicated web server to synchronize medical data. Web server tests [21] can be performed by capturing web packets and analyzing network traffic using software like Wireshark and tPacketCapturepro. Following are the security issues related to web security:

- Connection: During usage of apps, URLs are closely monitored and if the data is transferred through HTTP, the login data and sensitive information can be obtained through the URL, whereas if safer transport like HTTPS is used no such activity is possible.
- Authentication: The authentication process should be secure as a stronger password should be mandatory to prevent a user from a brute force attack.

5.5.4 PRIVACY POLICY INSPECTION

Since crucial medical data is being uploaded on an external server, it is quite important to inspect privacy policies to check for security concerns. We will be evaluating privacy policies on the following factors:

- Basic privacy policy information
- Completeness
- Invasiveness

5.6 CASE STUDY

A case study is an integral part of the research. As per the paper [10], it is especially important to undertake, understand, and derive results from a case study to summarize the effects that a normal user may face. It also helps to highlight minute details of any project. Thus, we are considering an application to understand deeply the process of working on an application, data mining, and threats that a user face.

5.6.1 APP SELECTION AND PREPARATION

We selected an application that is very commonly used in India and has about 1,65,000 downloads. It is a health and medicine app that has around four stars on the Play Store. Now, we downloaded this application and verified our mobile number. We also added name, date of birth, address, gender, and age as asked by the application. Now we will be testing how secure it is for a person to use this application.

5.6.2 Test Environment, Database, and Other Tools

Using the APK of this application, we did the static analysis and dynamic analysis of the application. The tool we used for the same is MobSF. Except for this, we undertook a manual analysis of the app considering factors like privacy policy and permissions.

5.6.3 Results of Testing

- Irrelevant information needed by the app – Information such as a microphone, camera, physical activity, and location is taken by the app which was of no use at that time.
- User monitoring and vulnerabilities – It is observed that the app is trying to keep an eye on the user's activity and there are some vulnerabilities present in the app which can be used by hackers or external organizations to take information from the user's device illegally.
- Excess advertisement – It was observed that after searching for a product on the application, a lot of advertisements based on that product were shown on many other platforms. It simply signifies that users of this app face identity threats. It can be tested using an add-on like AdMob.
- Inappropriate privacy policy – The privacy policy of this application very well states that the app will all browsing history of the user will be taken prior to visiting the app and they also record every conversation including video calls, consultations, and reports of the user. At some stages, the privacy policy looks incomplete and inadequate. These applications take your data more than what is asked and they declare it in their policies without any fear.

5.7 REVIEWED METHODOLOGY

Review methodology is adopted to validate the research gap and to motivate for conducting the survey. Under this methodology, a certain number of research papers are analyzed and results are proposed based on studies of different research papers. The review process is divided into four parts, namely review planning, literature research, conducting review, and compiling findings.

5.7.1 Review Planning

It is the process of researching and writing literature. Review planning of the chapter is well described in Figure 5.2.

5.7.1.1 Research Objective

The purpose of this chapter is to review the literature related to privacy and security issues of mHealthCare apps. Based on this objective, several contexts have been identified to consider every aspect of privacy.

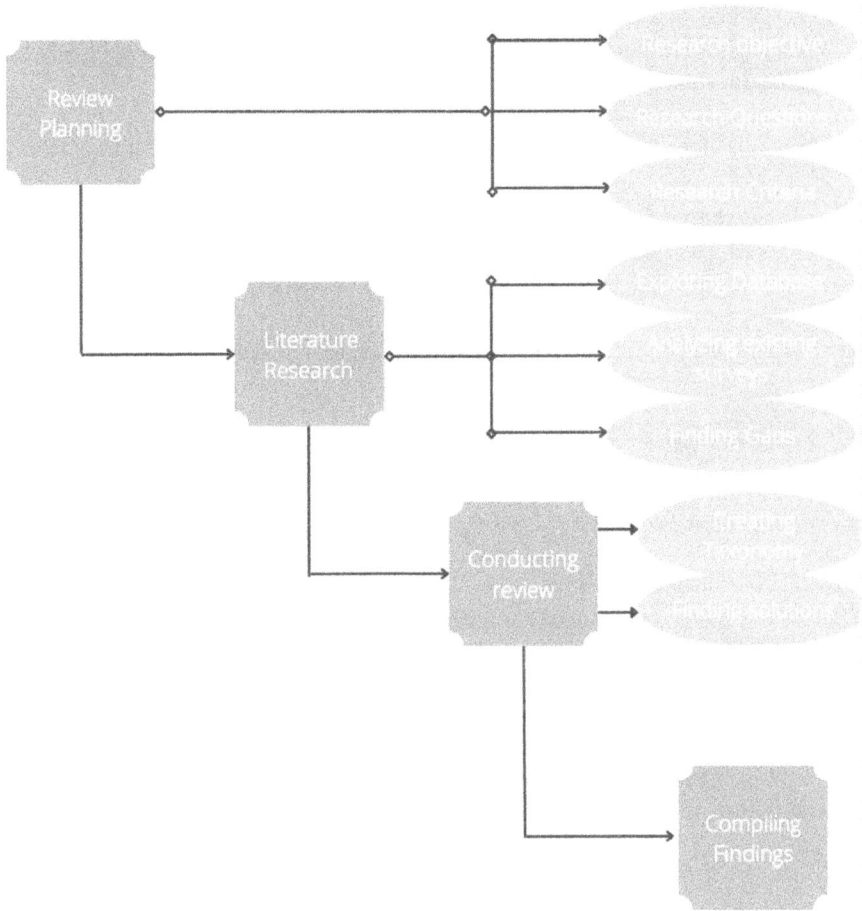

FIGURE 5.2 Classifying research methodology.

5.7.1.2 Research Questions

To achieve the objectives, we need to frame some research questions. The following are the research questions:

RQ1 What information is taken from the user and whether all that user information is of real use to the application?

RQ2 Is the information taken by the application not transferred to any third party?

RQ3 Are the privacy policies of healthcare apps complete and adequate?

RQ4 Can PHI be found on the dark web easily and if it happens what will be the approximate price of such priceless data?

RQ5 What do general people think of mHealthCare apps?

RQ6 What laws are there in our country to secure users from data thefts?

RQ7 Which organizations are responsible for ensuring proper treatment through mHealthCare apps?

RQ8 What solutions can we propose to decrease the loss of PHI?

These questions will be investigated and well answered using a literature review.

5.7.1.3 Research Criteria

The keywords such as "mHealthcare," "privacy," "security," and "issues" are found in every research paper's abstract, although the keywords have been selected based on the sections such as literature review, background, and taxonomy. The papers of the last 15 years having required keywords have been searched, studied, and analyzed.

5.7.2 LITERATURE RESEARCH

Literature research is the critical study of literature that is used for the purpose of analysis. It is the discussion of existing data within a particular phenomenon.

5.7.2.1 Exploring Database

The review methodology for this chapter involves searching appropriate articles from databases such as Google Scholar, IEEE eXplore, ScienceDirect, and Wiley.

5.7.2.2 Analyzing Existing Surveys

Security and privacy are major concerns for users of mobile healthcare apps; therefore, extensive research has been conducted in various domains to understand the security issues of healthcare apps.

5.7.2.2.1 Methodology

Our methodology to derive results is by analyzing research papers, survey papers, edited book chapters, and books consist of two parts – collection methodology and assessment methodology. We went through almost 50 papers and the most relevant and informative papers are considered for assessment.

5.7.2.2.2 Collection Methodology

To perform research that can change lives, we must have a collection of documents that tend to enhance our understanding and learning [13]. The literature required for surveys plays a key role in the validity and correctness of the same.

5.7.2.2.3 Identification Phase

For each database, titles and abstracts of every article were searched with keywords such as "health," "app," "mobile healthcare," "mHealthCare," "application," "security," "privacy," and "issues." The search was performed on May 10, 2022, and covered research articles written in English. Most of the articles [14] that we wished to take were from the past five years as there is rapid growth and development in the field of mHealth application and we wished to focus on recent literature as well as the current regulatory landscape.

5.7.2.2.4   Screening Phase

Screening of identified articles [14] is quite important to print concise research and the criteria for inclusion for articles is as follows:

- Articles in which there was a substantive focus on privacy and security issues were selected instead of those articles which just mentioned the same in the passing.
- Papers which had parameters such as threat modelling, challenges, evaluation techniques, and future work were given preference.
- Papers which focused on end user-centric mHealth interventions were thoroughly studied.

Papers were excluded from the collection if they fell under any of the following criteria:

- Papers which focused on a specific mechanism like a special type of attack like DoS attack.
- Paper that could be used by only one set of people like nurses/doctors or security professionals.

During the screening phase, papers were labelled as Yes, No, and Maybe. Yes meant inclusion, No meant exclusion, and maybe meant that paper is partial to our use. The papers tagged with Maybe were arranged in ascending of their usage and only a certain number of papers that were labeled with "Maybe" were selected depending upon the number of papers required after studying included papers.

5.7.2.2.5   Extraction Phase

At this phase, each article is evaluated in detail [14]. For easier collaboration and collective work, spreadsheets were used to record the credentials as well as to make annotations. This ordered data is used to do analysis.

5.7.2.2.6   Assessment Methodology

In this phase, qualitative analysis of systematic data is done to categorize the evaluation techniques and practices for the security and privacy of mHealth applications [13]. Thematic analysis is performed based on their primary contributions, that is:

- System's ability to fulfil stakeholder's security requirements
- Taxonomy of evaluation methods
- Analysis of design guidelines

5.7.2.3   Finding Gaps

Analysis of the work done before us helps us to establish a search gap. Every research paper has stressed on the fact that the privacy policy applications are not complete and inadequate but it has not been illustrated by any researcher what parts of the privacy policy make the applications a serious security hazard for its users. We have worked on this to select points from the privacy policies of applications that may even scare the people using that application.

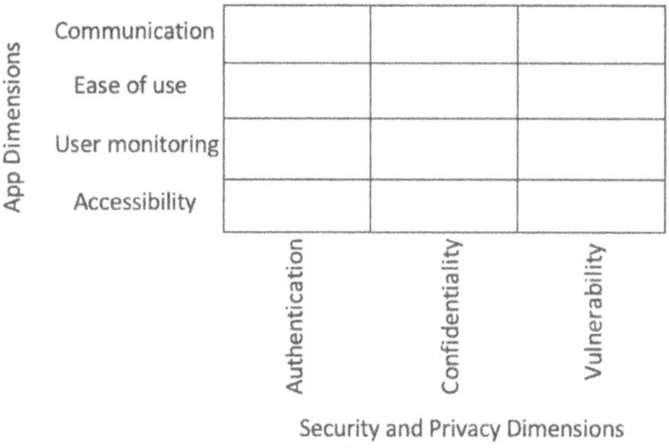

FIGURE 5.3   Dimensional views of the taxonomy of application [11].

5.7.3   CONDUCTING REVIEW

Under this section, we will be reviewing our systematic research which was done earlier and some preliminary results will be obtained.

5.7.3.1 Creating Taxonomy

To conduct taxonomy, we must examine the appropriate phases of each stage of our research. Such categorization will help to make an exact taxonomy.

We have drawn concepts and theories from prior literature to form a visual representation of dimensions as depicted in Figure 5.3

5.7.3.1.1   App Dimensions

We have divided the dimensions of the healthcare application into four parts, namely communication, ease of use, user monitoring, and accessibility as shown in Figure 5.4.

- Communication
  This incorporates the quality and modes of communication between the app developer and the user if any issue arises in the application and between the user and doctor if the user seeks a doctor's consultation in the app (if a doctor consultation is available).
- Ease of use
  In this, we analyzed the UI (User Interface) and UX (User Experience) of the application. The application's interface should be easy to use so that any novice user can use the application without any difficulties as most of people are not tech-savvy. Around 73% of the applications have an easy-to-use interface. Around 27% of applications have an interface which could be a bit tricky for novices.
- User monitoring
  Many mHealth applications monitor user activity like steps taken, distance traveled, etc., which is required for their proper functioning. Many fitness

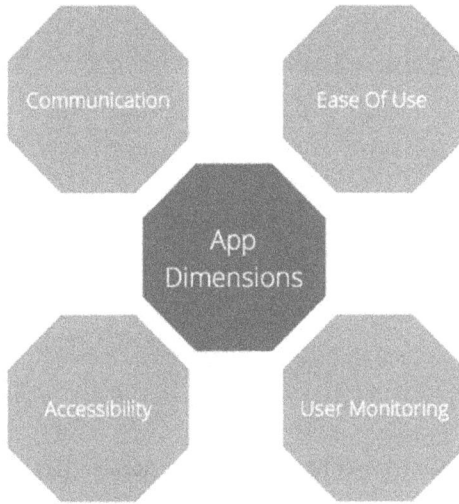

FIGURE 5.4 Application dimensions [11].

apps use this data to suggest physical activities to be done to meet their daily fitness goals.

- Accessibility
  Every app should have accessibility features for differently abled people like text-to-speech, color filters (for color blindness), etc. We found that most of the applications supported built-in Android accessibility features but only a few had their own accessibility features for differently abled people.

5.7.3.1.2 Privacy and Security Dimensions

Privacy and security dimension of the application has been divided into three parts namely- Vulnerability, Authentication and Confidentiality as depicted in Figure 5.5.

- Authentication
  Applications for which login is mandatory should verify that the email or phone number given by the user is not fake by using OTP verification. This prevents forgery and impersonation. Although most of the applications used OTP verification, there were some apps that were an exception to this. Upon our analysis, it was found that around 13% of apps either do not verify phone numbers/email or do not require a login. Furthermore, around 46% of the apps used one-factor authentication. And 40% of the apps require two-factor authentication.
- Confidentiality
  Users give their personal sensitive information to these applications to operate the application, so this information must be kept confidential and should not be shared with anyone. But on analyzing the privacy policies of apps, we found that around 13% of apps do not share data with third parties.

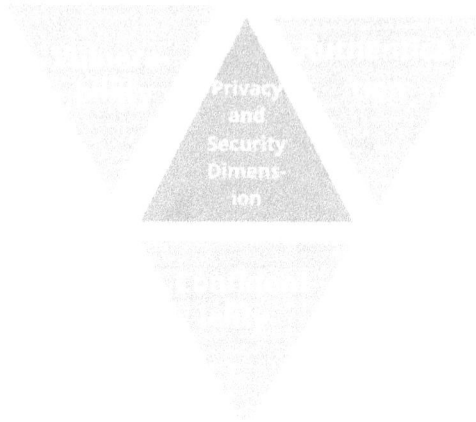

FIGURE 5.5   Privacy and security dimensions of applications [11].

Around 26% of apps share data with their partner companies for analytical purposes but anonymize the data. Around 33% were found to sell data to third parties and advertising agencies in the form of analysis and surveys. Furthermore, 26% of apps share data with third parties without anonymizing the data which is a serious threat to users' privacy.

- Vulnerability
  It is impossible for an application to not have any vulnerability, but every application should ensure proper encryption and industry standards so there is less chance of a data breach.

5.7.3.2   Finding Solutions

Prevailing solutions for respective security challenges are drawn from the database found on the defined taxonomy in Table 5.1.

5.8   EVALUATION

5.8.1   EVALUATION OBJECTIVES

To widen the spectrum of our research, we also conducted a google form to reach out people and know their views and awareness about security and privacy issues in mobile healthcare applications. We conducted this survey to find out about the satisfaction of people with the current situation of healthcare apps.

5.8.2   EVALUATION METHODS

5.8.2.1   Data Collections

For evaluation, we gathered data using a Google form. In the first section of the Google form, we asked people some ordinary questions about their name, age,

TABLE 5.1
Taxonomy of Healthcare Applications [11]

S.No	App Name	App Dimensions				Privacy and Security Dimensions		
		Communication	Ease of Use	User Monitoring	Accessibility	Authentication	Confidentiality	Vulnerability
1	APP I	◑	●	◑	◑	◑	●	○
2	APP II	●	◑	●	◑	◑	◑	◑
3	APP III	●	●	○	◑	●	○	●
4	APP IV	●	●	◑	◑	●	◑	●
5	APP V	●	●	◑	◑	●	◑	◑
6	APP VI	●	◑	◑	◑	◑	◑	○
7	APP VII	●	●	●	◑	●	◑	○
8	APP VIII	◑	◑	◑	◑	●	◑	◑
9	APP IX	●	●	◑	◑	●	○	◑
10	APP X	●	●	●	●	●	◑	●
11	APP XI	●	●	●	◑	◑	◑	◑
12	APP XII	●	●	◑	◑	◑	○	◑
13	APP XIII	◑	●	●	◑	◑	●	◑
14	APP XIV	◑	◑	◑	◑	◑	○	◑
15	APP XV	●	●	○	◑	●	◑	○

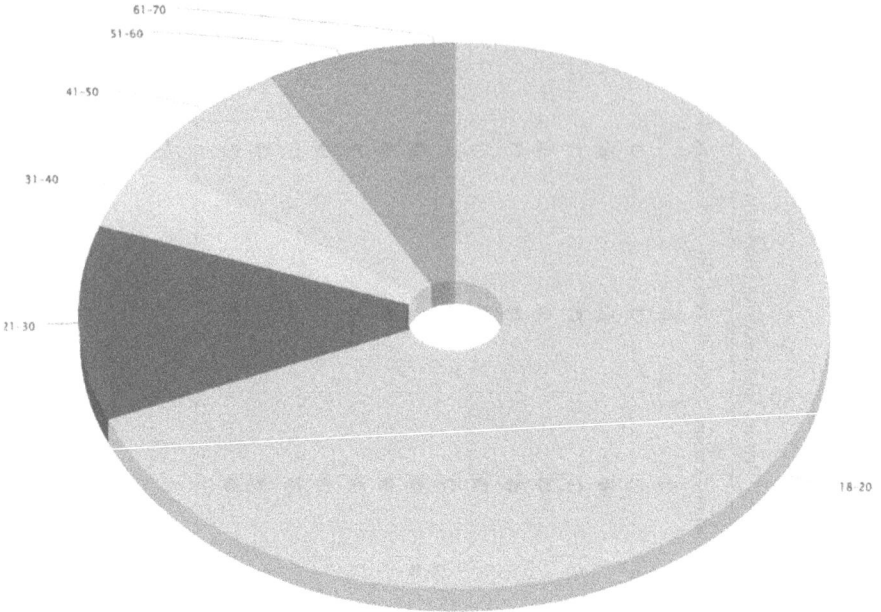

FIGURE 5.6   Age response in survey.

profession, in which area they reside, and whether they use mobile HealthCare applications or not to know what proportion and age group of people use mHeatlhCare
applications. In the second section, specific questions about HealthCare applications
were asked.

As it is evident from the Figure 5.6, most of the respondents (68.8%) lie in the
18–20 age group. It shows that people of this age group actively participated in the
survey and are aware of the privacy risks they pose.

Referring Figure 5.7, it is crystal lucid that the majority of the respondents (92.9%)
reside in urban areas; this was quite expected as the people living in urban areas are
more accessible to technology than people in rural areas because of the better communication and network facilities in urban areas.

As most of the respondents live in the age group of 18–20 years, it is obvious that
75% of the respondents are students. Although after students, software engineers
(6.3%) most actively participated in the survey as conveyed by Figure 5.8.

Although most of the respondents were from urban areas, almost 64% of
them have never used any mobile healthcare applications. Figure 5.9 shows
that even after the pandemic, where online applications were the only safe
option, most people still prefer face-to-face consultation rather than an online
consultation.

After this, the survey only continued for the people who have used healthcare
applications. Further on the questions asked by the users are depicted by Figure 5.10.

Where do you Reside

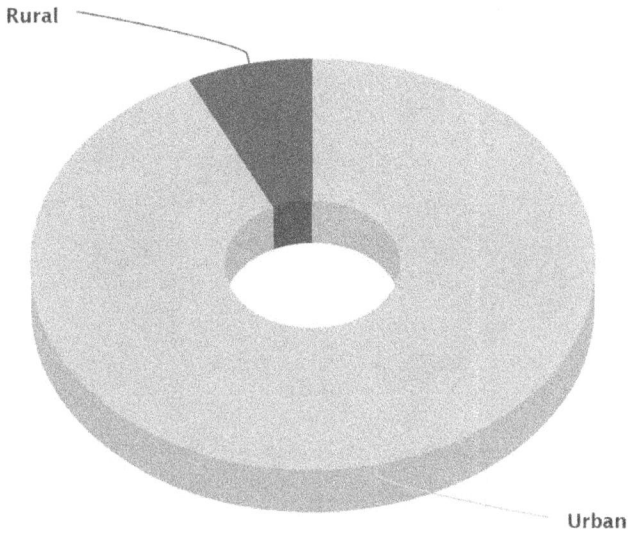

FIGURE 5.7   Response on the area of form fillers.

What is your Profession

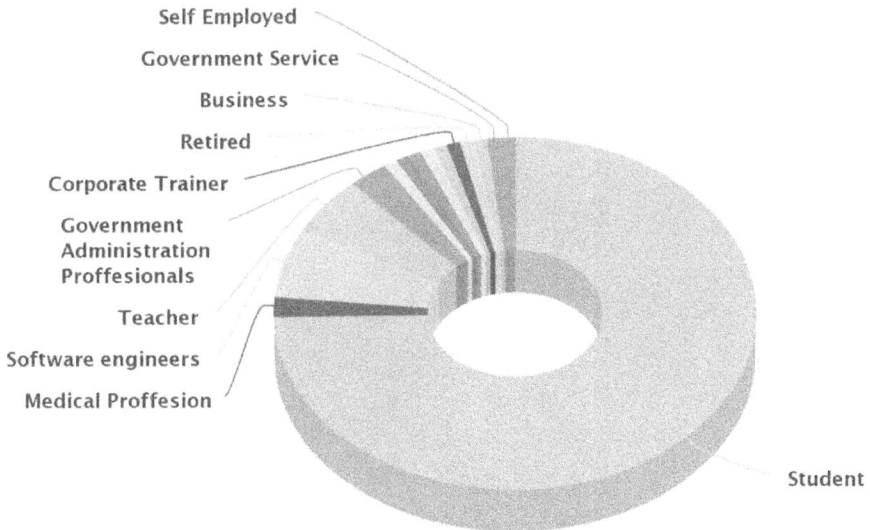

FIGURE 5.8   Profession response of the people who filled the form.

Have you Ever used any Healthcare Application

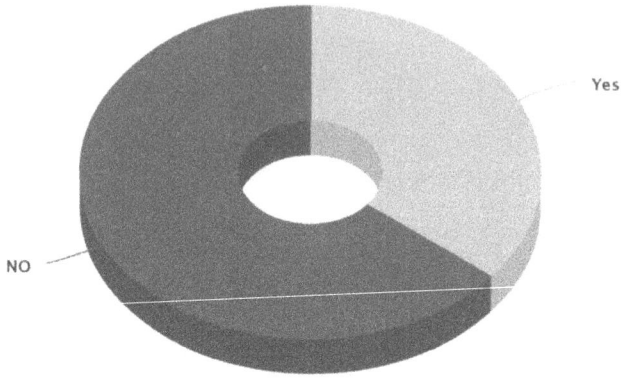

FIGURE 5.9 mHealthcare applications usage response of survey participants.

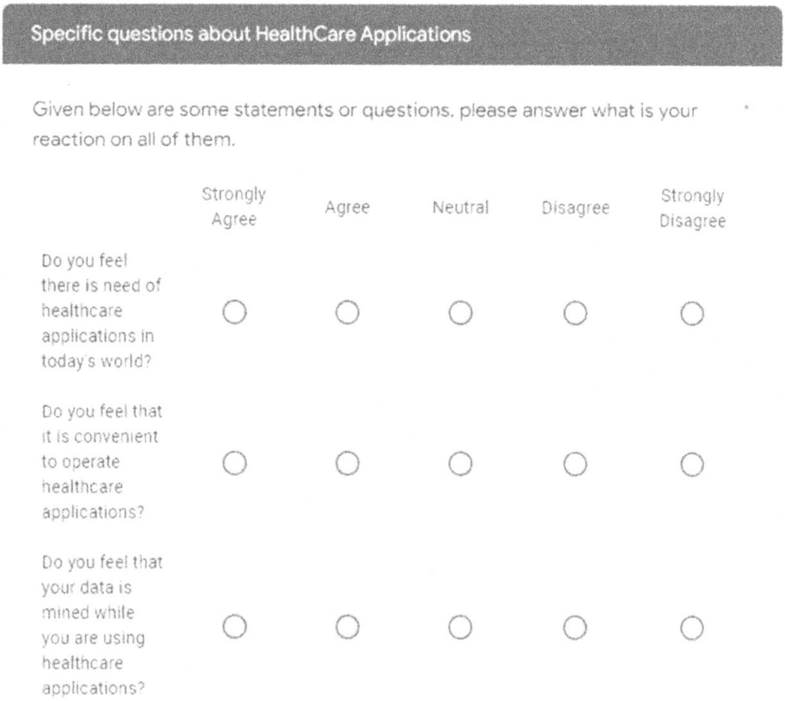

Specific questions about HealthCare Applications

Given below are some statements or questions, please answer what is your reaction on all of them.

	Strongly Agree	Agree	Neutral	Disagree	Strongly Disagree
Do you feel there is need of healthcare applications in today's world?	○	○	○	○	○
Do you feel that it is convenient to operate healthcare applications?	○	○	○	○	○
Do you feel that your data is mined while you are using healthcare applications?	○	○	○	○	○

FIGURE 5.10 Responses to general health questions asked from users.

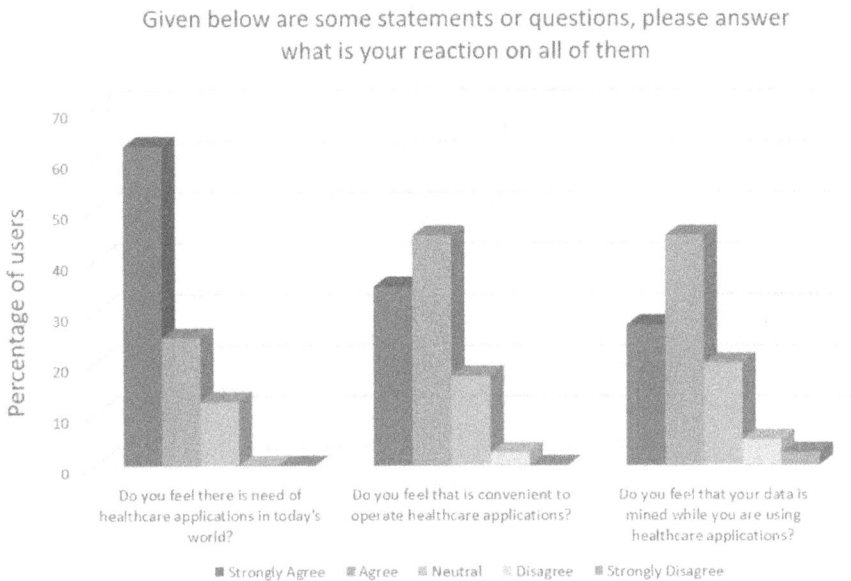

Given below are some statements or questions, please answer what is your reaction on all of them

FIGURE 5.11   General response of the participants in the survey.

As it is evident from the Figures 5.11 and 5.12, 60% of people strongly agree that there is a need for healthcare applications in today's world. Furthermore, more than half (72.5%) of the people think that healthcare applications are easy to use. Besides this, around 70% of people believe that their data is being mined. This shows that people are aware of the data breaches and privacy issues in healthcare apps.

It can be seen from Figures 5.13 and 5.14 that 40% of people do not have an idea about the doctor's qualifications, while 60% of people feel that a doctor is professionally qualified but there is a mixed response regarding the prescribed medicines. Most of the people stayed neutral regarding the satisfaction of consultancy. Most people did not like to show ailments under the cover parts on the camera. This might be because many people feel their data is being mined.

More than half of the respondents (57.5%) agree that permissions asked by the apps are not of their real use and they do not feel comfortable while giving those permissions. But it is evident from the Figure 5.15 that three quarters of people are honest while answering personal information. Most people feel that getting a consultation is easy in healthcare apps and are comfortable in asking queries after the examination, which might be the reason that three-fourths of people are honest while answering personal information.

As it is evident from the Figures 5.16 and 5.17 that more than half of the respondents believe that their data is being sold to third parties and leads to targeted advertisements and spam messages/calls which shows that people are quite aware of their data being used for advertisement purposes.

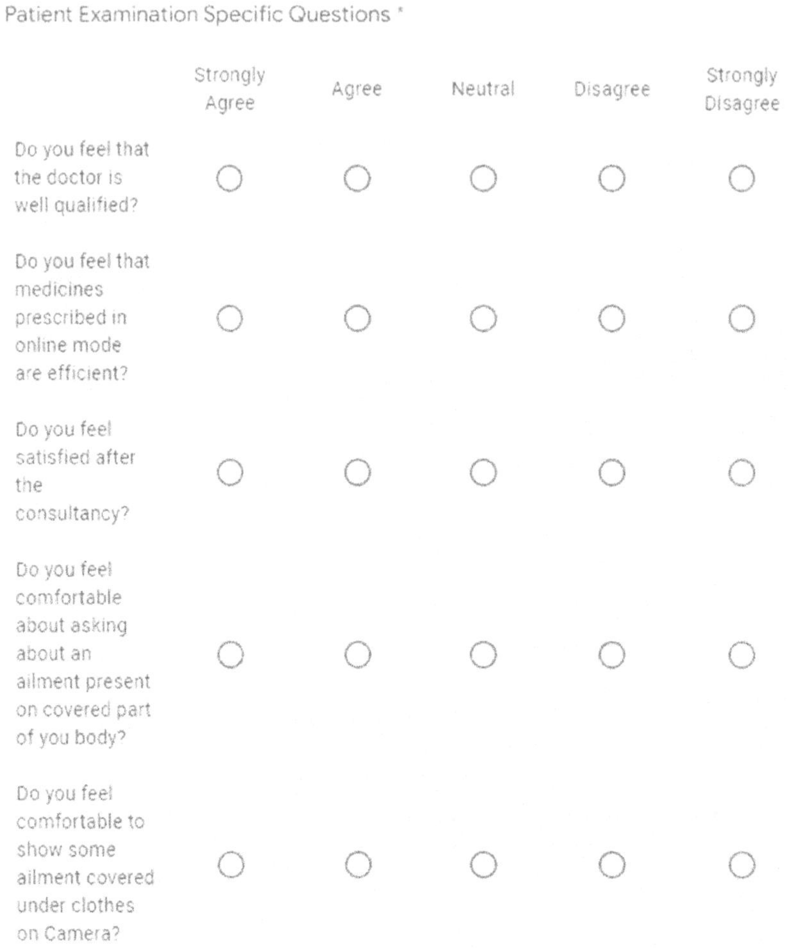

Patient Examination Specific Questions *

	Strongly Agree	Agree	Neutral	Disagree	Strongly Disagree
Do you feel that the doctor is well qualified?	◯	◯	◯	◯	◯
Do you feel that medicines prescribed in online mode are efficient?	◯	◯	◯	◯	◯
Do you feel satisfied after the consultancy?	◯	◯	◯	◯	◯
Do you feel comfortable about asking about an ailment present on covered part of you body?	◯	◯	◯	◯	◯
Do you feel comfortable to show some ailment covered under clothes on Camera?	◯	◯	◯	◯	◯

FIGURE 5.12   Specific questions asked by survey regarding examination of patients.

Figures 5.18 and 5.19 show that half of the respondents rated the use of health-care applications as three out of five. This is also reflected throughout the survey as most people need healthcare apps but they are aware of their data being sold and used for advertising purposes but at the same time they are quite honest while answering personal questions which means that they are quite helpless as they must use these applications for monitoring their personal health. This means that there is a lot of room for improvement in the privacy standards of these

Patient Examination Specific Questions

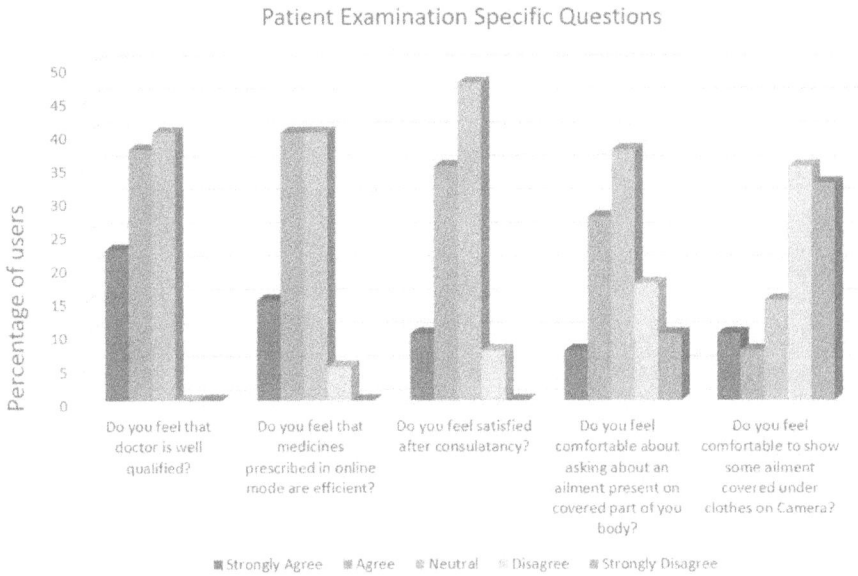

FIGURE 5.13 Response of the questions specific to patient examination.

applications and people are not satisfied with the current situation of mobile healthcare applications.

5.8.2.2 Security and Privacy Challenges

Numerous security and privacy challenges are faced by mobile healthcare applications. These applications require users to enter personal information which is not even of real use to the apps. As advertised from the graph, a few applications require weight, height, and even blood group. And most of the applications require user emails which are later used for spamming and advertisement purposes.

As it is evident from the Figure 5.20, a few applications require weight, height, and even blood group. And the majority of the applications require user emails which are later used for spamming and advertisement purposes.

Figure 5.21 depicts that more than 90% of the apps require the precise location of the user, which is a major privacy concern. Moreover, around 60% of the apps require access to read contacts, which is concerning as users' contact are of no real use to the delivery of any service of applications. Furthermore, 20% of apps require permission to read SMS, which is bothering as SMS contains sensitive information like OTPs.

Features in Android development terms mean the data that is fetched automatically without the user's consent. As it is seen from the Figure 5.22, 100% of the app fetch IP addresses, advertisement IDs, and Android IDs, which shows that these apps

Operation of the HealthCare Application *

	Strongly Agree	Agree	Neutral	Disagree	Strongly Disagree
Do you feel that all the permissions asked by the app are of their real use?	○	○	○	○	○
Do you feel comfortable to answer all those permissions?	○	○	○	○	○
Are you honest while answering options like name etc?	○	○	○	○	○
Do you feel that it is very easy to get doctor's appointment and consultation?	○	○	○	○	○
Do you feel the need for choosing a specific online doctor for your treatment?	○	○	○	○	○
Do you feel comfortable in answering your health related	○	○	○	○	○
Do you feel comfortable in sharing in all your health history with the doctor including some major disease information of your family member?	○	○	○	○	○
Do you feel comfortable in asking your queries after the examination by doctor?	○	○	○	○	○

FIGURE 5.14 Questions asked by users to review operation of mHealthcare apps.

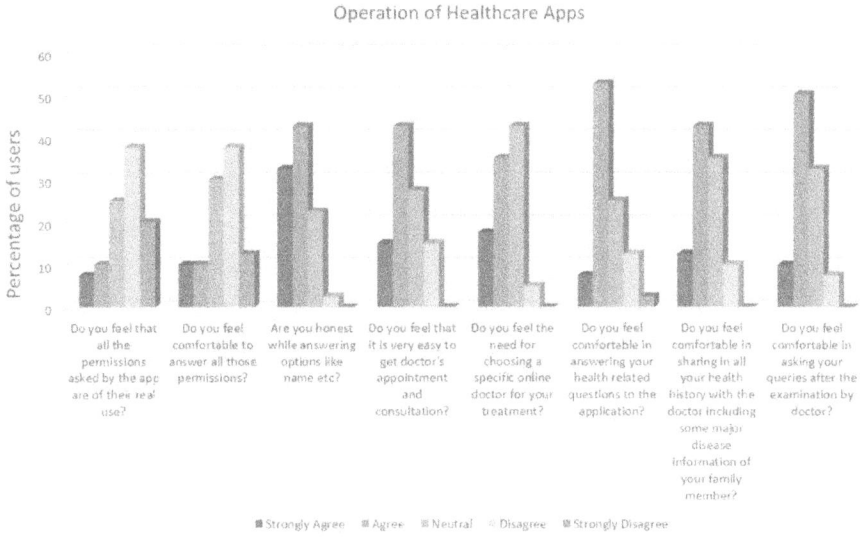

FIGURE 5.15 Comparative response on operation of mHealthcare applications.

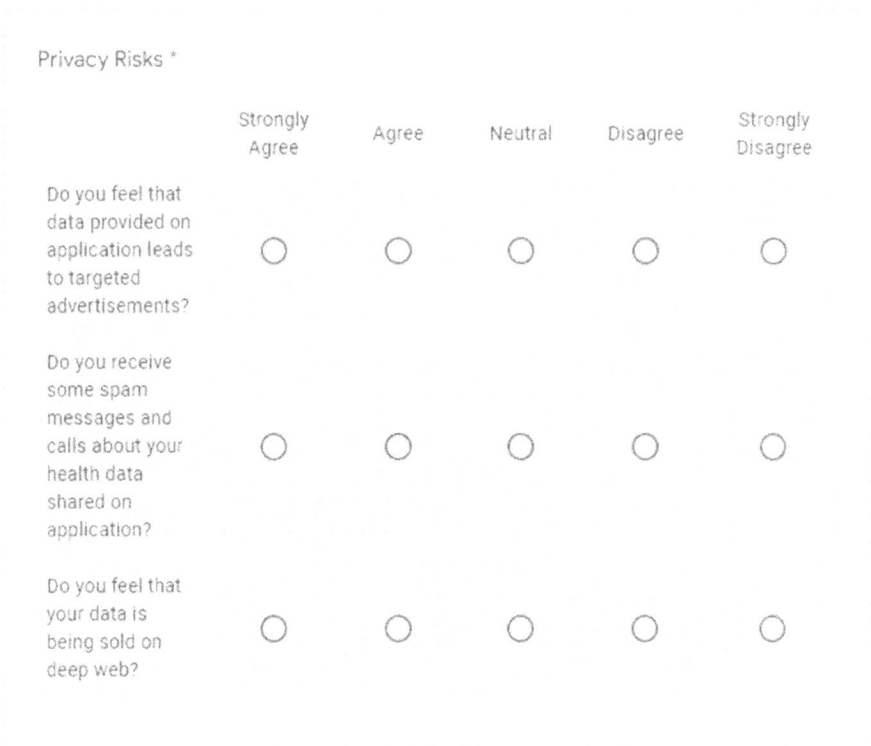

FIGURE 5.16 Questions to examine the awareness of users about privacy risks they pose.

Privacy Risks

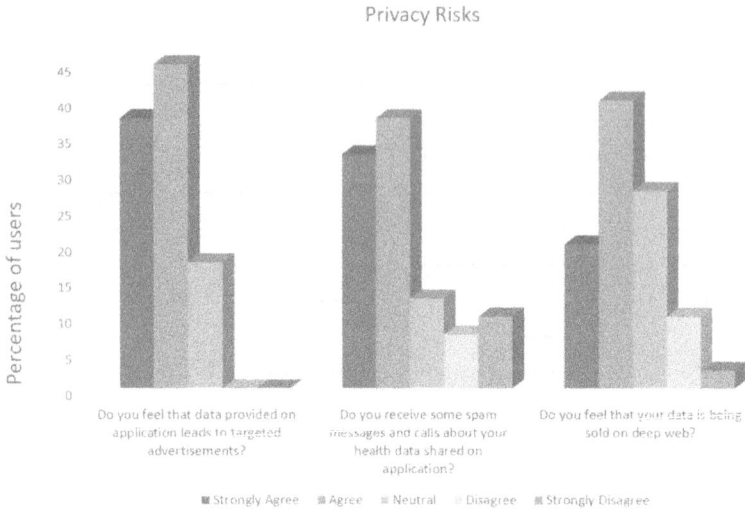

FIGURE 5.17 Opinion of the users about privacy risks faced by them while using mHealthcare applications.

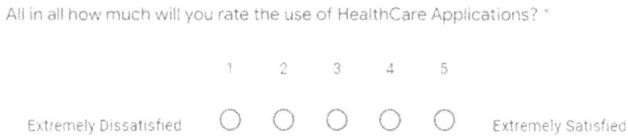

All in all how much will you rate the use of HealthCare Applications? *

	1	2	3	4	5	
Extremely Dissatisfied	○	○	○	○	○	Extremely Satisfied

FIGURE 5.18 Ratings of the use of healthcare applications.

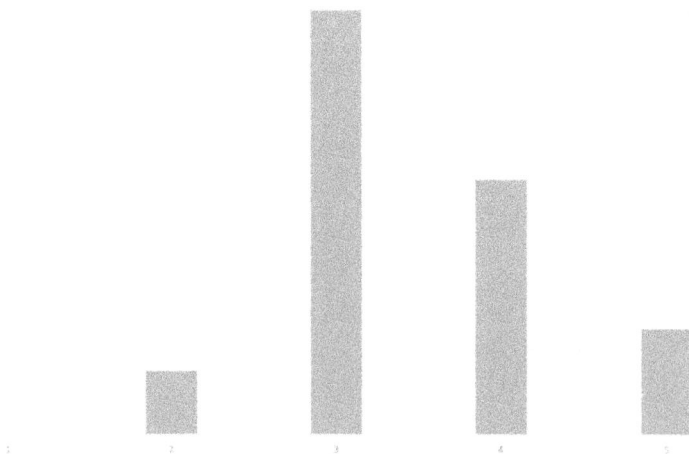

FIGURE 5.19 Rating of healthcare applications by their users.

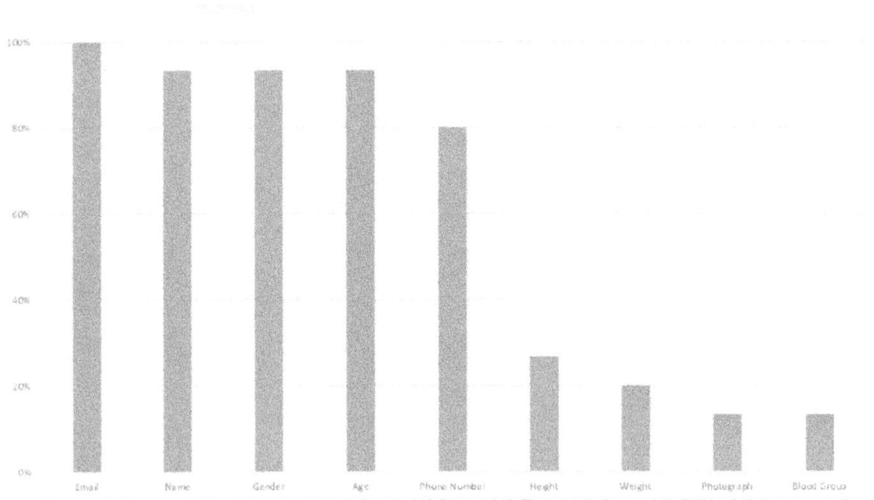

FIGURE 5.20   Percentage of apps requiring different registration credentials.

use targeted advertisements. Furthermore, around 90% of the apps record app usage patterns, and more than 60% of apps record browser history which is oftentimes sold to third parties in the forms of analysis and surveys and sometimes even sell the data deanonymized.

There is a lack of app standards in mobile healthcare applications. In some apps, there is even an absence of a privacy policy. These applications ask users for

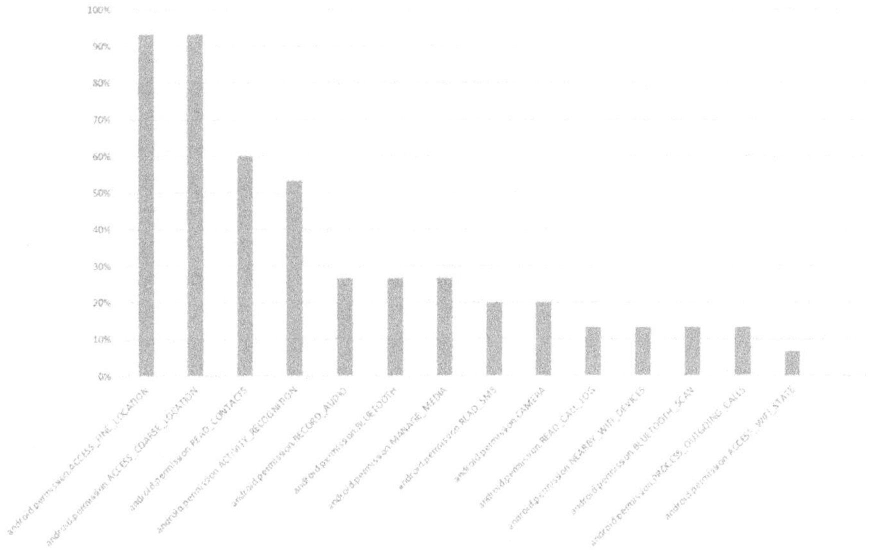

FIGURE 5.21   Permissions asked by apps.

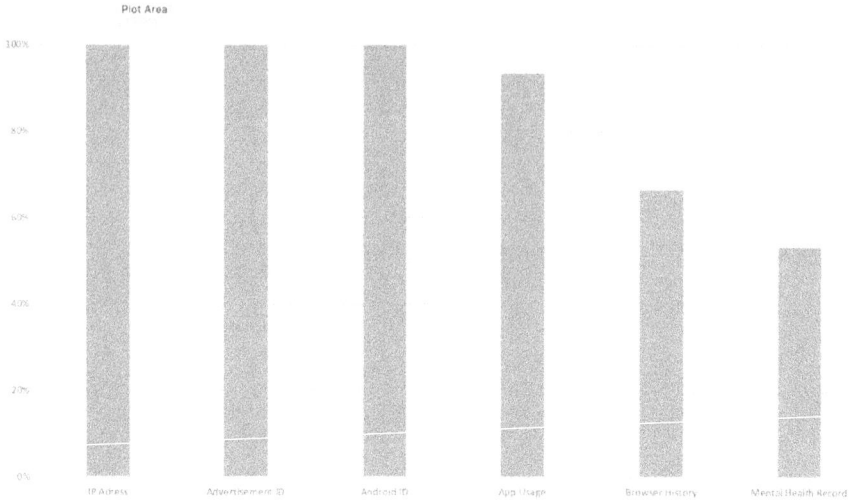

FIGURE 5.22   Percentage of apps verses features of apps [13].

permissions that are not even for their real use, and the user has no option but to give those permissions if he/she wants to use the apps. Although some apps are exceptions to this, most of them are in the same bowl.

5.8.2.3   mHealth Cloud Storage

Many mobile healthcare applications use commercially available cloud computing services like Microsoft Azure, Amazon Web Services (AWS), etc., as it is costly to set up the whole server, and then buy space in these commercially available servers. As their data is being stored on these servers, data is taken outside the company, and the data's privacy settings are beyond the control of the company. Therefore, there is a risk that their data is being mishandled or leaked by the service provider. As sensitive data is being transferred over the internet, there is a risk of it being intercepted en route.

5.8.2.4   Privacy and Security Issues in Digi Health Application of 6G

As digital healthcare is expanding, smart healthcare systems driven by AI will advance through unprecedented technology soon. Moreover, the increasing population might result in more emphasis on healthcare solutions than before. Body Area Networks (BANs) formed by smart embedded devices aid in personalized health management and monitoring. These BANs can garner data from multiple sensors and share it with other networks. As 6G will be the future for communication of data for health services, device authentication, secure transmission of data, and access of control for numerous of these embedded devices will be a hitch. While AI will be needed to handle and analyze the data from IoMT devices, AI models' data collection and model training must be standardized in a way that protects patients' data privacy.

Blockchain is a digital immutable database containing information that can be simultaneously used over a large network. Although blockchain technology seems to be highly secure as it shares data with all stakeholders and probably be used for data sharing in 6G networks, there remain some issues that are malevolent. Some of the malicious behavior attacks are transactions, privacy leakage attacks, double spending attacks, and vulnerability attacks. Some of the blockchain-based solutions proposed for these types of attacks include cryptographic algorithms and incentive strategies. Even though there are some low-level security algorithms like private blockchains, there exist some high-level security blockchains which can be used for the secure transaction of resources.

As the number of devices is rapidly rising, this will bring many security challenges. Nowadays, the communication protocols used by IoT devices are IEEE 802.15.4, CoAP, 6LoWPAN, etc. These protocols rely on encryption algorithms. But with the increasing computing power of next-generation computers and the development of quantum computing, they will not be able to keep up and will become obsolete at some point in time. To overcome this obstacle, virtualization can be used to create another layer of abstraction. This will not only be cost-effective but will also enhance the reliability of 6G networks. As the security of critical infrastructures like smart grids and medical systems is of foremost importance, AI-based security measures must be implemented which will continuously garner data and use that to minimize security risk. Thus, AI-based solutions should be practiced in the field of network security.

5.8.2.5 Mobile Devices Security Measures

Although we know it is impossible [31] to guarantee the privacy of users but the risk of a privacy breach can be reduced significantly by taking appropriate security measures. Security measures can be implemented on both users' as well as developers' end. Some implementable measures on the user's end are discussed in Table 5.2:

The possible implementable measures on the developers' end are discussed in Table 5.3:

TABLE 5.2
Measures by Users to Protect Themselves from Privacy Risks [15]

Measures	Explanation
Unique passwords	Users can protect their privacy by using a new and strong password for every platform.
Using a safe adblocker	Users can use a browser extension of a good adblocker which not only blocks the ads but also restricts them from fetching users' data.
Using an anti-tracker	Users can pair an adblocker with an anti-tracker extension to restrict most of the sites from collecting your data and some of the better trackers can even stop tech giants from collecting your data and show you personalized ads.
Using a secure network	The user should ensure that he is on a safe network, even when using Wi-Fi the user should try to use only verified and known Wi-Fi servers.
Accessing websites and apps using HTTPS protocol	Users should avoid apps and websites using the HTTP protocol as it is not a secured gateway, if not possible try to use an antivirus which provides online protection.

TABLE 5.3

Measures to Be Adopted by App Developers to Ensure Security to the Application Users [15]

Measures	Explanation
Two-factor authentication	Apps should do two-step authentications by asking for the user's name and password in the first step and OTP/biometric authentication in the second step.
SSL technology	Data should be processed and stored in an encrypted form and data should be transmitted via SSL (secure sockets layer). SSL technology encrypts the data shared between server and app.
Data wiping	Data should be erased whenever data capital requests and data should be removed after enough inactivity, data should be preserved in encrypted form
App testing and updates	The apps should be tested and updated before and after the market is released in the marketplace.

5.8.2.6 HealthCare Applications Infrastructure

The security engineering methodology produces a systematic manner for developing secure IT systems that are expandable, interoperation, and standard-based [9]. A thorough understanding of the security architecture will help the detection of security vulnerabilities in the preliminary stages of development. Security architecture necessitates addressing diverse, overlapping security architecture and requirements, inclusive of health information exchange, grid-based repositories, web-based services, and wireless health-based applications.

5.9 DISCUSSION

The effectiveness of research lies in the discussion of various important key factors of our research:

5.9.1 LEGAL DISCUSSION

Under this section, we will be discussing legal obligations and provisions for privacy and security issues faced by users:

Table 5.4 provides a tabular overview of provisions for privacy of application users in Indian Law.

5.9.2 DARK WEB – AN INSPIRATION FOR DATA THEFTS

The dark web is another side of the web whose access is not therewith common people and all sorts of illegal activities happen on this platform. It is like a normal website for hackers and advertisement providers. Content on the dark web is much more than the content on the web we browse. Advertising agencies buy data from these third parties and pay in the form of cryptocurrency. The dark web can be reached using VPN, virtual machinery, and Tor network. Sensitive data like credit card numbers, emails, and mobile numbers are easily accessible here and the Figure 5.23 proves the same.

TABLE 5.4
Indian Laws to Protect Privacy of Application Users

Laws	Explanation
Fair and reasonable processing	Personal data can be processed only for specific, clear, and lawful purposes.
Collection limitation	The collection of personal data shall be limited to such data that is necessary for processing.
Data storage limitations	Data should be retained only if the purpose is satisfied.
Accountability	The data fiduciary is completely responsible for any obligations on the act or process undertaken by it or its behalf.
Right to confirmation and access	The data principle has the right to either get confirmation about the status of data processing or a summary of the data processed.
Right to be forgotten	The data principle shall have the right to restrict data fiduciary from further processing or retention of personal data.
Transparency	The data principle should know which personal or sensitive data is processed or retained by the data fiduciary.
Personal data breach	The data fiduciary is responsible for notifying the data principle about any privacy breach and the nature of personal data subject to breach.

Thus, it can be well concluded that the dark web is a platform where personal identity data, personal health information, personal medical information, and personal financial data can be sold. In the absence of such a platform, all illegal activities will end on their own as people performing these anti-law activities will not be able to earn money by stealing the data. The government must think of steps to identify and punish such people.

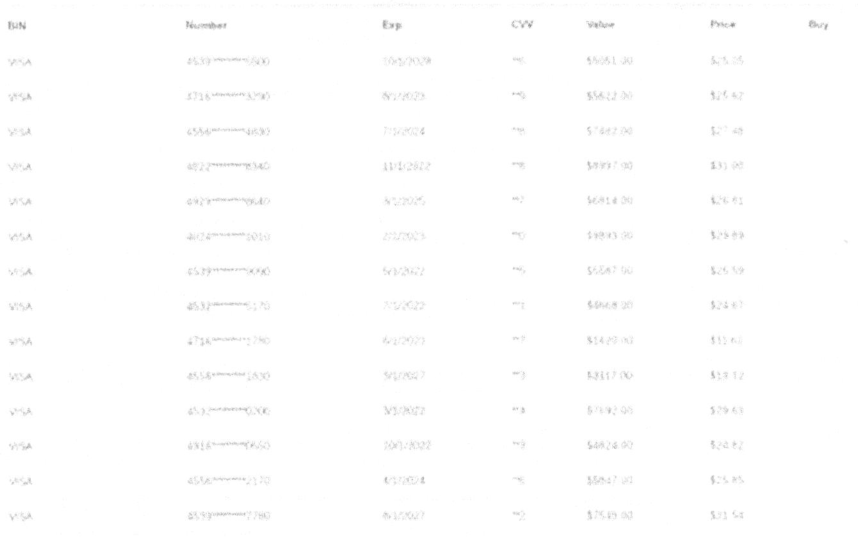

FIGURE 5.23 Data thefts on dark web.

TABLE 5.5
Role of Institutions to Ensure Appropriate Digi Health Services

Institution	Role
ICMR [20]	The Indian Council of Medical Research (ICMR), New Delhi, is one of the world's oldest medical research agencies. It is the highest body in India for the formulation, coordination, and promotion of biomedical research.
CDSCO [32]	Import Registration and Licensing, Approval of New Drugs and Clinical Trials Blood Banks, LVPs, Vaccines, r-DNA, Products, and certain Medical Devices (CLAA Scheme), Amendments to the D&C Act and Rules Prohibition of drugs and cosmetics Granting of Test Licenses, Personal Licenses, Export NOCs, and New Drug Testing Oversight and market surveillance are provided by the Inspectorate of the Centre, which is independent of the state authority.
IDPL [33]	By delivering excellent medications, IDPL contributed significantly to important national health programs such as the Family Welfare Program and Population Control (Mala-D & Mala-N), anti-malarial (Chloroquine), and dehydration prevention (ORS).
NCDC [34]	At the national level, the NCDC is involved in the design, promotion, coordination, and funding of cooperative development programs.

5.9.3 Roles of Institutions in Regulating Privacy and Healthcare-Related Issues

There are various institutions in India that are supposed to keep a check on medical services being provided to citizens using the applications present on the play store. The following Table 5.5 is a list of institutions responsible for regulating medical services in the nation:

5.10 RESULTS

Based upon the methodology, the experiments were carried out for 15 healthcare applications and the results are compiled to give a gist of the whole research that was carried out.

5.10.1 Manual Analysis

Permissions asked by every application are well analyzed by reading its privacy policy and running the application to identify what credentials it asks [13]. After conducting all this, we reached the following result:

In the above table, permissions are plotted against every app under the survey. Here the space left blank represents that the app did not ask for permission for that specific column. Number 1 represents that although permission is asked but turning off the permission does not turn off the app. Number 2 represents that permission is necessary for using the app.

From Table 5.6, it is evident that more than 50% of apps require location and physical activity whereas some apps have a phone, Wi-Fi or nearby devices as optional permission but no app has them as necessary permission.

TABLE 5.6
Permissions Asked by Applications [12]

App Name	WiFi	Location	Contact Details	Messages	Microphone	Bluetooth	Gallery	Camera	Call Logs	Nearby Devices	Phone	Physical Activity
APP I	1	2				1		2				2
APP II			1			1						
APP III		2	2	1					2			
APP IV		2										2
APP V		1	1		1			1				
APP VI		2					1					
APP VII		2	1	1	2	2				1	1	
APP VIII		2	2				2		1			
APP IX		1	2									2
APP X		2			1			1				2
APP XI		2	1		1						1	2
APP XII		2	1	2			1					2
APP XIII		2					1					1
APP XIV		2	2									1
APP XV		2				1				1		

TABLE 5.7

Features of the Applications [12]

App Name	IP Address	Advertisement ID	Android ID	App Usage (time, patterns)	Browser History	Mental Health Record
APP I	2	1	1			
APP II	2	2	2	2		
APP III	2	2	2	2	2	2
APP IV	2	2	2	2	1	2
APP V	2	2	2	2	1	
APP VI	2	2	2	2		2
APP VII	2	2	2	2	1	
APP VIII	2	2	2	2		
APP IX	2	2	2	2	1	1
APP X	2	2	2	2	1	2
APP XI	2	2	2	2	1	1
APP XII	2	2	2	2	1	
APP XIII	2	2	2	2		1
APP XIV	2	2	2	2	2	2
APP XV	2	2	2	2	2	

In Table 5.7, features are plotted against the apps and the legend remains the same as above.

Every single app in our survey takes IP address as a mandatory condition while most apps have IP address, Android ID, Advertisement ID, and App Usage as required conditions whereas only some apps have browser history as a necessary condition.

In Table 5.8, registration credentials are plotted against apps but the legend remains the same as above.

5.10.1.1 Static Code Analysis

Static analysis of the applications [13] was done using the MobSF application and it was well observed that every application was sending data to a third-party server and some apps even tried to check whether the device was rooted or not which is a feature quite irrelevant to their goals. So, it can be concluded that applications would have misused the device if it were rooted.

5.10.1.2 Dynamic Code Analysis

Dynamic analysis was performed using Wireshark [35] and since it was analyzed from the static analysis that data goes to a third-party server, we need to understand which type of data is of more important to a third party as depicted by Table 5.9. So, activity was done on the application and the following results were obtained:

Table 5.9 shows comparison of data and its risk factor.

TABLE 5.8

Registration Credentials Asked from the Users [12]

App Name	Height	Photograph	Weight	Name	Gender	Age	Email	Phone No	Blood Group
APP I							1		
APP II	2	1		1	2	2	1	1	
APP III				2	2	2	2	2	1
APP IV				2	2	2	2	2	1
APP V				2	1	2	2	2	
APP VI	2	1	2	2	2	2	2		
APP VII				2	2	2	2	2	
APP VIII				2	2	2	2	2	
APP IX				2	2	2	1	1	
APP X				2	2	2	2	2	
APP XI				2	2	2	2	2	
APP XII	1		1	2	2	2	2	2	
APP XIII				1	1	1	2	1	
APP XIV				2	2	2	2	2	
APP XV	2		2	2	2	2	2		

5.10.1.2.1 Bridge Results

The following results are required to complete our research in all senses and will help us to understand the research in a better way:

In the above Figure 5.24, the number of downloads is plotted against the percentage of apps. From the above graph, we can conclude that more than 50% of apps in our survey are well-known apps with more than 10 million downloads which very well suggest that the apps that we considered are one of the most popular apps and people are using these apps quite frequently.

The application records personal information and medical records from the user and delivers services and shares that information with the server, the privacy policy restricts both application and server from sharing information.

TABLE 5.9

Risk Factor of the Data Mined from the Applications Users

Data	Risk Factor
App usage history	Low
Personal information of the user	Medium
Vendor, product, and customer details	High
Complete details collected by the app	Remarkably high

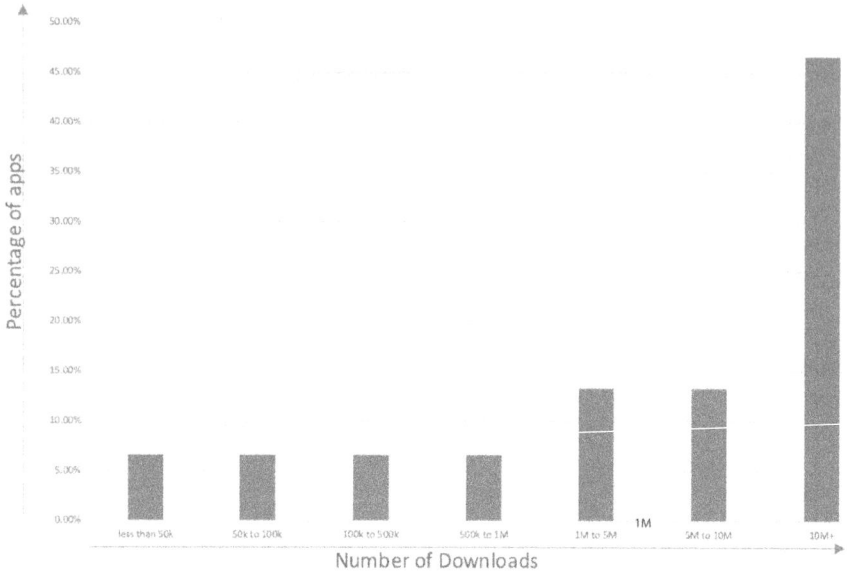

FIGURE 5.24 Number of downloads of the applications considered for the book chapter.

Any vulnerability in the server can cause privacy breaches and hence data leaks as explained in Figure 5.25 [13].

As shown in Figure 5.26, the data is first collected from the app through trackers and cookies. The collected data is then transferred to the client server for further processing and delivery of services. In a few apps, the data is further transferred to

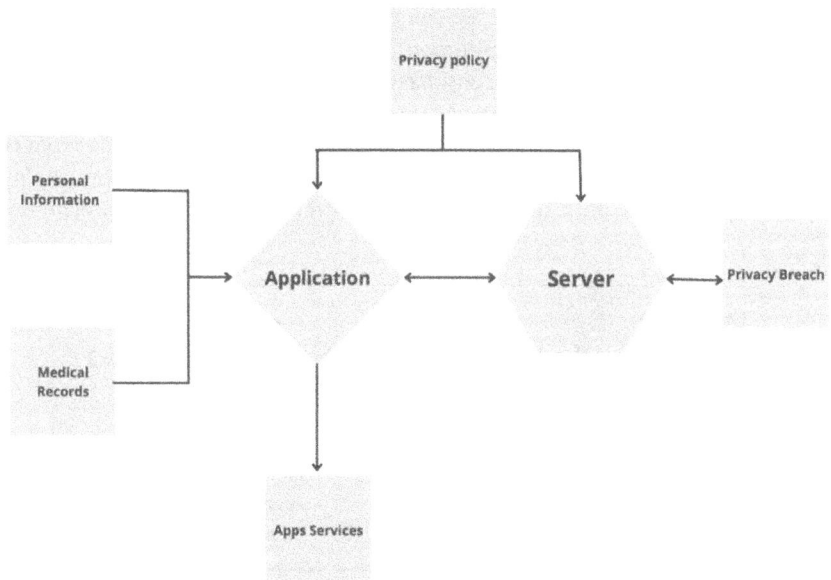

FIGURE 5.25 Setup describing privacy breach in mHealthcare applications.

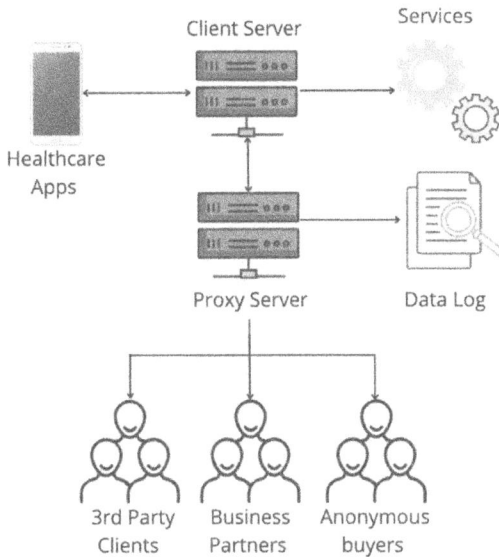

FIGURE 5.26 Scheme of interception setup [15].

a proxy server from where it is given to third-party clients or business partners and a log of collected data is maintained either for further analysis or to sell to anonymous buyers either in exact or in anonymous form.

5.11 CONCLUSION AND FUTURE WORK

Based on a methodical search, we have presented a scoping review that pinpointed research trends on security and privacy evaluation and design for mobile healthcare applications. We discovered a wide range of current information through literature reviews, background research, and threat analyses, which assisted us in formulating policy recommendations for mHealth applications. Additionally, we discovered laws that govern security and privacy issues for Indian citizens as well as requirements for institutions to monitor applications for healthcare. The proposed taxonomy establishes a framework for including the key components of mHealth applications. The success of the mHealth application depends on overcoming a number of obstacles, and there is scope for improvement based on the security and privacy they afford their users. Users also need to be aware of the game app developers, hackers and advertising agencies are playing with them. Concisely, our research is enough to let a user know about the privacy risks he/she poses and how to minimize the possibility of data theft.

Future work is simply the first step in a long journey toward analyzing security and privacy issues in mHealthcare applications. Further research and development are needed to cover the current limitations and to introduce improvements soon. A few suggestions for future work are listed next:

- Machine-learning algorithms like Decision Tree, Naive Bayes, Random Forest, etc. will be used to measure parameters like data collection, data usage, user rights, user content, data security, contact information, etc. [8].

- Development of a platform where recommendations about applications can be submitted to app developers.
- Development of material that can be used to spread awareness among the patients using mHealthcare applications.

ACKNOWLEDGMENT

We thank our Assistant Professor Sunita Kumari, GB Pant DSEU Okhla I Campus, Government of NCT of Delhi, for her research guidance and constructive comments that improved the quality of this chapter.

REFERENCES

1. https://www.mohfw.gov.in/pdf/Telemedicine.pdf
2. https://www.businessofapps.com/insights/privacy-and-security-in-mhealth-applications-guide
3. Mustafa, U., Pflugel, E., & Philip, N. (2019). A Novel Privacy Framework for Secure M-Health Applications: The Case of the GDPR. 2019 IEEE 12th International Conference on Global Security, Safety and Sustainability (ICGS3). doi:10.1109/icgs3.2019.8688019
4. Miloslava, P., Andrés, S., & Chatterjee, S., (2015). A Taxonomy of mHealth Apps – Security and Privacy Concerns 2015 ACM 48th Hawaii International Conference on System Sciences (HICSC). doi:10.1109/hicss.2015.385
5. https://www.wireshark.org/
6. https://play.google.com/about/developer-content-policy/, last accessed 15/10/2022
7. Iwaya, L. H., Ahmad, A., & Babar, M. A. (2020). Security and privacy for mHealth and uHealth systems: A systematic mapping study. *IEEE Access*, 8, 150081–150112. doi:10.1109/access.2020.3015962
8. Fan, M., Yu, L., Chen, S., Zhou, H., Luo, X., Li, S., … Liu, T. (2020). An Empirical Evaluation of GDPR Compliance Violations in Android mHealth Apps. 2020 IEEE 31st International Symposium on Software Reliability Engineering (ISSRE). doi:10.1109/issre5003.2020.0003
9. Harvey, M. J., & Harvey, M. G. (2014). Privacy and security issues for mobile health platforms. *Journal of the Association for Information Science and Technology*, D5(7), 1305–1318. doi:10.1002/asi.23066
10. Knorr, K., & Aspinall, D. (2015). Security Testing for Android mHealth Apps. 2015 IEEE Eighth International Conference on Software Testing, Verification and Validation Workshops.
11. Plachkinova, M., Andrés, S., & Chatterjee, S. (2015, January). A taxonomy of mhealth apps--security and privacy concerns. In *2015 48th Hawaii International Conference on System Sciences* (pp. 3187–3196). IEEE.
12. Adhikari, R., Richards, D., & Scott, K. (2014). Security and privacy issues related to the use of mobile health apps. ACIS.
13. Papageorgiou, A., Strigkos, M., Politou, E., Alepis, E., Solanas, A., & Patsakis, C. (2017). Security and privacy analysis of mobile health applications: The alarming state of practice. doi:10.1109/ACCESS.2018.2799522
14. Nurgalieva, L., O'Callaghan, D., & Doherty, G. (2020). Security and privacy of mHealth applications: a scoping review. *IEEE Access*, 8, 104247–104268.
15. Mitchell, S., Ridley, S., Tharenos, C., Varshney, U., Vetter, R., & Yaylacicegi, U. (2013). Investigating Privacy and Security Challenges of mHealth Applications (ICSTW). doi:10.1109/icstw.2015.7107459

16. Kiah, M. M. (2018). A Security Framework for MHealth Apps on Android Platform.
17. Abdel Hakeem, S. A., Hussein, H. H., & Kim, H. (2022). Security requirements and challenges of 6G technologies and applications. *Sensors*, 22, 1969. doi:https://doi.org/10.3390/s22051969
18. Lu, Y. (2020). Security in 6G: The prospects and the relevant technologies. *Journal of Industrial Integration and Management*, 5(03), 271–289. doi:10.1142/s24248622205001651
19. Treacy, C., McCaffery, F., & Finnegan, A. (2015). Mobile Health & Medical apps: Possible Impediments to Healthcare Adoption.
20. Zhou, X., Demetriou, S., He, D., Naveed, M., Pan, X., Wang, X. F., Gunter, C. A., & Nahrstedt, K. (2013). Identity, Location, Disease and More: Inferring Your Secrets from Android Public Resources. In Proceedings of the 2013 ACM SIGSAC conference on Computer & Communications Security (CCS '13). Association for Computing Machinery, New York, NY, USA, 1017–1028. https://doi.org/10.1145/2508859.2516661
21. https://www.openssl.org/, last accessed 15/10/2022
22. https://stackoverflow.com/questions/31951616/how-to-run-mallodroid-script
23. https://www.mwrinfosecurity.com/products/drozer/
24. https://docs.oracle.com/cd/E24191_01/common/tutorials/authz_cert_attributes.html, last accessed 15/10/2022
25. https://www.imperva.com/learn/application-security/man-in-the-middle-attack-mitm/, last accessed 15/10/2022
26. https://play.google.com/store/apps/details?id=com.denper.addonsdetector
27. https://play.google.com/store/apps/details?id=com. Antivirus, last accessed 15/10/2022
28. https://play.google.com/store/apps/details?id=com.avast.android.mobilesecurity
29. https://play.google.com/store/apps/details?id=com.googlecode.droidwall.free
30. http://developer.android.com/tools/help/adb.html
31. https://cloudian.com/guides/data-protection/data-protection-and-privacy-7-ways-to-protect-user-data/, last accessed 15/10/2022
32. https://cdsco.gov.in/opencms/opencms/en/About-us/Introduction/, last accessed 15/10/2022
33. http://www.idplindia.in/about.php, last accessed 15/10/2022
34. https://www.ncdc.in/index.jsp?page=promotional-developmental=en, last accessed 15/10/2022
35. https://developer.apple.com/app-store/review/guidelines/, last accessed 15/10/2022

6　6G-Enabled IoT for e-Healthcare Systems

Emergence and Upgradation

Richa Gupta and Deepshikha Yadav

CONTENTS

6.1　Introduction 122
    6.1.1　6G 122
    6.1.2　Artificial Intelligence Takes Over 123
    6.1.3　By 2030, the Evolution Rate of Self-Driving Cars May Be as High as 20–30% 124
    6.1.4　Advanced Robotics in Making 124
    6.1.5　By 2024, Minimum 10% of People Will Be Wearing Smart Clothing 124
    6.1.6　Travel Can Become a Reality 124
    6.1.7　Cloud Computing 125
    6.1.8　Augmented Reality Smart Glasses 125
    6.1.9　Human–Computer Interfaces 125
    6.1.10　Gene Technology 126
    6.1.11　Internet of Things 126
6.2　Future Trends for Wireless Healthcare with 6G 126
    6.2.1　6G Communication Technology for Smart Healthcare Systems 127
        6.2.1.1　Smart Healthcare 127
    6.2.2　Associated Technologies of 6G 128
6.3　The Next Decade Is IoT's Decade 129
    6.3.1　Medical Wearables Benefits 129
    6.3.2　Remote Health Monitoring 131
    6.3.3　Intelligent Wearable Devices 131
6.4　Assistances of IoT in Medical Facilities 132
6.5　Internet of Everything (IoE) 133
    6.5.1　Virtual Touch on Internet: Haptic Technology 133
    6.5.2　Clever Medical Technologies 134
6.6　How Secure is Data in 6G? 138
6.7　Challenges of 6G Technology 139
6.8　Conclusion 140
References 140

DOI: 10.1201/9781003321668-6

6.1   INTRODUCTION

The advancement in technology has visible impact in every sphere of society, changes in communication means being one of them. We are fortunate to live in a period where science and technology are assisting us in improving our lives and reevaluating how we carry out our daily activities. Our ability to create further is made possible by the technologies we are already familiar with and exposed to. Technologies of the present and the future will undoubtedly impact how we live in the future and contribute to that development.

Information transfer is getting faster day-by-day. It's getting faster because we're connecting more people and doing more things than ever before. Today, it's not just about how much information we can share, it's about how much we can share at once. Figure 6.1 shows a brief insight of different generations of communication protocols evolved since the 1980s [1]. The given hierarchical view shows the proportional increase in the data transfer speeds since the past three decades. The prominent applications implemented for each listed generation gives an idea about the practical implementation of these technologies. Following is a list of more technologies that will have a profound impact on people's lives during the next ten years and beyond.

6.1.1   6G

The 6G technology will represent the following significant development in data and information transfer technology. The 6G revolution will centre on how to link and manage billions of units in the future—from macro to micro to nano. Even when compared to the brand-new 5G networks that are now being deployed, 6G will offer a significant performance improvement. Using terahertz (THz) bands from 100 Giga hertz to 10 THz, 6G will have an air latency mostly less than 100 ps and a maximum data rate of 1 terabit per second (shown in Figure 6.2). The benefits of 6G over 5G include being 50 times faster, 100 times more dependable, offering better coverage,

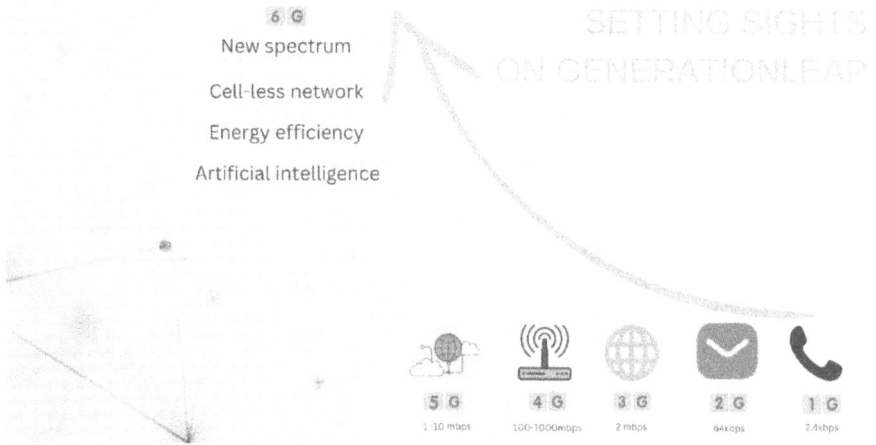

FIGURE 6.1   Evolution of communication technologies.

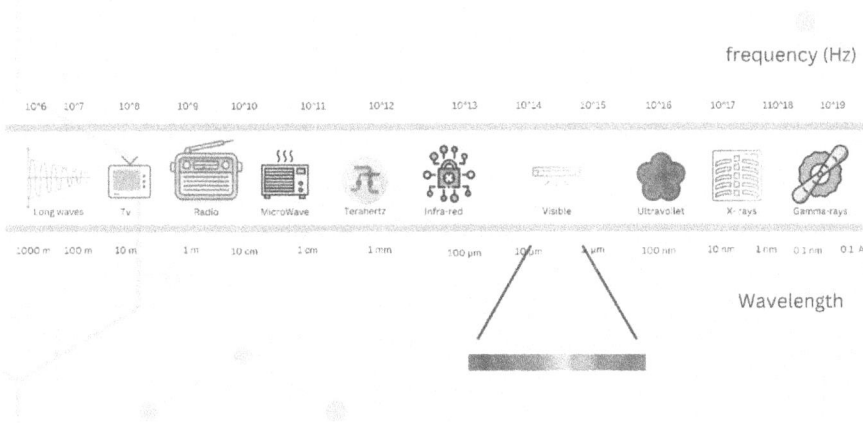

FIGURE 6.2 Frequency spectrum.

and supporting 10 times more devices per square. The power of 6G will change how we work and interact in the commercial environment. Imagine being able to summon accurate mobile holograms at the press of a button. It is possible to converse with a collaborator as though they were both seated at the similar table. Long-haul trips and sizable in-person conferences can be eliminated when meetings are conducted entirely virtually.

The healthcare industry is where 6G is being used in a surprising way. The research community can employ 6G to diagnose and prescribe treatments across continents and will provide speedier rescue efforts to regions with wider coverage. In localised communities across the nation, doctors can coach and oversee assistance to provide quicker and more effective medical care. Given the popularity of online gamers, who frequently test the boundaries of augmented worlds, 6G can offer a wide range of capabilities. Digital games and contests can become fully immersive Extended Horizon adventures with the speed of 6G, supporting sophisticated wearables, helmets, and even implants.

6.1.2 ARTIFICIAL INTELLIGENCE TAKES OVER

Artificial intelligence is employed in numerous various sectors, including machines, robotics, mobile voice help, and many more. Technological advances like Big Data, automation, and IoT have been primarily driven by AI. Additionally, business executives are now utilising AI for planning policies and strategies as well as incorporating AI into decision-making processes in the future. AI technology is catching on like wildfire in a variety of fields, including medicine, business, and the robot industry. Brands are interested in this innovation because low error rates and great productivity are crucial, and it has already begun to have an impact on the world. According to the database business Statista, there were 2,028 AI companies operating in the United States as of 2018. According to recent trends and statistics, a few reports indicated that the number of AI start-ups could reach 9,000 by the close of 2030.

6.1.3   By 2030, the Evolution Rate of Self-Driving Cars May Be as High as 20–30%

Since the price of gasoline and diesel has suddenly increased due to its rapid depletion of natural resources, people are being compelled to switch to a new form of transportation. The market for electric cars, hybrid, hydrogen fuel cells, and just a variety of other fuelling options with self-driving technology will expand by 2030 [2], if these variables are taken into consideration. Unfortunately, there are also more fatalities on the road. With the technology, there is no pollution and increased safety. Tesla reportedly knocked on India's door last year in 2020, and according to Indian analysts, self-driving cars would account for up to 5–10% of the global auto market by 2030. There are currently more than 1,500 autonomous vehicles operating on US highways.

6.1.4   Advanced Robotics in Making

Technologies like AI, machine learning, detectors, motors, hydraulics, and innovative ingredients will alter how goods and services are delivered. Advanced robot construction, operation, and maintenance will experience a rise in tech skills. The first robot, Sofia, was granted citizenship by the Saudi Arabian government and is now the most sophisticated humanoid robot ever created. Researchers and professionals are working to create a sensation that may be implanted in robots so that they can recognise human feelings and needs. In the US, a lot of businesses and restaurants employ robots, but by 2030, these machines will be smarter and more prevalent. Tata Motors is one automaker that employs machine robots in its automobile manufacturing facilities. By 2030, robots may replace up to 20 million industrial jobs worldwide, according to the analysis firm Oxford Economics.

6.1.5   By 2024, Minimum 10% of People Will Be Wearing Smart Clothing

Experts forecast that during the next five years, at least 10% of the world population will dress in clothing with a chip. You have access to this chip, which is utilised to transmit the most information via the Internet. The American clothing company Tommy Hilfiger has created a new range of apparel with intelligent Bluetooth chips integrated into them. These clothes connect to a mobile game and app from the company and let users collect loyalty points as they go from one location to another. The fabric will connect to an app while it is worn, and the app will push users to play games, run, and engage in other activities in order to accrue reward points.

6.1.6   Travel Can Become a Reality

Space tourism is becoming a possibility because of quick technological advancements. We shall be going to space in not too many more years. Suborbital tourist vehicles are now being developed by a large number of competitors, like Blue Origin, SpaceX, Virgin Galactic, and so on. Though human space travel is just getting started, how far it develops for future generations will depend on the opportunities it offers to the planet. On the contrary, several businesses are rethinking space elevators now that humans have already decided to travel to space via the shuttle. When a lot of scientists from Shizuoka University announced in 2018 that they would conduct an operation at the International Space Station, the concept of space elevators took a step ahead. According to some reports, the first commercial space exploration will be introduced in 2050, while a few businesses may test the first tourist spacecraft by 2030 [3].

6.1.7 CLOUD COMPUTING

The ability to store, use, and access computing resources that are developed on the Internet can be referred to as cloud computing technology. Anyone can use a private, public, or hybrid cloud. About 70% of American businesses already use the cloud, and much more are anticipated to do so. Cloud computing helped milk producers including Amul, Brewster, Chitale Dairy, and many others increase output and employee satisfaction. The business uses RFID (Radio Frequency Identification) labels to collect all information about the well-being of its cows. After evaluating this information, they send information to staff members, telling them to change a cow's diet in accordance with the needs, and provide medication or inject a vaccination (if required). It will be challenging to recall a time before cloud computing existed by 2030 because of how pervasive it would be. The largest players in the cloud computing business at the moment are Microsoft Azure and Google Cloud Platform.

6.1.8 AUGMENTED REALITY SMART GLASSES

Artificial Reality (AR) Google Glass and Microsoft Hololens are two popular examples of the new class of wearable glasses known as "smart glasses." The actual and digital worlds merge thanks to smart glasses. We can verify the details on your smart glasses rather than using your phone to do so. One brand-new type of media device is smart glasses. They cover more complex technologies like Microsoft's Hololens as well as simpler ones like Google Glass, which simply has one prism. We can consider smart glasses to be the "Eye phone" of today. According to the most recent report, the market for such eyeglasses will start to grow in 2025, and by 2030, it will explode.

6.1.9 HUMAN–COMPUTER INTERFACES

Wearable technology and human–computer interfaces are created to enhance human performance physically and possibly mentally and to help us live longer, healthier lives. The term "wearable," however, does not necessarily refer to something you strap to your wrist or another part of your body; it also includes robotic prosthetics, smart running shoes that can analyse your gait and efficiency, even autonomous smart wearable used in industrial settings. Many people are of the opinion that technological advancements like these may eventually lead to the creation of fully augmented humans, transhumans, or "humans 2.0," in which the human body is modified to resemble a sports vehicle in order to attain improved physical and mental performance. This would revolutionise medicine and eventually perhaps even call into question what it means to be a human.

6.1.10 GENE TECHNOLOGY

Experts forecast that over the next five years, at least 10% of the worldwide people will dress in clothing with a chip. You have access to this chip, which is utilised to transmit the most information via the Internet. This could have an impact on a plant's number of leaves or colour, while it could have an impact on a person's height, eye shape, or risk of contracting diseases. This creates a virtually limitless number of opportunities. The field of medicine is where gene editing is being used extensively. The correction of DNA abnormalities, which can result in major ailments like cancer or heart disease, is one of the most fascinating ongoing efforts. Human genome editing is currently prohibited in many nations, including the majority of Europe, because its long-term effects remain unknown.

6.1.11 INTERNET OF THINGS

Another fascinating area of upcoming technology is IoT. Many "things" today have Wi-Fi built into their design, enabling connections to both the Internet and other devices. The Internet of Things, known as IoT, is the future of technology which has already paved the way for devices like smartphones, household appliances, vehicles, and numerous other things to access the Internet and share data. As consumers, we already benefit from and use IoT. Businesses will gain a lot today and in the upcoming days. But IoT could aid businesses in making choices that are healthier, more effective, and more informed as data is collected and analysed. Along with other advantages we haven't yet thought of, it can facilitate predictive maintenance, speed up medical treatment, enhance customer service, and more.

6.2 FUTURE TRENDS FOR WIRELESS HEALTHCARE WITH 6G

Through mobile, terrestrial, and satellite connectivity, 6G will offer more extensive and comprehensive coverage. The goal of 6G is to create a unified communication system that combines compute, navigation, and sensing. In the area of security, 6G would address the security, confidentiality, and privacy of vast data generated by sensors and devices. Whenever it comes to modernising contemporary lives, society, and industry, 5G will have certain drawbacks. For instance, hologram transmission is not possible due to the reduced data rate. As a result, the time is right to consider the potential of 6G communication technology. The future healthcare system must also be imagined to certify the welfare of society's inhabitants, as seen in Figure 6.3 [4]. Additionally, an emergency services is just a medical transporter with priority access to the roads and oxygen that is provided by the regular car. Additionally, the senior people are woefully inadequate in light

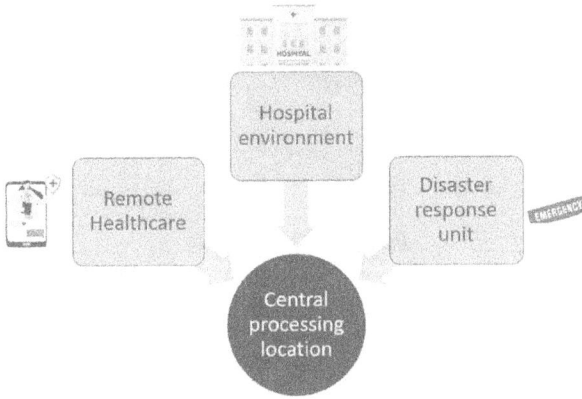

FIGURE 6.3 Wireless healthcare structure.

of the current situation. Elderly patients require intensive attention from medical professionals. But it's no longer accessible.

A large percentage of patients pass away in ambulances on route to the hospital or till they get there. Additionally, healthcare systems do not currently use the strategy for detecting accidents. To provide medical care promptly and on-site, the detection and alert system needs real-time detection. Furthermore, a lack of technological infrastructure makes it impossible to control epidemic and pandemic outbreaks like COVID-19.

6.2.1   6G COMMUNICATION TECHNOLOGY FOR SMART HEALTHCARE SYSTEMS

6.2.1.1   Smart Healthcare

Smart Healthcare: The Future of Healthcare is Connected and Intelligent. In the future, our healthcare will be smarter and more connected.

- 6G is a big part of this future.
- 6G will allow your doctor and healthcare team to have instant access to your health information, which will make it possible for them to provide better, more personalised care.

We're in the midst of a healthcare revolution. We're no longer just treating the symptoms of a disease – we're preventing them from happening in the first place. Our healthcare system is becoming more digitised, more connected and more personalised as shown in Figure 6.4. This is where smart healthcare comes in. Healthcare is going through a digital revolution. We're seeing the rise of wearable technologies that can monitor our health, and artificial intelligence that can detect diseases before they become a problem.

The IoT is becoming even more intelligent and is able to collect data and respond to our needs. The world of healthcare is changing, and the Internet is at the centre of it.

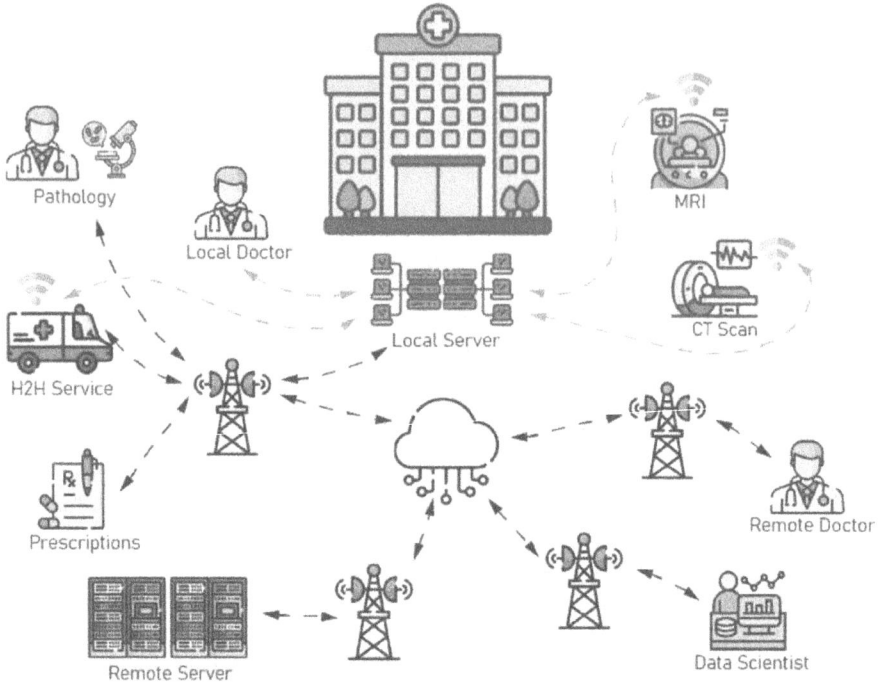

FIGURE 6.4   Components of smart healthcare system.

Just as the 5G revolution has reshaped the way we live, the 6G era will change the way we do things. The first 6G-enabled devices are already available in Asia, and the first 6G networks are live in certain parts of the world. In the next few years, you'll be able to get 6G in your home and business. You'll be able to have the same access to high-speed wireless Internet in your home or office as you do in a public place, like an airport or shopping mall.

Future healthcare will require 6G communication technology at tremendous data rates (1 Tbps), outstanding operational frequency of at least one THz, least end-to-end latency of one millisecond, excellent dependability (10–9), and great mobility (1,000 kmh). In telesurgery, real-time communication is crucial.

For sophisticated healthcare systems, hologram transmission and augmented/virtual reality will both be beneficial. On the other hand, 5G or B5G will not be able to support intelligent healthcare. The 5G era will see a significant advancement in the usage of intelligent healthcare. Rural connectivity, however, still presents a challenge for 5G communication and healthcare.

6.2.2   Associated Technologies of 6G

Supporting technologies are necessary for 6G communication technology to live up to its promises. As an intelligence communication technology, 6G's communication technology must incorporate AI. The Internet of Everything (IoE), which will be useful in many ways, will also be facilitated by 6G. Edge technology is also required for 6G networks to bring cloud applications closer to smart technologies. A multitude of technologies make up 6G communication technology as a result.

6.3 THE NEXT DECADE IS IoT's DECADE

Disease diagnosis and therapy could experience a revolution within the next ten years or more. By offering special details and insights to business sponsors, doctors, and patients, IoT wearables are changing the way we receive healthcare. Medical, biotech, and biomedical research organisations may improve their choices and achieve a competitive advantage thanks to the information collected via IoT devices. Real-time monitoring and treatment of diseases will evolve as a result of advances in IoT and its constant collaboration with the pharmaceutical and healthcare industries. The following are current IoT developments:

- Wearables for heart attacks
- Glucose tracker
- Sensors for stroke patients
- Asthma monitoring
- Movement disorders
- Coagulation monitoring
- Depression monitored through an app
- Smart eye lenses
- Health monitoring
- Cancer cure
- Pose rectification
- Hearing support
- Sleep observing
- Premature detection of Alzheimer's
- Hospital in-house 24-hour care
- Respiratory disease recognition
- Imitation kidneys
- Lung intensive care

Figure 6.5 depicts some of the possible healthcare applications which can utilise the IoT-based services [5] for better and more efficient medical facilities in near future.

6.3.1 MEDICAL WEARABLES BENEFITS

Individuals can obtain the knowledge they need to improve their health outcomes with the help of IoT-enabled medical devices. Healthcare wearables increase awareness of essential facets of a person's health status. Benefits comprise:

- Real-time fitness specialist care,
- Alerts and alarms to monitor susceptible patients' well-being status,

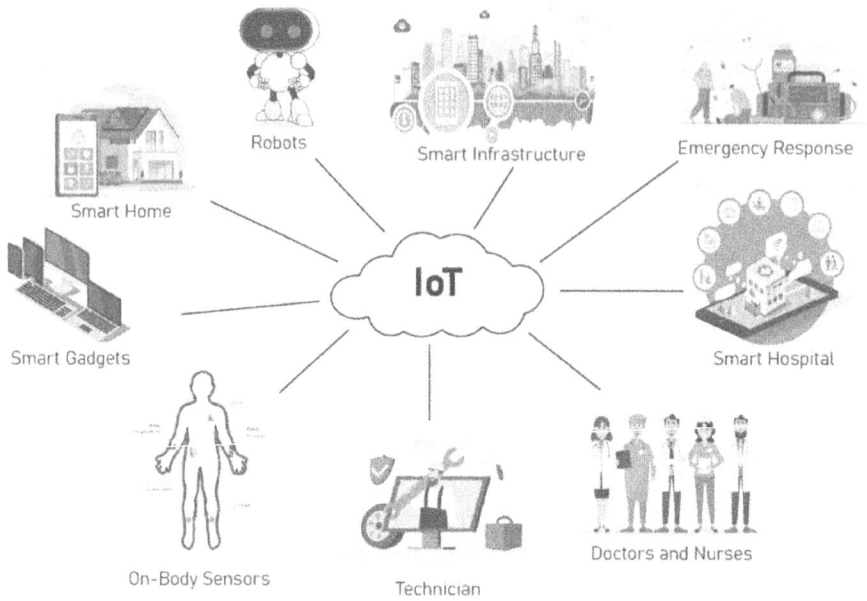

FIGURE 6.5 IoT-based healthcare technologies.

- Patient–physician facts distribution,
- Community media sharing,
- Wearable technology that tracks health information.

Some of the medical wearable devices used for health monitoring are shown in Figure 6.6.

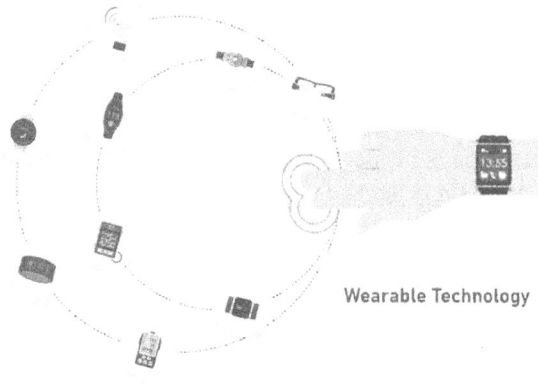

FIGURE 6.6 IoT-based healthcare technologies.

6.3.2 REMOTE HEALTH MONITORING

Vitals and health data can be remotely monitored with wearable medical equipment. Wearable medical technology enables professionals to stay in touch with patients. Patients gain more knowledge about their health, which improves therapy results. Wearable medical technology enables providers to deliver better treatment, boost productivity, and lower operational costs.

6.3.3 INTELLIGENT WEARABLE DEVICES

Connected wearable technology provides a workable alternative to help disease management systems and improve health assessment services. The healthcare industry is greatly benefiting from wearable technology [6]. As seen in Figure 6.7, patients who are carrying these devices can monitor variables including blood pressure and body temperature. A doctor can receive this information and use it to treat the patient quickly and effectively. Internet-connected smart wearable devices provide cognitive and emotional data to testing and monitoring organisations. These gadgets can monitor your body's weight, nutrition, blood pressure, health issues, and blood testing. The test results will be delivered promptly. Additionally, IWD gains knowledge from a person's body history and suggests the next line of treatment, such as exercising or walking. IWD will keep track of each individual's past behaviour, diet, and health. In the situation of a deficiency, IWD can, therefore, offer nutritional guidance. Hospital visits will be cut down by the early detection of minor physical issues like deficiencies. As a result, hospitals will spend less money on care for

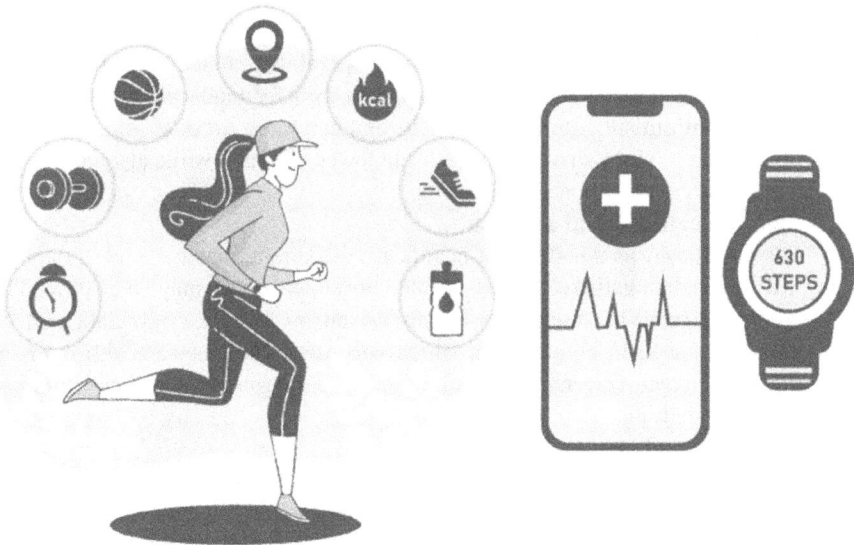

FIGURE 6.7 Health monitoring in real time.

less straightforward illnesses. Additionally, IWD will evaluate samples of blood and transfer them to experts for review. Therefore, IWD can be utilised to identify disease at an early stage. IWD can consequently enhance health outcomes and lengthen human lifespan. It is also essential for services provided to the elderly who require intense care. Future IWDs will be handheld devices with many functionalities. All capabilities will be in one device.

Such devices will initially be expensive, but as time goes on, the cost will drop, making them affordable for the average individual to buy.

6.4 ASSISTANCES OF IoT IN MEDICAL FACILITIES

With the improvement in demand for real-time exact remote health monitoring, amalgamation of IoT with medical facilities seems to be offering numerous opportunities.

1. **Parallel monitoring and reporting**

   In the case of a health emergency like cardiac arrest, diabetes, or asthma attacks, real-time monitoring via connected devices can stop a million fatalities. Using linked devices to gather relevant medical and health-related data, a smart medical gadget coupled with a smartphone application can evaluate a patient's symptoms in real time [7]. The IoT-connected device gathers and communicates health-related data, including ECGs, measurements of weight, blood pressure, oxygenation, and blood sugar, among other things. Anyone who has the appropriate sharing access authority can access the data because it is stored in the cloud.

2. **End-to-end connectivity and affordability**

   IoT can help automate medical and patient healthcare processes through healthcare mobility solutions. The expense of providing healthcare services is significantly reduced thanks to interoperability, machine-to-machine connection, information sharing, and data transfer made possible by the IoT. By minimising unnecessary visits and using resources of higher quality, this technology-driven approach can lower expenses while also improving resource allocation and planning.

3. **Data assortment and analysis**

   It's not as easy as it sounds for healthcare workers to manage a lot of data. Real-time data gathered by IoT-enabled portable devices may be examined and segregated by mobility solutions driven by IoT. Less raw data will, therefore, need to be gathered, which will allow for crucial health informatics and data-driven insights, ultimately reducing errors and accelerating decision-making.

4. **Tracking and alerts**

   Real-time surveillance and alerts in life-threatening scenarios can turn into a lifesaver to safeguard a critically ill patient's health with regular updates and real-time alerts for correct monitoring, analysis, and diagnosis. Healthcare mobility solutions permitted by IoT-enabled real-time monitoring, notification, and tracking.

5. **Remote medical assistance**

It is a terrible situation when one patient requires medical attention but is unable to get a doctor due to barriers like distance or ignorance. IoT-enabled logistics services that offer patients adequate medical treatment when they're on the go are at the base of the problem [8]. Patients can take prescription medications at home thanks to public healthcare systems connected to them via IoT devices.

6.5 INTERNET OF EVERYTHING (IoE)

The IoE links people, things, information, and processes into a seamless interconnected system with the goal of enriching experiences and promoting improved decision-making. The IoE worldview envisions a world in which numbers of equipment, devices, and everyday things are equipped with sensors, allowing them to connect and grow more intelligent [9]. What does the IoE mean for businesses, organisations, and people? The primary goals of the IoT are to transform data into actions, facilitate data-driven decision-making, and provide new capabilities and richer experiences.

6G follow 6CâAˇZ´ s for communication. The five key functions in this case are capture, communication, caching, cognition, computation, and control.

- Without it, holographic communication in the medical field is impossible.
- The gathered information is transformed into digital form, which will then be locally cached and instantly transmitted to distant sites.
- Digital data may be converted to time-dependent signals and reassigned to other devices for processing in some instances.
- However, cognition assists in the formulation of workable decisions based on the intake of digital data before computing.
- These are smart choices that improve the usability of computing.

In order to aid in smart device control in the healthcare industry, computed data is provided to smart devices. Large data rates will be necessary to provide tactile sensations in intelligent healthcare devices. IoE will need a lot of capacity to link lakhs of intelligent devices, capture tactile sensations, and turn them into digital data in order to enable 6G. When 6G becomes a commercially viable option, a newer era of Big Data, known as Big Data 2.0, will start. "Big Data 2.0" refers to the use of a supercomputer to manage and analyse immense quantities of small-scale data produced by medical devices.

6.5.1 Virtual Touch on Internet: Haptic Technology

With the application of force, motion, or vibration, haptic technology simulates touch. A virtual touch can be transmitted from one user to another using the tactile Internet, whether they be robots or humans. High-speed connectivity is crucial for tactile Internet along with the use of ERLLC for real-time tactile data collection [10]. One such model is shown in Figure 6.8. With the use of this technology, telesurgery,

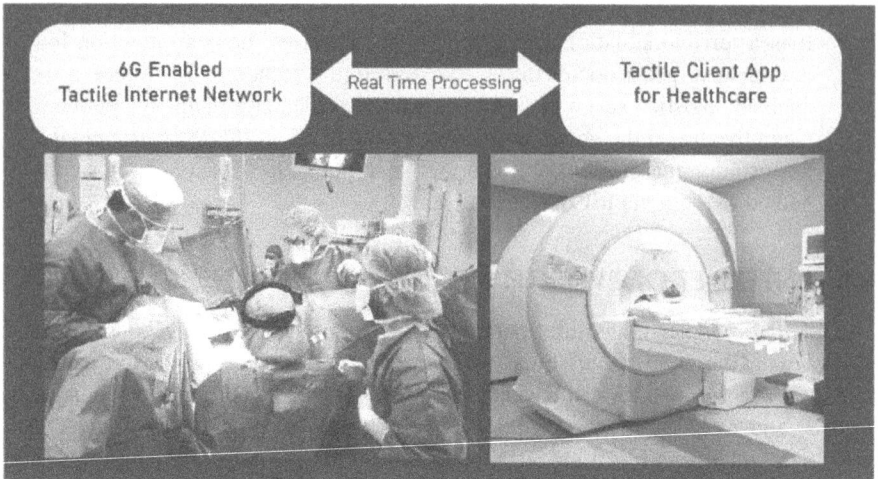

FIGURE 6.8   Tactile internet model example.

or remote patient monitoring, will be conceivable. Additionally, doctors won't have to physically be present to diagnose patients through touch. Three categories of haptic human–computer interaction (HCI) exist: desktop, surface, and wearable.

A desktop HCI system will allow a distant physician to carry out surgery or make diagnostics using a virtual tool. Instead of being three-dimensional, surface HCI movement is two-dimensional. Use a horizontal device, such as a smartphone or tablet, to send commands. The robot can be designed to converse with the patient by waving the hands on the screen. In wearable HCI, the remote doctor, for instance, uses a haptic glove. Tactile/haptic technologies will also aid in the provision of medical treatment in the event of an emergency. In the event of natural calamities like the COVID-19, all nations are required to enter lockdown and cease all interactions with the outside world. Tactile/haptic technology will be relevant in these scenarios. Complex surgeries can be completed out remotely by qualified doctors deploying robots. During epidemics and pandemics, medical personnel pose significant risks. They run the risk of contracting the serious or contagious illness if individuals don't take safeguards. Tactile and haptic technology enable robots to engage with or help patients while medical staff is present remotely. The Internet's 6G increase, speed, low-latency technology enables all of this.

6.5.2   CLEVER MEDICAL TECHNOLOGIES

The Innovative Internet of Medical Things (IIoMT) can arise inside the 6G communication paradigm and meet a set of purposes for people's well-being [11]. IIoMTs are AI-powered clever machines that can decide things according to their own using communication technologies. Together with IIoMT, IoE can advance, making it possible for medical devices to link to the Internet, including MRI and CT scans. The scanner will inspect the electronic devices and send the data to distant areas via

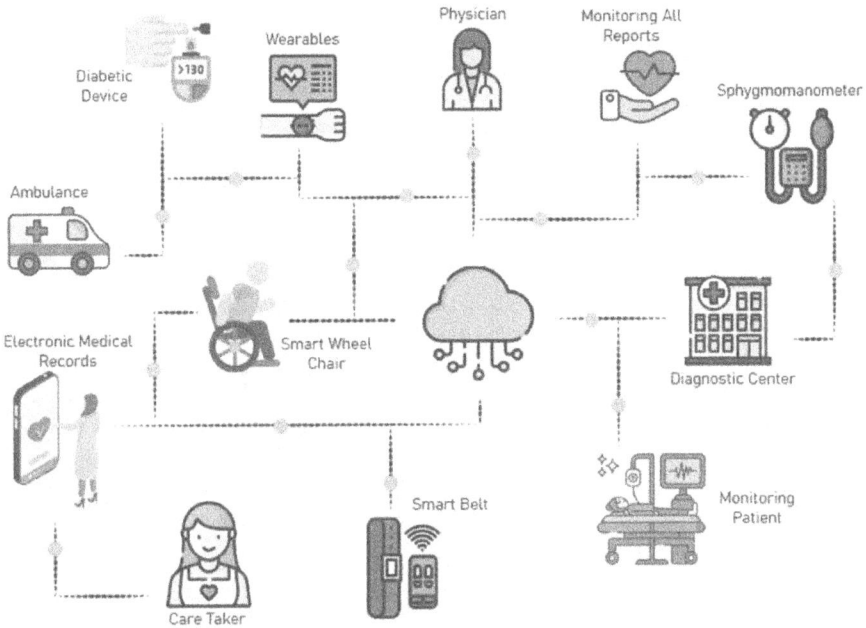

FIGURE 6.9 Intelligent interconnected healthcare model.

6G technology. A pathologist can promptly assess this data. In order to facilitate better and faster decision, almost all medical devices will then be able to link to the Internet (as shown in Figure 6.9). The IIoMT will indeed be able to deal with constraints relating to time, space, and money as a result. For illustration, doctors who function in distant areas can readily treat cancer patients. Usually, it takes time to ascertain if a person with cancer has a benign or malignant cancer. However, 6G communication can promptly make it possible to discover cancer in real time. Neither patients nor surgeons are mandated to go to specialised hospitals. Time and funds are both crucial. Accordingly, remote experts will coordinate with regional technical experts to assist and help cancer patients. Early cancer identification can virtually eliminate cancer patient mortality risk. Nonetheless, such sensors ought to be developed. Not just cancer but a plethora of ailments fall under this context, for instance, medications for cardiac diseases.

1. **A reader for analysing blood sample**

   As the global disease index rises, people are working to create new and improved health monitoring tools that are accurate and automatic. Due to manual sample collection, there is still a recurrent risk that medical staff would become exposed to numerous infections. In the wake of the most recent COVID-19 pandemic, the worst-case scenario has been revealed. Blood may be used to identify the majority of diseases because it is crucial to human health. Traditional blood sampling involves drawing blood from a person's body using needles. Nevertheless, a number of research

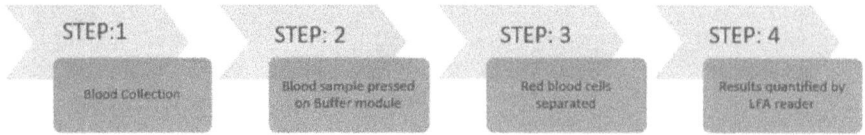

FIGURE 6.10   Blood sample collection system.

towards needle-free blood-sampling apparatus are now being conducted. For instance, modern needle-free techniques are recommended for diabetic patients whose blood sugar levels need to be monitored. Figure 6.10 demonstrates how a wearable Sample Reader sensor can be created to analyse the patients' medical parameters without the requirement for a needle stick. Such blood sample devices have the potential to transform the medical field.

These sample sensors can keep track of a number of blood-related characteristics, including the counts of white blood and red blood cells. Through the use of 6G technology, the data collected by these intelligent sensing devices may be transported remotely to a healthcare facility for real-time data updating and monitoring. These gathered samples can be automatically transmitted to testing facilities with the patient's permission for in-depth analysis and consistent report production. As a result, the need for manual involvement when analysing blood samples will be significantly reduced. This ability can be crucial for providing older patients with close attention and precise monitoring. In fact, such gadgets can easily monitor the parameters in times of epidemic and medical emergency to reduce manual exposure during pandemic periods.

2. **Hospital-to-home services**

Emergency medical services typically place a priority on expedited oxygen delivery and patient road transportation. According to predictions, all automobiles in the near term will be powered by artificial intelligence [12]. We are unable to offer complete emergency hospital services at this time owing to a lack of clever technologies and extremely quick communication networks. As a result, the impact of emergency service and ambulance services on our lives is minimal. To address these issues in the medical industry, the hospital-to-home concept is being promoted. We can increase access to better and faster medical care by including amenities like oxygen and an emergency signal in every passenger car. This can be useful in clinical cases if prompt medical care is necessary to save a person's life. These technologically enhanced services aim to improve ambulance services and take the place of standard facilities with cutting-edge methods. This will make it easier for hospitals to connect with individuals who really need immediate medical care at home when there is a life-threatening emergency. Artificial intelligence and quicker communication technologies are required to create such intelligent cars. As a result, hospitals and physicians will depend less on medical facilities. In a nation where the population has a significant impact on the provision of ineffective services, the integration of intelligent gadgets and high-speed information transfer will strengthen medical facilities. Another feature of these systems is the availability of mobile traffic and the ability to update real-time data while moving. Such mobile networks can give precise and reliable data for managing ambulances and potentially take the place of the present antiquated methods. For instance, information about the tragic event of a traffic collision and its precise position can be given to a nearby paramedic for prompt intervention. The device may act as a makeshift hospital that can begin caring for patients even before a medical team gets there. If speedier modes of communication are not accessible, such quick and efficient services cannot be provided. Here, emerging technologies like 6G connection may prove useful in altering the way management systems are currently running.

3. **Telesurgery**

The use of assisted technologies in surgery and medicine is gaining ground more quickly. One such discipline is telesurgery, sometimes known as "remote surgery," where surgery is carried out using robots and medical professionals from a distance [13]. In systems like these, accurate and exact real-time data transport are two essential components. 6G can greatly aid in the development of this procedure because it is a profitable concept for future medical technology. It also requires a fast connection speed and URLLC because its dependability is totally based on communication. 5G and B5G do not totally meet these standards. Because of this, cutting-edge technology like 6G is a crucial tool for making these facilities accessible and cheap. 6G communication is a real-time programme that enables audible and tele-assisted discussion during surgery. People can actually afford to speak with those who are world-class authorities in the topic in question. Procedures could be more accurate and have higher success rates since they include direct communication. In situations where the patient cannot travel longer distances, such solutions can be quite valuable. These strategies can help us reach every nook and cranny for the betterment of society in remote areas with sparse medical services.

4. **Pandemic situation**

An effective communication system is essential in pandemic and epidemic circumstances. Typically, such circumstances arise as a result of a sickness that affects large populations. As a result, there is a professional medical personnel shortage. First and foremost, those who work in medicine are most at danger for contamination, and second, under such circumstances, people also fear for their lives. A real-life example of that occurred during the most recent medical crises. It also made clear the difficulties and obligations that must be met in such circumstances. In these circumstances, 6G technology can be helpful in a variety of ways. In order to obtain samples from sick people, for instance, the blood specimen collection system that was mentioned previously in the chapter may be of significant assistance. Additionally, health professionals can readily monitor and consult in such situations due to the job's extremely contagious nature. This will lead to better and quicker services during emergencies as well, when people's ability to move around and engage in normal activities is severely constrained.

There are currently millions of COVID-19 virus carriers, which calls for billions of further testing. It can be difficult to maintain accurate and up-to-date information for such a vast number of people. This raises another issue with regards to large-scale data management and storage services. Since time is so important in stopping the development of a disease like COVID-19, updating the information is absolutely necessary. The recent global catastrophe requires the swift approval and deployment of comprehensive, sophisticated healthcare management systems.

5. **Precision medicine**

The development of a personalised drug or therapy for the benefit of a patient's condition is known as precision medicine. Doctors and researchers group patients based on a shared criterion to provide precision medicine. Precision medicine will tremendously benefit from the development of 6G technology. It also requires AI in order to deliver individualised healthcare. Clinical trial participants' health information is necessary for improved therapy development. For instance, research into cell therapy is being attempted to treat fatal illnesses. IWD can be used by doctors and academics to gather data. Real-time data collection will be used to provide more accurate health statistics. Additionally, the study may be carried out anywhere on the earth. A person's geographic location affects their immune system. As a result, isolating the targets of observation will alter their surroundings. The research will then be impacted by this. As a consequence, the doctor or researcher will employ IIoMT to keep an eye on subjects who are being monitored globally.

6.6   HOW SECURE IS DATA IN 6G?

For its users' confidentiality, a trustworthy communication network primarily relies on security and privacy. This necessitates the deployment of far more enhanced security in 6G. Data transmission through a network in the healthcare industry must be done with a high degree of protection [14]. A patient's death might occur as a result of any alteration with medical information. Therefore, safeguarding health information from hackers is crucial. With this technology, very high levels of privacy and encryption procedures are promised. In this THz communication generation, the employment of technologies including artificial intelligence, quantum computing, and machine-learning algorithms may protect the data from security threats. Since we are employing the THz frequency range, jamming and eavesdropping difficulties are instantly resolved. The secrecy of sensitive data is another point that 6G communication emphasises. Due to inadequate security procedures, it should not be permitted for such highly confidential information to leak. Additionally, administrators are not permitted to view this private data. Privacy, which is among the most important aspects of healthcare, is another theme of 6G. Edge technology will be used in 6G to enhance privacy. The edge nodes are nearer to the intelligent devices. The very same edge nodes also analyse the computed data. Due to the memory constraints of edge nodes, content is not condensed in one place. Edge protects its users' privacy as an outcome. The edge nodes' data filtering is still another critical factor. Only the most vital information is transferred to the cloud after being screened at the edge nodes. Likewise, it implies that the cloud will have less user-specific records. While the current frenzy for cloud storage offers reliability for smaller data sets, it is unable to guarantee the integrity of bigger data blocks. A high amount of anonymity for healthcare information is now provided by blockchain technology. For processing and conserving patient health data, it creates a safe environment. It is anticipated that 6G, together with all the other sophisticated technologies mentioned before and others, would significantly enhance cognitive data management systems in the near future.

6.7 CHALLENGES OF 6G TECHNOLOGY

Figure 6.11 shows the challenges encountered by researchers while attempting to implement 6G wireless functionalities. Since this technology is still in research and development phase, we cannot surely list and mark particular drawbacks or disadvantages of 6G. These details need to be withheld until practical 6G systems are installed for trial and testing phase.

1. The characteristics of 6G include multi-connectivity and cell-less design. As a result, faultless scheduling is necessary for multi-network integration and connectivity (THz, VLC, mmwave, sub-6GHz). In a cell-less design, the UE connects to the RAN rather than a particular cell. The hardest issue in this case is conceiving a fresh network configuration.

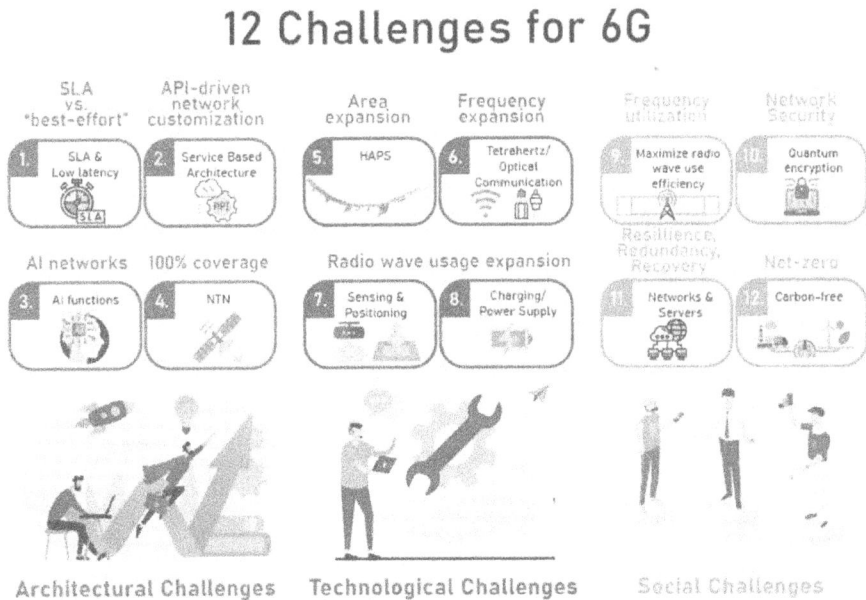

FIGURE 6.11 Challenges for 6G.

2. Knowing that THz is used for part of its communications, the constraints of THz (Terahertz) frequencies might be viewed as shortcomings of 6G wireless technology. The term "terahertz frequency" refers to the electromagnetic (EM) wave spectrum with a wavelength of 30–3000 micrometres that falls between 0.1 and 10 THz. Terahertz waves can be widely used in space communications and are ideally suited for use between satellites. Coverage is heavily impacted by the shadow sensitivity of the THz signal. Additionally, lower terahertz frequencies undergo increased free space fading. A massive issue in THz is ultra-large-scale antenna, which mandates ultra-high bandwidth and strong quantitative resolution.
3. Processing power is a crucial concern in the deployment of low-cost, low-power 6G products. Given that only a small portion of 6G communications exploit visible light wavelengths, identical restrictions appear to apply to 6G wireless systems as well. Visible light has a wavelength range of 390–700 nm. To manage a large range of connections and subnetworks in a cost- and energy-efficient approach, a 6G strategy is indispensable. To do this, it is essential to optimise the circuitry in interface and endpoint equipment as well as the layout of the connectivity protocol stack. Strategies for gathering energy-related information are applied to fulfil its requirements.

6.8 CONCLUSION

In order to anticipate for the issues posed by the projected sharp rise in wireless data traffic, corporate and academic groups have begun work on the sixth generation of wireless data transmission (6G). Aside from providing a slew of new services, 6G technology enables bitrates of up to Tbps with a congestion of less than 1 ms. In order to foster future 6G in the following parameters efficacy, intellectual ability, channel capacity, confidentiality, secrecy, and anonymity, research begins by establishing a vision and the main aspects geared at achieving this goal. Then, we briefed about a variety of possible issues with 6G technology and prospective solutions to support 6G in the future. International research endeavours that strive to create a future 6G vision surrounding this effort.

REFERENCES

1. B.G. Evans and K. Baughan. (2000). "Visions of 4G." *Electron. Commun. Eng. J.*, 12(6): 293–303.
2. X. Krasniqi and E. Hajrizi. (2016). "Use of IoT technology to drive the automotive industry from connected to full autonomous vehicles." *IFAC-PapersOnLine*, 49(29): 269–274.
3. C.M. Hall. (2019). "Constructing sustainable tourism development: The 2030 agenda and the managerial ecology of sustainable tourism." *J. Sustain. Tour.*, 27(7): 1044–1060.
4. A. Ahad, M. Tahir, M.A. Sheikh, K.I. Ahmed, A. Mughees and A. Numani. (2020). "Technologies trend towards 5G network for smart health-care using IoT: A review." *Sensors*, 20(14): 4047.
5. V. Jagadeeswari, V. Subramaniyaswamy, R. Logesh and V. Vijayakumar. (2018). "A study on medical Internet of Things and Big Data in personalized healthcare system." *Health Inf. Sci. Syst.*, 6: 1–20.

6. D. Nahavandi, R. Alizadehsani, A. Khosravi and U.R. Acharya. (2022). "Application of artificial intelligence in wearable devices: Opportunities and challenges." *Comput. Meth. Prog. Bio.*, 213: 106541.

7. M.H. Kashani, M. Madanipour, M. Nikravan, P. Asghari and E. Mahdipour. (2021). "A systematic review of IoT in healthcare: Applications, techniques, and trends." *J. Netw. Comput. Appl.*, 192: 103164.

8. B. Haque, D. Jacquline Mon and D. Gracia. (2021). "A literature survey on the applications of internet of things." Przegląd Elektrotechniczny, 97.

9. X. Fan, X. Liu, W. Hu, C. Zhong and J. Lu. (2019). "Advances in the development of power supplies for the internet of everything." *InfoMat*, 1(2): 130–139.

10. M. Sreelakshmi and T.D. Subash. (2017). "Haptic technology: A comprehensive review on its applications and future prospects." *Materials Today Proceedings*, 4(2): 4182–4187.

11. T.N. Nguyen, Q.-D. Ngo, H.-T. Nguyen and G.L. Nguyen. (2022). "An advanced computing approach for IoT-botnet detection in industrial Internet of Things." *IEEE Trans. Industr. Inform.*, 18(11): 8298–8306.

12. E. Sulis, I.A. Amantea, M. Aldinucci, G. Boella, R. Marinello, M. Grosso, P. Platter and S. Ambrosini. (2022). "An ambient assisted living architecture for hospital at home coupled with a process-oriented perspective." *J. Ambient. Intell. Humaniz. Comput.*, 1–19.

13. C. Huang, S. Hu, G.C. Alexandropoulos, A. Zappone, C. Yuen, R. Zhang, M.D. Renzo and M. Debbah. (2020). "Holographic MIMO surfaces for 6G wireless networks: Opportunities, challenges, and trends." *IEEE Wirel. Commun.*, 27(5): 118–125.

14. M. Wang, T. Zhu, T. Zhang, J. Zhang, S. Yu and W. Zhou. (2020). "Security and privacy in 6G networks: New areas and new challenges." *Digit. Commun. Netw.*, 6(3): 281–291.

7 Machine Learning in Healthcare Cybersecurity

Role of Human Activity Recognition and Impact of 6G in Smart Healthcare

Neha Gupta, Suneet Kumar Gupta, and Vanita Jain

CONTENTS

7.1 Introduction 143
7.2 Literature Review and Statistical Analysis... 145
    7.2.1 Statistical Analysis 147
        7.2.1.1 HAR Applications.. 147
        7.2.1.2 Hyperparameters... 148
        7.2.1.3 Popular DL Models.. 148
7.3 Smart Healthcare HAR Devices.. 149
    7.3.1 Smartphones and Wearable Devices 149
    7.3.2 Video Sensors 151
    7.3.3 RFID.. 151
7.4 Applications of HAR in Smart Healthcare.. 152
    7.4.1 Smart Health to Overcome Lifestyle Diseases 152
    7.4.2 Smart Health in Assisting Rehabilitation Tasks 152
    7.4.3 Smart Health for Personal Life-Log 152
7.5 Discussion.. 152
    7.5.1 Short Note on the Impact of 6G in Smart Healthcare 152
    7.5.2 6G Applications in Healthcare 153
    7.5.3 6G Challenges... 153
7.6 Conclusion 153
References... 154

7.1 INTRODUCTION

Over recent years, human activity recognition (HAR) has risen as a topic of significant importance and research. HAR can be simply defined as the task of measuring a person's activity (physical) with the help of objective technology. This task is challenging owing in terms of complexity and diversity of human activities, which can be simplified by sub-categorizing. HAR has become an interesting research field with time, especially because of the advancement in the usage of electronic devices like smartphones, video cameras, and environmental sensors in our daily lives [1, 2]. Adding further, the progress of deep learning and other algorithms has made it possible for researchers to use HAR in many fields including sports, health, well-being, etc. [3, 4]. For example, HAR is one of the most promising resources for helping elderly people living alone by supporting their cognitive and physical function through daily actions [5, 6].

Another domain that is proving to emerge manifolds in the industry of information technology is the Internet of Things (IoT). IoT can be applied effectively in the modern healthcare field, by actively monitoring the daily activities of patients and elderly people [7–9]. This enables the role of HAR with IoT significant for smart healthcare devices. One major asset provided by IoT to the healthcare-monitoring system is the technology of wearable sensors. In addition, the incorporation of IoT with health care has led to the development of smart applications like m-Healthcare and other monitoring systems [10]. For health monitoring, the patient can use sensor devices (stand-alone sensor, smartwatch, or smartphone sensors). These devices have fitted gyroscope and accelerometer sensor, that sends sensor data to a server that listens to that to enable continuous activity monitoring [7–9]. Changes to these structures exist, especially with modern smart devices having the skills to do activity recognition as well as self-monitoring [10, 11]. These have better processing units, bigger memories, and better senses.

In the case of nursing activities, observing the pattern and paying attention to methods are some of the ways that are beneficial in increasing the effectiveness of health care. One such instance can be including only the essential activities in the exercise routine of the patient in order to aid earlier discharge and avoid excessive and unnecessary work. Various researchers have adopted such practices with the use of mobile sensors like accelerometers, gyroscopes, etc. in related fields of healthcare and nursing activities. As per Mairittha et al., it was found that several key features are required for effective activity recognition such as a user-friendly interface of an application, recording target persons, interface for recognition and feedback, detailed records, and the functionality of offline database and operation [12]. Based on applications and modality, HAR can be categorized as video-based HAR systems and sensor-based HAR systems. In video-based HAR systems, cameras are used to record images or videos to monitor human behaviour, while sensors in the body and surrounding areas are used by HAR-based sensory systems to capture and record human activity data [13, 14]. Due to the privacy invasion caused by the installed cameras in the participants' surroundings, requests to monitor daily activities are governed by sensor-based systems [15]. In addition, another benefit of nerves is their proliferation.

Figure 7.1 depicts the broad overview of smart healthcare-based HAR framework for the purpose of health monitoring and evaluating a person's health in an m-Health ecosystem. In healthcare systems like these, automatic action recognition and monitoring helps the medical specialists to monitor their patients with continuously generated data. At first, the smartphone that a person is carrying acquires and analyses the signals of the physical activities performed by the user and then uploads this activity information through the wireless and wired networks for the intelligent health information analysis. Intelligent and interactive health data analysis is becoming more significant as the healthcare systems are transitioning to value-based and

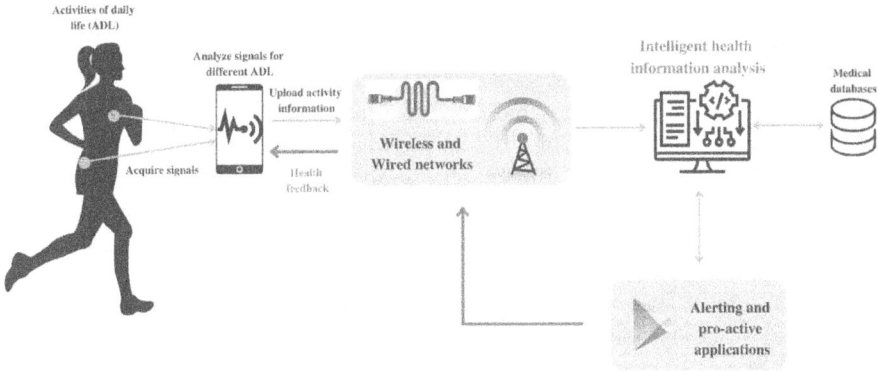

FIGURE 7.1 An overview of a smart healthcare-based HAR framework for health monitoring.

intelligent systems for enhancing the health outcomes and care quality. This intelligent health data analytics is inspired by innovative and intelligent techniques emerging from Big Data and artificial intelligence. Medical databases along with alerting and proactive applications are a part of the intelligent health information analysis used in smartphone-based HAR. After analysing the health data, the health feedback is transferred from the applications to the wired and wireless network which further updates it on the person's smartphone.

As a result of the rapid growth of smart devices with various sensors, it is possible to insert sensors into portable devices, such as phones, watches, mirrors, as well as intangibles, such as vehicles, furniture, and walls. Nowadays, sensors are widely installed in our environment, recording information about human activity, and do not invade the privacy of the user by any means. In this chapter, we have performed the detailed literature review and statistical analysis in the next section. Further, in the second section, a detailed description about smart healthcare devices is provided, in the third section, we have discussed the applications of HAR, and in the fourth section, we have proposed the future on smart healthcare in terms of 6G.

7.2 LITERATURE REVIEW AND STATISTICAL ANALYSIS

In the last decade, numerous researches have been carried in the domain of HAR using a variety of approaches. In this section, we aim to highlight some of the deep-learning HAR techniques suggested in the time that relates to our proposed approach. In a study illustrated by Almaslukh et al., earlier work on HAR was limited to a specific position which restricted the user's activity. Some researchers proposed position-independent and position-aware HAR which enabled users to freely attach their smartphones to any part of their body which in turn reduced the hassle and increased the efficiency of the process. Attaching the smartphone to any part of the body helps reduce the restriction of motion and provides better results as the data fetched is of random activities done by the user which helps determine the realistic data [16].

According to the literature, there were two methods that are majorly used to develop a HAR model, which enable the free attachment of a phone to any on-body position. The first one is position-independent HAR. In this approach, mixed sensors were used in building the model. This method trained the model using the data gathered from various source including different postures. Additionally, some special handcrafted features were also used which restricted the variation in motion data in a different position for the same activity. Some domain experts suggested that the restriction of one activity in different positions is the limitation of handcrafted features. Generalization with different settings for the same problem cannot be done as the features are shallow. The second approach is position-aware HAR. It is based on building two or more classifiers. The first classifier is used to recognize the specific position of the sensor. Meanwhile, the second classifier is used to recognize the position-specific activity but having limitations: this method is highly expensive to run on such a small device as a smartphone.

Nweke et al. surveyed various ways of HAR models such as smartphone or on-body sensors-based HAR systems. They have also categorized the DL methods used in HAR models in terms of generative approach, discriminative approach, and the hybrid approach which combines the advantages of both generative and discriminative [17]. The limitation of this survey was that it was limited to the HAR models based on either device sensors or the body-worn sensors. Whereas Li et al. presented different neural networks for radar-based activity recognition. His survey, however, was only limited to techniques such as CNNs and RNNs. The scope can be expanded to tackle specific challenges such as deep transfer learning and multimodal fusion [18].

In 2019, Kim et al. used SVM based on micro-Doppler signatures for HAR and used handcrafted features. A decision-tree structure was employed, and a gesture recognition system was built using 60 GHz mm-wave radar. They have adopted random forest classifier for identifying real-time gesture recognition. The authors have also proposed an improved DTW algorithm for hand gesture recognition with a terahertz radar which was completely capable of exploring the properties of range profile and Doppler signatures [19]. A mobile application named FonLog can be used as a tool for data collection to detect human activities in nursing homes and other healthcare areas. The app consists of various features like recording activity targets, recognition feedback, detailed records, a user-friendly interface, and functionality of offline operation that can help collect the data of various activities effectively [12].

The model proposed by Torres et al. uses the approach of a single triaxial accelerometer which doesn't impose any strict restrictions on the smartphone's location though it does take into consideration some typical locations where the users carry their smartphones [20]. Yet, it serves as a relevant example to exhibit the role, challenges, and a few main potential effects that these smartphones have now and will have in the future in m-Health.

The works of Ogbuabor et al. tend to research the role of physiological sensors including the gyroscope, magnetometer, accelerometer, and their conjunction for automated HAR model which is based on neural networks [21]. According to experimentation performed on each individual physiological sensors, they draw the analysis that individual sensor can be used for capturing and identifying the human actions. But the results are improved when they combined data of each sensor for capturing and recognizing the human action. However, merging of many sensors together may lead to significant difficulties due to the restrictions on the smartphone's battery. Action recognition requires continuous signals from the smartphone. The study by

Mairittha et al. proposes a mobile application named FonLog which can be used as a data collection tool in action recognition of humans for nursing services [12]. This app has the necessary characteristics for efficient data collection which is gathered by the feedback from nursing staff which includes recording action targets, instant activity, recognition feedback, detailed records that are customizable, and offline functionality.

The model proposed by D'Angelo et al. introduces a technique that focusses on enhancing the performance of the tracking application used for the COVID-19 virus with the help of HAR and a classifier based on convolutional neural networks is provided for the same [22]. In the proposed method, the raw accelerometer data of a smartphone is organized to form an HAR-image which is further used as fingerprints of the in-progress activity. The analysis and experimentation of real-time data shows that the HAR-images can be used as a better source for human activity recognition. An IoT technology-based intelligent m-Healthcare system devised by Radhwan et al. that used data-mining techniques which is proposed to provide extensive human activity recognition has been proposed in this research [23]. A reliable and accurate IoT technology-based human action recognition model is developed with a client-dependent data-mining strategy for offline human action recognition.

7.2.1 STATISTICAL ANALYSIS

7.2.1.1 HAR Applications

HAR models aim to identify various activities performed by different individuals based on a series of data collected by the sensors. The foundation for many possible applications in sports, fitness, surveillance, daily life activities, and health is activity recognition. Nearly 30% of Chinese, European, Canadian, and American citizens will be older than 60 by 2050, according to a Goldstone report. With the global growth of medical research and technology, life expectancy is rising, and as a result, the demand for medical assistance is also increasing. Examining various models created for the purpose of HAR revealed that 30.2% of them, or the bulk of them, were utilized for health-monitoring reasons.

The intelligent environment is one of the most popular applications of HAR with smart home being one of its examples. A smart home creates an environment equipped with sensors that improve the safety of residents and enhance their living standards. Almost 23.3% of the studied models were created for the current trend towards smart houses. With the increase in life expectancy, the need for assistance in the lives of older people is also rising, and it was seen that 18.6% of the models were built for this purpose. Initially, surveillance systems were run by people, but as the number of deployed cameras increased, efficiency levels dropped. In response, vision-based security and surveillance systems were put into use, with 11.6% of the studied models being seen to be useful in this capacity. The World Health Organisation (WHO) reports that falls are the second-most common cause of unintentional injury and death worldwide. Elderly people who fall also frequently develop functional dependencies. Nearly 16.3% of the models studied were built for the purpose of fall detection. Figure 7.2 (a) shows the statistical analysis of popular HAR applications.

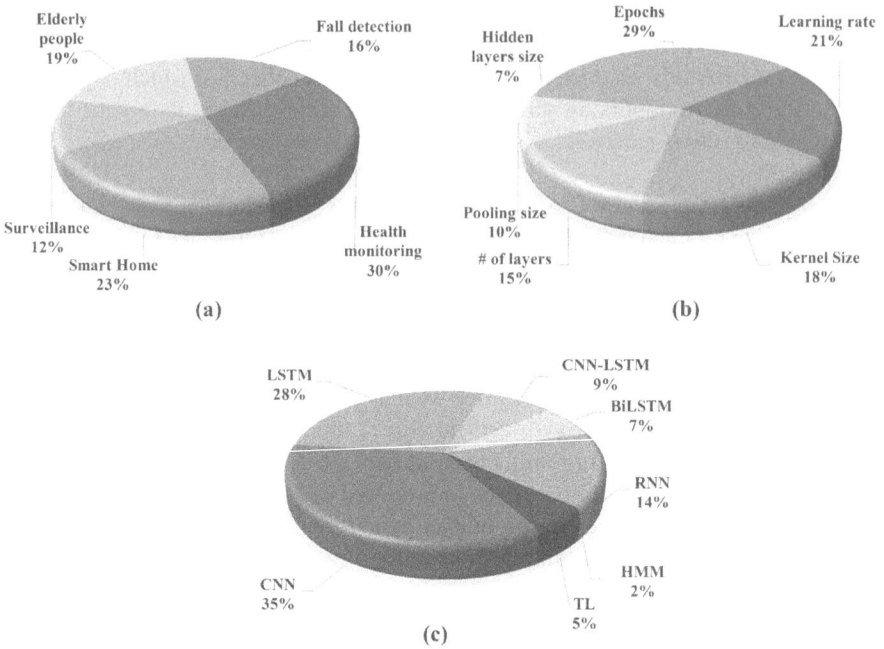

FIGURE 7.2   (a) HAR applications, (b) hyperparameters used, and (c) DL models.

7.2.1.2 Hyperparameters

A parameter in a machine-learning model is an internal variable of the model whose value can be calculated from the data. In contrast, a hyperparameter in a machine-learning model is a variable external to it whose value cannot be determined by the data. Figure 7.2 (b) illustrates the analysis of most used hyperparameters adopted by researchers in DL-based HAR models.

Hyperparameters are those parameters whose values are set before the learning process starts and they specify how a network is to be trained. Based on the study that we conducted on some HAR models, it was seen that the number of epochs was the most used hyperparameter. Nearly 29.5% of models used epochs as one of their hyperparameters. Learning rate was the second-most used hyperparameter in these models. Kernel size was used in 18% of these models, while a number of layers were used as a hyperparameter in 14.8% of them. Almost 9.8% of models used pooling size as one of its hyperparameters, whereas time step and neurons in hidden layers were used in only 6.6% of the models.

7.2.1.3 Popular DL Models

Sensors for the recognition of human activity are classified into three main categories: vision sensors, environmental sensors, and radio frequency sensors. Vision-based sensors are essentially dependent upon the visual perception of the environment. The environment sensors include device sensors and wearable sensors. While the latter is equipped with a set of sensors like an accelerometer, magnetometer, and gyroscope, and uses the approach of directly interacting with the human body to recognize human actions, the former attaches sensors to commonly used devices and performs human action recognition on the basis of user's interaction with the environment and these devices. Radio-frequency sensors are basically device-free sensors that receive signals that are affected by human activities in the channel. As a result of these activities, the received signal may exhibit distinct features that can be exploited for HAR purposes. According to studies on various HAR models, 16.7% of the models utilized vision sensors, 27.3% used radio frequency sensors, and the remainder, or 56.1% of the models, which is a significant fraction of HAR models, employed environment sensors. Figure 7.2 (c) illustrates the usage of various DL techniques used by researchers while implementing their HAR models.

7.3   SMART HEALTHCARE HAR DEVICES

7.3.1   SMARTPHONES AND WEARABLE DEVICES

HAR is done in different stages like collecting the data, pre-processing and training the data, and then finally recognizing the type of activity through various methods [24]. One common method is capturing the data through smartphones and on-body or body-worn sensors. Body-worn sensors are usually embedded into the wearable devices or attached directly to the body to detect the kind of activity being performed by the user. Sometimes, users might refrain from adapting to wearable sensor techniques. In such cases, smartphone sensors are considered. Device sensors capture data with the help of commonly used built-in physiological sensors such as accelerometer, magnetometer, and gyroscope on smartphone devices [2, 10]. Smartphones and wearable devices are a good choice and consist of a large number of high-precision sensors that are integrated into these devices [25]. Many devices are present that can be used to capture different motions and activities performed by the user, but the methods or principles stay nearly the same. (1) Changes in the data with respect to different movements or actions performed by the user are recorded using sensors like an accelerometer and gyroscope. (2) This data is then sent to desktops or other systems for computation using some complex algorithms. (3) Data processing is done based on the number of parameters which finally helps in analysing and recording the kind of activity being done by the user [25].

Smartphones and wearable devices tend to offer many benefits as compared to other practices in case of HAR. No complex or expensive setup is required to predict the activity; built-in sensors are used to note down the motion [26]. Triaxial or 3-axis accelerometers are generally used for detecting activities like walking, jogging, and running, to name a few [26, 27]. Built-in sensors can capture more continuous data and signals which help in delivering accurate results [28]. We can easily get information regarding the user's linear acceleration, velocity, direction, and the electromagnetic radiation with the help of accelerometer, gyroscope, and magnetometer sensors present in the smartphones and wearable devices [29]. In addition, the user is always in the range of the sensor to capture continuous data, unlike in the case of video sensors [25, 30]. Contrary to the advantages stated, some researchers feel that while smartphones and wearable devices are a fairly good choice for activity recognition, there can be certain limitations too [31]. Both smartphones and wearable devices need frequent charging or changing of batteries. Also, the user might not always have wearable device wrapped around the body, especially in case of an elder person as the user, but if used consistently, it can prove to be beneficial [32].

Overall, smartphones and wearable devices are considered to be a much better choice as they maintain the user's privacy, provide continuous measurement of data, and produce more accurate results because of the presence of in-built sensors that work around a number of parameters in the 3-dimensional space [33]. There can be broadly two ways of deploying wearable devices for HAR: Using a 3-axis accelerometer or body area network (BSN) [34] and sensors used in combination with other sensors like temperature sensors, gyroscopes, etc. [35]. With time, researchers have started to prefer smartphones as the ideal solution for the accurate recognition of activities [31]. This is because of the cognitive and computing power, exceptional processing capabilities, easy deployment option, and robustness of smartphones [8].

Smartphones also consist of a variety of sensors like accelerometers, gyroscopes, and magnetometers and have wireless connectivity, which makes them very useful for purposes like smart home monitoring [36]. Smartphones consist of inertial sensors that use appropriate sensing resources to obtain HAR information. Because of the presence of high-quality built-in sensors, wearable devices are automatically able to filter external magnetic interferences. They are able to estimate the acceleration and angular velocity accurately [26]. Sensor-based identification is much preferred because of its many benefits like small size, ease to carry, high sensitivity, and anti-interference ability. Sensors identify the physical states and characteristics using inertial measurement units (IMU) sensors like accelerometers and gyroscopes, and magnetic field sensors which are altogether used to identify the activity [37].

The usage of smart devices like smartphone and smartwatch makes them the perfect choice for smart healthcare application. Smartphones are becoming widely popular in terms of activity recognition, step counting, calculating temperature, heart rate, blood pressure, etc. [21]. This is because of the presence of accurately functioning built-in sensors like accelerometers, gyroscopes, magnetometers, barometers, and many more. Out of all the various types of sensors embedded in smartphones, accelerometers and gyroscopes are most used for HAR. Accelerometers are the triaxial (x, y, z) sensors used to measure acceleration, which is nothing but the change in velocity of any object. The values extracted from the sensor in terms of x, y, and z coordinates can be used to determine the acceleration of a user. However, the raw data collected from this sensor must be processed to its much more accurate form with the help of a classifier. While the x coordinate deals with the lateral movement of the device, the y axis provides information on the vertical movement. Any movement described in and out of the plane that is defined by the x and y axes is taken care of by the z axis.

Gyroscope sensors are necessary for measuring the orientation of the device by calculating the actions such as roll, yaw, and pitch gestures of the phone around the x, y, and z axis, respectively. As per the results of research carried out by [21], where the performance of the proposed model was evaluated for both accelerometer and gyroscope data separately, and then their combined results passed to the classifier and for better understanding of results confusion matrix was generated.

7.3.2 VIDEO SENSORS

One very effective and most direct approach to HAR is to use video-based model which involves video cameras for data gathering. Cameras are utilized for recording videos and images to distinguish participants' behaviour. Cameras provide rich and unique sets of information that are way better than other sensors. They offer continuous monitoring of actions with clear features which enables intelligent analysis and predictions throughout the process. This method provides ground truth, which can be used to check the results and improve the accuracy of machine learning in the real world.

Over the period, many authors introduced different methods of classification of video-based HAR. One such model was proposed by Nweke et al. which involves the late fusion technique [17]. This model combines frames by linking the first and last frames in the clip. Early fusion was another method that was introduced which extracted all the local features from the same patches and locally linked them before encoding. Some more authors have proposed various methods for classifications: a combination of CNN and LSTM, pose detection with LSTM, and slow-fast networks of videos [38].

There are basically three types of HAR problems:

- The first is simple activity recognition where a short video clip is provided to the model which gets processed and predict the singular global action being performed.
- The second is temporal activity recognition where a long video clip consisting of a set of different actions is passed at different intervals to the HAR model. One of the two parts of this architecture localizes each individual action into temporal partitions. Whereas the second part focuses on classifying each video proposal.
- Lastly, there is spatio-temporal detection in which the video clipping contains multiple actions performed by multiple people. Each person is detected and localized in the video and the performed activities of each individual are classified [39].

7.3.3 RFID

RFID stands for radio frequency identification. This approach have many applications in smart home environment such as health monitoring of elderly people living alone, exercise monitoring, etc. In this approach, RFID tags are placed at different positions near the participant's body or in a person's environment. These tags are used to track the vertical as well as the horizontal positioning of a person accurately in a smart space or home. RFID uses an analysed dataset against a set of reference position datasets [40]. Li et al. proposed an RFID-based HAR model for trauma resuscitation which is a quick-paced and highly dynamic process to treat severely wounded patients immediately after injury. The authors proposed this model to monitor the trauma-effected person regularly which helps in improving the documentation rates and compliance of attending physician arrival [41].

7.4   APPLICATIONS OF HAR IN SMART HEALTHCARE

7.4.1   Smart Health to Overcome Lifestyle Diseases

Over the period of last few years, an increased growth is observed in the occurrence of chronic diseases like stroke, cardiac failure, diabetes, and hypertension [21, 42]. This is partly because of the adaptation of certain physical habits and activities in an individual's daily life. Obesity, for example, which results from the combination of many factors, is considered an epidemic that greatly impacts physical health. Such lifestyle diseases demands continuous monitoring of physical activities; therefore, there is the need of an intelligent mobile applications to monitor the movement and activities of a user. These applications can suggest and guide the user to perform certain actions and help prevent chronic medical conditions [21].

7.4.2   Smart Health in Assisting Rehabilitation Tasks

One of the major applications of HAR is "assistance in rehabilitation services." With the virtual assistance provided by smartphone, a person or patient can perform several exercises at home instead of going to any kind of rehabilitation centre. The data gathered using smartphone sensor can be used to accurately estimate the activities of a patient daily such that a therapist is able to track progress and observe the quality of care needed. The system captures the physical activity being performed by the user which can be classified based on a comparison of accuracies with the previously learned metrics under the supervision of a specialist. Such techniques also help in reducing the cost of healthcare expenditure [17, 43, 44].

7.4.3   Smart Health for Personal Life-Log

With the commencement of HAR techniques using smartphone sensors, remote monitoring of patients or telemonitoring has become possible. Smart healthcare solutions help in analysing patients far away from the facility of health service providers in a person-specific, time-saving, and cost-effective manner. To provide personalized and real-time support, these systems must be able to collect sufficient information and provide the desired mechanisms. Therefore, mobile-based life-log solutions for a person are necessary to conceptualize routine tasks such as data sharing, containing, and mining to speed up an application's development cycle [11, 12].

7.5   DISCUSSION

7.5.1   Short Note on the Impact of 6G in Smart Healthcare

The 6G technology has a great potential to change the future of healthcare sector relatively better than the current 5G systems. AI being very important for smart healthcare will depend on the 6G connections, which will transform our way of life. 6G will solve the two most significant problems to smart healthcare, time and location. 6G is a well-anticipated communication technology that is expected to take over the entire market from around 2030 onwards. 6G will solve the space–time barrier that our current healthcare system is not able to.

7.5.2 6G APPLICATIONS IN HEALTHCARE

The role of artificial intelligence-based healthcare solutions with 6G offers a rich set of increased specialist care ways to track health conditions of a patient and helps in developing automated warnings in case of an emergency. It also provides relevant and 24-hour engagements with healthcare personnel. There are certain 6G technologies that can be utilized in smart healthcare solutions.

i. *In-body, on-body, off-body communications* – It involves the remote monitoring of a patient's health with the help of ICT-based monitoring tools. The body layer contains all forms of communications [45].
ii. *Human bond communications* – It offers enhanced services like patient monitoring, diagnosis, assistance, and treatment. This technique detects and data is collected through human senses [46].
iii. *Visible light communications* – VLC is a type of optical wireless technology. Light rays are used as a tool to deliver data. It can be used to take data from the body and for broad communication between users [47].

7.5.3 6G CHALLENGES

Some of the challenges faced by 6G technology are mentioned next:

i. Security and privacy – Strong authentication systems and cryptographic algorithms are required which can offer shorter key length [45]
ii. Technological aspects – Critical data is retrieved and circulated to the process of communication between body layers. There are several nodes and each of them has notably diverse communication requirements [45]

7.6 CONCLUSION

This chapter revolves around the role of HAR in smart healthcare systems, and discussed the impact of 6G with enhanced smart health solutions. Further, we have discussed the various devices which are used to gather the health-related data such as smartphone or other wearable device sensors, video cameras, and RFID devices. Also performed the statistical analysis of previously proposed studies in terms of HAR applications, hyperparameters used, and DL models. With the evolution of IoT-based devices, growth is monitored through the smart healthcare applications. In this chapter, we have provided the insight about various HAR-based smart health applications such as health monitoring, cost-effective personalized application to patients remotely, and remote-assistive care to elderly living alone, etc. For providing health report to medical professional, 6G offers secure and efficient medium. The features offered with 6G are the future for HAR applications which in turn benefit the smart healthcare domain.

REFERENCES

1. F. Fereidoonian, F. Firouzi, and B. Farahani. "Human activity recognition: From sensors to applications." In *2020 International Conference on Omni-layer Intelligent Systems (COINS)*, August 2020, pp. 1–8. doi: 10.1109/COINS49042.2020.9191417.
2. N. Gupta, S. K. Gupta, R. K. Pathak, V. Jain, P. Rashidi, and J. S. Suri. *Human activity recognition in artificial intelligence framework: A narrative review*, no. 0123456789. Netherlands: Springer, 2022.
3. D. Ravi, C. Wong, B. Lo, and G. Z. Yang. "Deep learning for human activity recognition: A resource efficient implementation on low-power devices." *BSN 2016 – 13th Annu. Body Sens. Networks Conf.*, pp. 71–76, 2016. doi: 10.1109/BSN.2016.7516235.
4. G. S. Nambissan, P. Mahajan, S. Sharma, and N. Gupta. "The variegated applications of deep learning techniques in human activity recognition." In *2021 Thirteenth International Conference on Contemporary Computing (IC3-2021)*, pp. 223–233, August 2021. doi: 10.1145/3474124.3474156.
5. G. De Leonardis et al. "Human activity recognition by wearable sensors." *2018 IEEE Int. Symp. Med. Meas. Appl. Proc.*, in press, 2018. doi: 10.1109/MeMeA.2018.8438750.
6. L. Yao et al. "Compressive representation for device-free activity recognition with passive RFID signal strength." *IEEE Trans. Mob. Comput.*, vol. 17, no. 2, pp. 293–306, 2018. doi: 10.1109/TMC.2017.2706282.
7. G. M. Weiss, K. Yoneda, and T. Hayajneh. "Smartphone and smartwatch-based biometrics using activities of daily living." *IEEE Access*, vol. 7, pp. 133190–133202, 2019. doi: 10.1109/ACCESS.2019.2940729.
8. S. Yao, S. Hu, Y. Zhao, A. Zhang, and T. Abdelzaher. "DeepSense: A unified deep learning framework for time-series mobile sensing data processing." *26th Int. World Wide Web Conf. WWW 2017*, pp. 351–360, 2017. doi: 10.1145/3038912.3052577.
9. I. Y. Nebogatikov and I. P. Soloviev. "Human activity recognition by wearable sensors in the smart home control problem." *J. Phys. Conf. Ser.*, vol. 1864, no. 1, 2021. doi: 10.1088/1742-6596/1864/1/012112.
10. J. R. Kwapisz, G. M. Weiss, and S. A. Moore. "Activity recognition using cell phone accelerometers." *ACM SIGKDD Explor. Newsl.*, vol. 12, no. 2, pp. 74–82, 2011. doi: 10.1145/1964897.1964918.
11. H. Ding et al. "FEMO: A platform for free-weight exercise monitoring with RFIDs." *SenSys 2015 – Proc. 13th ACM Conf. Embed. Networked Sens. Syst.*, pp. 141–154, 2015. doi: 10.1145/2809695.2809708.
12. N. Mairittha, T. Mairittha, and S. Inoue. "Demo: A mobile app for nursing activity recognition." *UbiComp/ISWC 2018 - Adjun. Proc. 2018 ACM Int. Jt. Conf. Pervasive Ubiquitous Comput. Proc. 2018 ACM Int. Symp. Wearable Comput.*, pp. 400–403, 2018. doi: 10.1145/3267305.3267633.
13. L. Sun, K. Jia, D. Y. Yeung, and B. E. Shi. "Human action recognition using factorized spatio-temporal convolutional networks." *Proc. IEEE Int. Conf. Comput. Vis.*, Inter, pp. 4597–4605, 2015. doi: 10.1109/ICCV.2015.522.
14. D. R. Beddiar, B. Nini, M. Sabokrou, and A. Hadid. "Vision-based human activity recognition: A survey." *Multimed. Tools Appl.*, vol. 79, no. 41–42, pp. 30509–30555, 2020. doi: 10.1007/s11042-020-09004-3.
15. C. Pham, N. N. Diep, and T. M. Phuong. "E-shoes: Smart shoes for unobtrusive human activity recognition." *Proc. - 2017 9th Int. Conf. Knowl. Syst. Eng. KSE 2017*, pp. 269–274, January 2017. doi: 10.1109/KSE.2017.8119470.
16. B. Almaslukh, A. M. Artoli, and J. Al-Muhtadi. "A robust deep learning approach for position-independent smartphone-based human activity recognition." *Sensors (Switzerland)*, vol. 18, no. 11, 2018. doi: 10.3390/s18113726.

17. H. F. Nweke, Y. W. Teh, M. A. Al-garadi, and U. R. Alo. "Deep learning algorithms for human activity recognition using mobile and wearable sensor networks: state of the art and research challenges." *Expert Syst. Appl.*, vol. 105, pp. 233–261, 2018. doi: 10.1016/j.eswa.2018.03.056.

18. Y. Jia, Y. Guo, G. Wang, R. Song, G. Cui, and X. Zhong. "Multi-frequency and multi-domain human activity recognition based on SFCW radar using deep learning." *Neurocomputing*, vol. 444, pp. 274–287, 2021. doi: 10.1016/j.neucom.2020.07.136.

19. Y. Kim and B. Toomajian. "Hand gesture recognition using micro-doppler signatures with convolutional neural network." *IEEE Access*, vol. 4, pp. 7125–7130, 2016. doi: 10.1109/ACCESS.2016.2617282.

20. C. Torres-Huitzil and A. Alvarez-Landero. *Recognition in Smartphones for Healthcare Services*. Cham, Switzerland: Springer, 2015. doi: 10.1007/978-3-319-12817-7.

21. G. Ogbuabor and R. La. "Human activity recognition for healthcare using smartphones." *ACM Int. Conf. Proceeding Ser.*, pp. 41–46, 2018. doi: 10.1145/3195106.3195157.

22. G. D. Angelo and F. Palmieri. "Enhancing COVID – 19 tracking apps with human activity recognition using a deep convolutional neural network and HAR – images." *Neural Comput. Appl.*, 2021. doi: 10.1007/s00521-021-05913-y.

23. Subasi, A., Radhwan, M., Kurdi R., and Khateeb, K. "IoT based mobile healthcare system for human activity recognition," *2018 15th Learning and Technology Conference (L&T)*, Jeddah, Saudi Arabia, pp. 29–34, 2018. doi: 10.1109/LT.2018.8368507.

24. E. Sansano, R. Montoliu, and Ó. Belmonte Fernández "A study of deep neural networks for human activity recognition." *Comput. Intell.*, vol. 36, no. 3, pp. 1113–1139, 2020. doi: 10.1111/coin.12318.

25. W. S. Lima, E. Souto, R. El-Khatib, R. Jalali, and J. Gama. "Human activity recognition using inertial sensors in a smartphone: An overview." *Sensors (Switzerland)*, vol. 19, no. 14, pp. 14–16, 2019. doi: 10.3390/s19143213.

26. S. Wan, L. Qi, X. Xu, C. Tong, and Z. Gu. "Deep learning models for real-time human activity recognition with smartphones." *Mob. Networks Appl.*, vol. 25, no. 2, pp. 743–755, 2020. doi: 10.1007/s11036-019-01445-x.

27. M. M. Hassan, M. Z. Uddin, A. Mohamed, and A. Almogren. "A robust human activity recognition system using smartphone sensors and deep learning." *Futur. Gener. Comput. Syst.*, vol. 81, pp. 307–313, 2018. doi: 10.1016/j.future.2017.11.029.

28. A. Ferrari, D. Micucci, M. Mobilio, and P. Napoletano. "Trends in human activity recognition using smartphones." *J. Reliab. Intell. Environ.*, vol. 7, no. 3, pp. 189–213, 2021. doi: 10.1007/s40860-021-00147-0.

29. J. W. Lockhart, T. Pulickal, and G. M. Weiss. "Applications of mobile activity recognition." *UbiComp'12 – Proc. 2012 ACM Conf. Ubiquitous Comput.*, pp. 1054–1058, 2012. doi: 10.1145/2370216.2370441.

30. H. M. Ali and A. M. Muslim "Human activity recognition using smartphone and smartwatch." *Int. J. Comput. Eng. Res. Trends*, vol. 3, no. 10, p. 568, October 2016. doi: 10.22362/ijcert/2016/v3/i10/48906.

31. M. Straczkiewicz, P. James, and J. P. Onnela. "A systematic review of smartphone-based human activity recognition methods for health research." *NPJ Digit. Med.*, vol. 4, no. 1, pp. 1–15, 2021. doi: 10.1038/s41746-021-00514-4.

32. K. Moore et al. "Older adults' experiences with using wearable devices: Qualitative systematic review and meta-synthesis." *JMIR mHealth uHealth*, vol. 9, no. 6, pp. 1–19, 2021. doi: 10.2196/23832.

33. A. Jalal, M. Uddin, and T. S. Kim. "Depth video-based human activity recognition system using translation and scaling invariant features for life logging at smart home." *IEEE Trans. Consum. Electron.*, vol. 58, no. 3, pp. 863–871, 2012. doi: 10.1109/TCE.2012.6311329.

34. J. Cui and B. Xu. "Cost-effective activity recognition on mobile devices." *BODYNETS 2013 - 8th Int. Conf. Body Area Networks*, pp. 90–96, 2013. doi: 10.4108/icst.bodynets.2013.253656.

35. J. Wang, Y. Chen, S. Hao, X. Peng, and L. Hu. "Deep learning for sensor-based activity recognition: A survey." *Pattern Recognit. Lett.*, vol. 119, pp. 3–11, 2019. doi: 10.1016/j.patrec.2018.02.010.

36. S. Sun, Z. Cao, H. Zhu, and J. Zhao. "A survey of optimization methods from a machine learning perspective." *IEEE Trans. Cybern*, vol. 50, no. 8, pp. 3668–3681, 2020. doi: 10.1109/TCYB.2019.2950779.

37. F. Attal, S. Mohammed, M. Dedabrishvili, F. Chamroukhi, L. Oukhellou, and Y. Amirat. "Physical human activity recognition using wearable sensors." *Sensors (Switzerland)*, vol. 15, no. 12, pp. 31314–31338, 2015. doi: 10.3390/s151229858.

38. C. Feichtenhofer, H. Fan, J. Malik, and K. He. "SlowFast Networks for Video Recognition." 2018 [Online]. Available: http://arxiv.org/abs/1812.03982.

39. H. S. Koppula, R. Gupta, and A. Saxena. "Learning human activities and object affordances from RGB-D videos." *Int. J. Rob. Res.*, vol. 32, no. 8, pp. 951–970, 2013. doi: 10.1177/0278364913478446.

40. K. Chen, D. Zhang, L. Yao, B. Guo, Z. Yu, and and Y. Liu. "Deep learning for sensor-based human activity recognition: Overview, challenges and opportunities." *arXiv*, vol. 37, no. 4, 2020.

41. X. Li, Y. Zhang, I. Marsic, A. Sarcevic, and R. S. Burd. "Deep learning for RFID-based activity recognition." *Proc. 14th ACM Conf. Embed. Networked Sens. Syst. SenSys 2016*, pp. 164–175, 2016. doi: 10.1145/2994551.2994569.

42. M. Maniruzzaman et al. "Accurate diabetes risk stratification using machine learning: Role of missing value and outliers." *J. Med. Syst.*, vol. 42, no. 5, p. 92, May 2018. doi: 10.1007/s10916-018-0940-7.

43. P. Gupta and T. Dallas. "Feature selection and activity recognition system using a single triaxial accelerometer." *IEEE Trans. Biomed. Eng.*, vol. 61, no. 6, pp. 1780–1786, 2014. doi: 10.1109/TBME.2014.2307069.

44. M. Devanne, H. Wannous, S. Berretti, P. Pala, M. Daoudi, and A. Del Bimbo. "3-D human action recognition by shape analysis of motion trajectories on Riemannian manifold." *IEEE Trans. Cybern.*, vol. 45, no. 7, pp. 1340–1352, 2015. doi: 10.1109/TCYB.2014.2350774.

45. F. Al-Jawad, R. Alessa, S. Alhammad, B. Ali, and M. Al-Qanbar. "Applications of 5G and 6G in smart health services.", *IJCSNS International Journal of Computer Science and Network Security*, vol. 22, no. 3, pp. 173–182, 2022.

46. A. Vergütz, N. G. Prates, B. H. Schwengber, A. Santos, and M. Nogueira. "An architecture for the performance management of smart healthcare applications." *Sensors*, vol. 20, no. 19, p. 5566, September 2020. doi: 10.3390/s20195566.

47. S. Nayak, R. Patgiri, and S. Member. "6G communication technology: A vision on intelligent healthcare." In: Patgiri, R., Biswas, A., Roy, P. (eds) *Health Informatics: A Computational Perspective in Healthcare. Studies in Computational Intelligence*, vol. 932, pp. 1–9, 2021. doi: https://doi.org/10.1007/978-981-15-9735-0_1.

8 6G-Enabled IoT Wearable Devices for Elderly Healthcare

Shubham Gargrish, Sharad Chauhan,
Meenu Gupta, and Ahmed J. Obaid

CONTENTS

8.1 Introduction 157
8.2 Related Work 159
8.3 A 6G-Enabled Wireless Healthcare Service 161
8.4 Importance of IoT in Healthcare 162
8.5 Technology That Supports 6G 162
     8.5.1 Artificial Intelligence 162
     8.5.2 Virtual Reality and Augmentation (VR/AR) 163
     8.5.3 Human–Computer Interaction (HCI) 163
     8.5.4 Hospital-to-Home Services 164
8.6 The New 6G Business Model 164
8.7 Discussion 165
8.8 Conclusion and Outlook 165
8.9 Future Findings 166
References 167

8.1 INTRODUCTION

To lower health risks globally, an enhanced healthcare system is a key requirement. Healthcare outlines a set of guidelines that a society must adhere to in order to preserve the basic requirements of people. Any healthcare system's effectiveness is based on the services it offers, the viability and accessibility to those services, and the citizenry's usability, acceptance, and trustworthiness [1]. Despite living in the twenty-first century and having access to all of today's advanced technological resources, the globe will still be threatened by the COVID-19 pandemic in 2020. Even before the basic characteristics of the virus were understood, its propagation was rapid and cryptic. Due to its standout characteristics and promising future applications, 6G communication technology is luring many academics. From 2030 onwards, we shall see traces of the revolution in a variety of disciplines [2]. Numerous 6G features have already been debated in prestigious forums, and numerous 6G communication technology requirements are constantly being gathered [3, 4]. Additionally, Chen et al. [5] highlight problems and difficulties

DOI: 10.1201/9781003321668-8

with 6G communication technology. For timely implementation, 6G communication technology has already been launched in several nations. The 6G initiative was first started by Finland in 2018 [6]. Second, the 6G scheme was launched in 2019 by the US, South Korea, and China [7]. Japan just started a 6G research scheme for 2020 [8]. Additionally, numerous 6G algorithms have been created [9, 10]. Launching the 6G project is now crucial if we want to shun declining behind other nations. In contrast, B5G has not yet been invented and 5G communication technologies have not yet been deployed worldwide. In order to alter current lifestyle, society, and industry, 5G and B5G will have a number of downsides [11, 12]. For instance, the decreased data rate makes it unable to allow holographic communication. Therefore, this is the best moment to consider the potential uses of 6G communication technology in the future. In order to make sure the welfare of society's citizens, it is also essential to consider the future of healthcare [13].

The existing healthcare system offers just the most basic amenities, and time and space are its main obstacles. This cannot be avoided in the present situation, but it won't be a problem in the near future. A regular car can also provide ambulance service, which is only a means of transporting patients with access to oxygen and priority in the flow of traffic [14]. In addition, the service for the elderly in the present is very inadequate. Medical staff must provide rigorous care for the elderly as shown in Figure 8.1. It is still not available, though the majority of patients pass

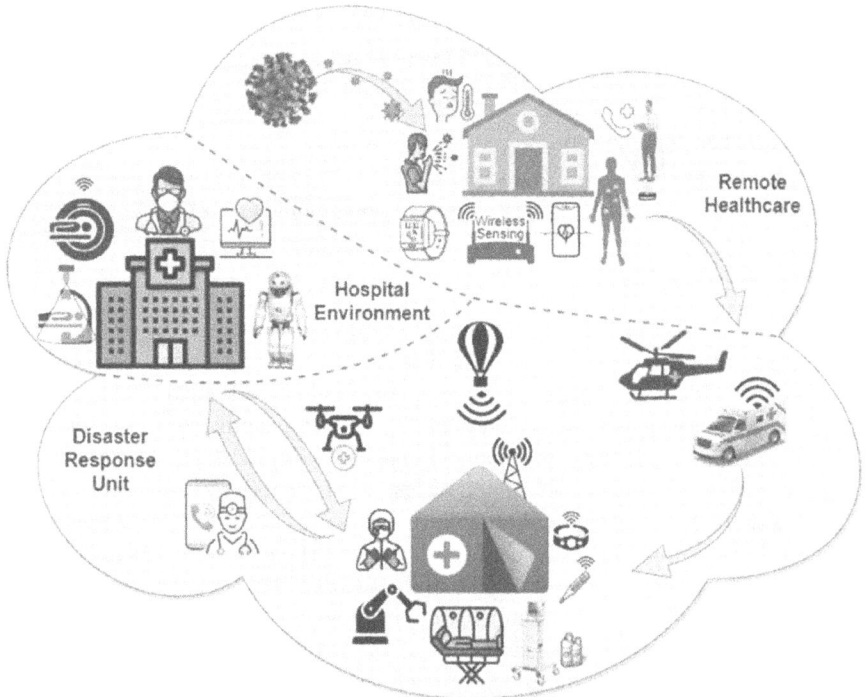

FIGURE 8.1   Current landscape of intelligent healthcare system.

away in ambulances either en route to the hospital from their homes or even before they arrive [15]. Additionally, present healthcare systems do not have the accident detection system. To deliver medical care promptly and on-site, the accident detection system needs real-time detection [16, 17]. Additionally, due to a deficiency of sophisticated infrastructure, epidemic and pandemic outbreaks like COVID-19 cannot be forbidden. In hindsight, a virus of that type will reappear. Therefore, creating an intelligent healthcare system is crucial.

Elevated data rate (1 Tbps), high-operational frequency (1 THz), low back-to-back delay (1 ms), high dependability (109), sky-scraping mobility (1,000 km/h), and wavelength of 300 m are the prerequisites of 6G communication technique for the future of healthcare [18]. Particularly, real-time communications are needed for telesurgery. The development of intelligent healthcare systems will also be aided by augmented/virtual reality and holographic communication. However, intelligent healthcare will not be supported by 5G or B5G. Smart healthcare will be largely adopted in the 5G communication age, moving forward one step. In rural areas, connectivity is still a big problem for both healthcare and 5G technology [19]. Figure 8.1 shows the landscape of intelligent health services and how technology in communication enhances their performance.

There are seven sections in this chapter. Various related works in healthcare development and implementations are described in the next section. A concise discussion of 6G technology in healthcare is presented in the second section. The example of fictitious Internet of Things healthcare services is expanded in the third section. The proposed model's technique is presented in the fourth section. The anticipated outcomes of this model are detailed in the fifth section. The model's flaws and difficulties are highlighted in the sixth section. The chapter ends with a conclusion in the last section, which also covers potential future enhancements.

8.2   RELATED WORK

Any medical professional's top priority should be speedy and trouble-free right to use the healthcare data in order to construct a successful and strong healthcare system and prevent disastrous situations [20]. Life expectation has amplified by more or less 64 percent over the past 55 years, and by 2023, there will be more people in their sixties than children under five [21, 22]. This demonstrates that the number of seniors is rising annually. Chronic lifestyle diseases are most common in people aged 55–59 years old. The enhancement of the healthcare sectors has been the subject of numerous research projects. This section discusses a few of them. Four relevant layers – the "sensor layer," "networking layer," "internet layer," and "application service layer" – are coordinated by a K-healthcare model that is put forward in [23]. Implementing a cloud IoT platform for remote patient monitoring with serious concerns has also been discussed. Numerous studies and research projects have been carried out in recent years to assist and innovate healthcare for elderly patients in rural areas. In [24], the authors examine several healthcare systems based on a range of viewpoints and characteristics, including disease management, different types of chronic and critical diseases, patients of varying ages, etc. Then, they demonstrated and reviewed various IoT-based healthcare solutions, some of which were integrated with already-in-use tools including sensing, networking, and data processing. The authors of [24] present an alternative viewpoint on the 6G-based medical system. They have suggested several potential future projects and uses for 6G technology in the medical industry. For instance, telesurgery based on holographic communication may be enabled in the near future with the support of 6G technology. They also depict a business plan that shows how the hospital can act as a patient's health insurance intermediary and how to cut costs overall. An overview of IoT-based healthcare systems and their numerous uses, including monitoring children, managing surgeries [25], managing chronic diseases, and motion sensors, is presented by the authors as shown in Figure 8.2. Additionally, they have researched how IoT devices can be managed for healthcare purposes based on their network connectivity, battery life, and other factors [26].

Every generation of mobile technology's design has had an impact on the development of automated systems based on the demands of the end users. 5G technology is integrated into everything from cloud devices to driverless vehicles operating in aircraft and on roadways. Because of network advancements, enormous amounts of data may be sent at very high speeds. The transition from 1G to 6G network technologies is shown in Table 8.1. Technology plays a significant role in many different fields thanks to its many applications, such as the IoT, some custom-made communication, wearable health devices, sensors with robotics, integrating intelligence with networks, holographic telepresence, ground-breaking network structural design, industry 4.1, telemedicine, and others.

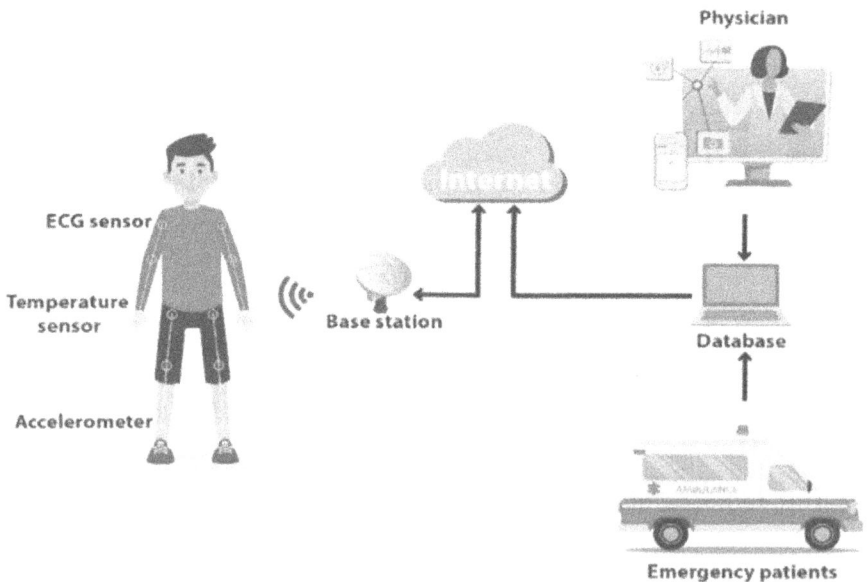

FIGURE 8.2   The older healthcare system flow.

TABLE 8.1
Transition from 1G to 6G Network Technologies

Requirements	5G	6G	B5G
Processing Delay	100 ns	50 ns	≤ 10 ns
Range of Mobility	100 < 500 km/h	500 km/h	1000 km/h
Data Rate	1 Gbps	100 Gbps	1 Tbps
Category of Application	• eMBB • URLLC • mMTC	• Reliable eMBB • URLLC • mMTC • Hybrid (URLLC+eMBB)	• MBRLLC • HCS • MPS
Operating Range Frequency	3–300 MHz	500 MHz	1 THz
Wavelength	3 mm	1 mm	300/μm
Streaming Rate	Tremendously high rate Streaming	Enormously high rate Streaming	Security
Satellite Amalgamation	Partial	Partial	Full
XR Amalgamation	Partial	Full	Full
AI Amalgamation	Partial	Full	Full

8.3 A 6G-ENABLED WIRELESS HEALTHCARE SERVICE

By offering an integrated smart health service, 6G technology will soon rule the healthcare industry. This chapter will cover this AI-driven communication technology's fundamental characteristics. Large data throughput, high capacity, high-mobility rate, low latency, and wavelength of around 300 m are the key needs of 6G for healthcare systems. It is anticipated that 6G technologies will utilize 3D architecture, including space–time frequency, and will be fully supported by satellite. As a result, 6G will get beyond the major obstacles that prevent the majority of remote patients from receiving care – geographic barriers. Additionally, it can broadcast real-time data thanks to the robust connectivity capabilities between sensors and other devices. AI algorithms and edge technologies are both a part of the integrated 6G technology schema. It is possible to create edge intelligence (EI) by combining these technologies. Edge computing with ML, DM, and highly developed networking capabilities that are related to the field of computational intellect is known as edge intelligence (EI). The 6G network can be used to implement this distributed smart computer paradigm as a self-reliant data dispensation, analysis, and decision-making component. A wavelength of about 300 m is needed for 6G communication technology's 1 Tbps data efficiency rate, 1 THz frequency, and 1,100 km/h mobility collection. With the help of these significant and promising 6G characteristics, users can operate quickly in real-time and receive complete help from the medical system right now. The implementation of smart healthcare in recent years has demonstrated that certain factors must be taken into account to meet user reliability standards. The 6G technology, on the other hand, is an example of an AI-based intellectual system that can be independent, computed itself, and manual awareness-based on any serious and unwanted situation. Since 6G-based AI-integrated network, real-time communication, a crucial component of contemporary healthcare, will be possible. An efficient healthcare system requires real-time communication, which AI can deliver with great accuracy and performance. Deep-learning algorithms (DL), which do not require data preprocessing, are generally thought to be present in 6G. Real-time data processing is possible. An AI system called deep reinforcement learning (DRL) has recently been used in health technology. Reinforcement learning and deep neural network (DNN) benefits are combined in DRL, which has the potential to revolutionize 6G technology. Additionally, 6G can play a noteworthy role in the integration of communication channels, offering improved dependability, Big Data analytics, and the management of epidemic and pandemic crises.

8.4   IMPORTANCE OF IoT IN HEALTHCARE

A technology model known as the Internet of Things (IoT) unites physical items, sensors, and other components into one cohesive, shared network. It has been made possible by the application of improved technological advancements, radio frequency classification, spectrum sharing, and Big Data analytics. To recover necessary and crucial information, investigate data, and finish each other's jobs, network things, items, and devices can connect with one another [27]. The majority of IoT gadgets are equipped with sensors, actuators, built-in microcontroller chips, communication networks, and a collection of common protocol stacks. Numerous devices are anticipated to be used for detecting, controlling, and processing those models in order to improve the implementation of the applications of cyber-physical IoT. IoT-based medical module sensors are often designed to track and gather data from the user or patient before sending it to the cloud for online archival storage [28]. These are real-time data in the majority of cases. As a result, IoT offers a healthcare monitoring platform that can measure patient attributes in a widespread and pervasive way. The third-generation joint venture project standards, which will help peer-to-peer networking, are heavily reliant on the device-to-device communication archetype. It provides a cost-effective answer to the problems with health management.

8.5   TECHNOLOGY THAT SUPPORTS 6G

To deliver on its sayings, 6G communication technique needs accompanying technologies. Since 6G is an AI-driven communication technology, its communication technology must be integrated with AI. Additionally, 6G will enable the Internet for Everything (IoE) and will advance several industries. Additionally, edge technology is required for 6G technology in order to offer cloud functionalities to intelligent devices. So, there are numerous technologies that make-up 6G communication technology.

8.5.1   ARTIFICIAL INTELLIGENCE

A genuinely AI-driven communication network will be 6G [29]. Every part of network communication will become intelligent with 6G, enabling the system to be self-aware, self-calculating, and self-deciding in a given situation. With 6G, the entire planet will be covered, including space, atmosphere, and ocean. This is only possible by giving the various components of communication "intelligent AI." AI algorithm implementation results in great performance and accuracy in communication networks. Synchronized communication, which is crucial for modern healthcare, can be provided via communication that is really AI-driven.

Healthcare powered by AI enhances clinical diagnostics and decision-making [30]. AI is needed in the healthcare industry to do jobs instantly. Data preprocessing is not necessary for DL. Concurrent data can be provided as input because it does the computation using original health data. Additionally, while computing a sizable number of network characteristics, it exhibits great accuracy [17].

8.5.2 VIRTUAL REALITY AND AUGMENTATION (VR/AR)

The use of AR makes actual objects appear more virtual. Additionally, it combines a variety of sensory faculties, including auditory, visual, haptic, and somatosensory. Real-time interactivity and precise 3D representations of both virtual and actual things are also features of AR. VR is made-up of computer created information or virtual world in which nothing is actually real. To deliver high-quality service, high data rates are necessary, to broadcast high resolution videos, as well. Furthermore, real-time voices and prompt control responses demand very low latency [31]. However, 6G will create new opportunities for its application in the medical sector. AR will make it possible to see into a patient's body with not a single scrape. Additionally, medical professionals can change the depth of the chosen body part. For improved visibility, the specified body part might also be made larger. The use of 6G will allow clinicians to view patients remotely. For improved diagnosis, holographic communication and augmented reality can be integrated. Doctors can practice medical operations in virtual reality without using actual patients. When doing risky, complex operations or surgeries, it will be highly beneficial. These will all be intelligent devices with 6G Internet connectivity. As was said before, a fluid and high-resolution presentation visualization for distant medical education or diagnostics can be generated using 6G.

8.5.3 HUMAN–COMPUTER INTERACTION (HCI)

Haptic technology applies pressure, motion, or vibration to the user to simulate a physical touch. The use of tactile Internet allows one user to physically touch another user, who could be a robot or a person. To capture the tactile in real-time, tactile Internet needs fast communication speeds and ERLLC. Telesurgery, or remote surgery, will be performed using this technology. Using touch instead of being physically present will aid doctors in making diagnoses. Three categories of haptic human–computer interaction (HCI), including wearable, surface, and desktop, have been established. The desktop HCI will enable the remote physician to do surgery or make a diagnosis using a virtual instrument [32]. The movement is 2D rather than 3D in surface HCI. A cell phone or tablet with a flat screen serves as the commanding device. The robot can be instructed to interact with the patient by stirring the hand on the monitor. The remote doctor uses a haptic glove, for example, in wearable HCI. Healthcare will also benefit from tactile and haptic technology following a catastrophe. For instance, the COVID-19, when all nations are on lockdown and communication with the exterior environment is forbidden or natural calamity.

8.5.4 HOSPITAL-TO-HOME SERVICES

Currently, ambulance services only provide transportation for patients who need oxygen and are a major safety problem on the road. It is not intelligent enough to serve as an emergency service. As a result, our quality of life is not significantly impacted by the ambulance systems. Any conventional car can handle the same issues if oxygen and an emergency signal are preserved. A new kind of ambulance service is necessary to improve living. The need for H2H services will increase once ambulance systems are restored. Hospitals can now rapidly and urgently contact families thanks to advancements in communication technology. Future intelligent vehicle development will be solely AI-driven.

H2H will, therefore, be put into use as a remote hospital on an intelligent platform for smart cars with a minimal dependency on healthcare facilities, including doctors and nurses. This mobile hospital will take the role of ambulance systems. For illustration, a mobile hospital can be summoned in real time to the scene of an accident. The mobile sanatorium will then start attending to the patients before it gets to the hospitals [33]. A mobile hospital can also find any emergency situation in real time and save lives. It will also enhance contemporary lifestyles. Particularly important in services for the elderly, the result is that 6G connectivity transforms modern lives through H2H services [34].

8.6 THE NEW 6G BUSINESS MODEL

The traditional hospital business model needs to be revised since 6G will transform business. Currently, the hospital receives direct payment from the patient for the costs of treatment either by the client or the health insurance plan. The medical coverage policy is run by a business. The business creates a system of hospitals. This medical facility accepts cashless payments and expenses are deducted from the company. Most diseases and the elderly are not covered by the insurance's medical services [35]. The hospital is described in this business model and when it comes to treatment and payment, insurance is a separate entity to the hospital. The insurer will cover the cost of the money that was paid to the hospital. The excessive amount must be covered by the patients. As a result, medical insurance and hospital services are highly inadequate and do not protect our lives. In actuality, neither the hospital nor the insurance provider is liable for our care from the time of birth until death [36].

Medical indemnity and hospital services are, therefore, woefully insufficient and do not safeguard our life. Actually, from the moment of our birth to the moment of our death, neither the hospital nor the indemnity companies are responsible for our healing and medical care. The insurance yearly as well as monthly based premium will be paid directly to the hospital. The insurance funds will be used to run the facility. From birth till death, the hospital will take care of the patient's health.

To contact the hospital, a patient can dial the H2H service. The enduring will be shifted to any partner hospital after the hospital has confirmed the HIH identification. The patient will receive top-of-the-line care [37]. The patient is not required to pay any medical bills following hospital release. This policy will also include coverage for quality of life (QoL), which includes IWD correlation and monitoring, H2H services, telesurgery, surgical procedure, pregnancy, delivery, and vaccinations, ICU services, NICU services, aged care, personalization, and meticulousness medication covers all illnesses and mishaps, such as cancer, flu, and neurological. There will be no limit on how many treatments a patient can receive. Additionally, the policy will pay for OPD as well as any other medical costs, including pathology and medication costs, so there won't be any bills or claims to deal with.

8.7 DISCUSSION

The proposed model prioritizes a particular group of patients, including those from rural and remote areas, pregnant women, people who are dealing with life-threatening conditions like cancer and dialysis, as well as people who have lifestyle diseases like high blood pressure, diabetes, and asthma.

In this section, the expected result is examined fictitiously. The statistics of men, women, and children will be made clear in the patient group's outcomes. Clustering the patient data requires a significant statistical representation. The following are some input parameters that must be taken into account:

   i. Diagnosis
   ii. Data sharing
  iii. Treatments
  iv. Task scopes
   v. Non-data sharing
  vi. Prescription and drug dose

Different analysis and verification platforms can categorize evaluation matrices. Data collection and analytics can be used to dig up veiled information, as to how serious a patient's health is or what requirements and required steps they wish at that specific time, after gathering a significant amount of data from the targeted patients. The sensor devices, which may be integrated into smartphones or function independently, will sense and gather these data. Then, using the 6G technology's standard network protocol, these data will be delivered via a cloud technology for archival storage. The platform of cloud will include a hierarchical structure to protect data privacy and an auto-update feature to process data quickly.

8.8 CONCLUSION AND OUTLOOK

Intelligent and smart healthcare must help in improving quality of life. Specifically, intelligent healthcare was made up of H2H, HIH, and IIoMT. High-quality mobile connection, integration with AI, and support from both edge and cloud computing are requirements for any IIoMT. BSR sensors are essential to IIoMT. BSR sensors have not yet been created. Numerous healthcare-related problems can be resolved with BSR. Therefore, the research society must pay close attention to the BSR sensor. IWD will be a ground-breaking medical device that comes with various sensors, including BSR. Numerous diseases will be automatically diagnosed with its assistance, and a person's health will be significantly improved. Additionally, an individual does not require to go for regular check-ups such as blood work, sugar levels, blood pressure, etc. IWD sends personal health information to the health monitoring center on a regular basis to check for any abnormalities. A senior can be watched over without the assistance of medical personnel. Elderly care requires extensive care, and by integrating IWD with the medical system, the person will be automatically taken care of without the need for medical staff involvement. IWD will also learn about a person's eating habits, medical background, body type, degree of pollution in the area, and any other deformity.

The current ambulance service merely acts as a patient transportation with a few basic medical supplies. This service ought to be changed to H2H offerings. H2H service has the potential to save a billion lives, and hence it needs to be implemented right now on intelligent vehicle. Additionally, the accident mortality rate can be employed for decreased H2H service. Also, smart healthcare needs the hospital to adopt a new business strategy. Currently, the business model of direct payment and health insurance hospitals requires better technology support. Only certain disorders are covered by the health insurance. It does not include several illnesses like COVID-19, the Ebola virus, delivery, and pregnancy. The HIH business plan is going to be really free of charge and without any hassles.

IoT is successfully influencing the healthcare market, primarily in industrialized nations, and has several applications across various fields. But because it hasn't yet been used, 6G technology's features in this field still need to be better understood. This chapter looked at a few papers connected to IoT-based healthcare architecture contribution to research based on 6G technology. Also briefly described is how, within the next several years, 6G technology will improve the health market. The fundamental prerequisites for 6G technology, as well as its functions and characteristics, are also covered. With its promised features and faster speeds, 6G will be crucial in the healthcare industry level of accuracy. There are several connections between 6G and IoT. In fact, they'll launch a personalized healthcare support system in the next ten years. The entire medical system will become more adaptable as a result, and resources won't be wasted. Global evolution will result from healthcare policy's dynamic adaptation. The rationalized health charges will be implemented in order to stop the inefficient distribution of hospital services.

8.9   FUTURE FINDINGS

This suggested strategy can enable a home hospital service and lessen the burden of patients they encounter while receiving treatment for serious illnesses. It will lessen the need for human involvement and enable quicker virtual communication. Patients can contact with the medical server and receive the quickest responses for any type of assistance. This model would lessen the need for human resources, and remote patients might receive better care from the medical staff. Distance-related barriers will be lessened.

Although this system has several advantages, it also has certain drawbacks, including a high-deployment cost, acceptance among stakeholders, and lack of knowledge. It could use some improvement, and more study in this area is possible. While combining two technologies has its problems, each node – administrators from the medical-ICT sector as well as users – must contribute in order for the healthcare sector to enter a new era of innovation.

REFERENCES

1. Chinmay, C., Roy S., Sharma, S., and Tran, T.A. (2020). *Environmental sustainability for green societies: COVID-19 pandemic*. Singapore: Springer Nature. ISBN: 978-3-030-66489-3
2. Chanda, P.B., Das, S., Banerjee, S., and Chinmay, C. (2021). Chapter 9: Study on edge computing using machine learning approaches in IoT framework, CRC: green computing and predictive analytics for healthcare, 1st edition. In: *Green Computing and Predictive Analytics for Healthcare*, pp 159–182. CRC Press.
3. Yeole, A. and Kalbande, D. (2016). Use of internet of things (IoT) in healthcare. In: Proceedings of the ACM symposium on women in research 2016 – WIR '16, pp. 71–76.
4. Nayak, S. and Patgiri, R. (2020). 6G communication technology: A vision on intelligent healthcare. [online] arXiv.org. Available at: https://arxiv.org/abs/2005.07532. Accessed 7 December 2020.
5. Chen, S., Liang, Y., Sun, S., Kang, S., Cheng, W., and Peng, M. (2020). Vision, requirements, and technology trend of 6G: how to tackle the challenges of system coverage, capacity, user data-rate and movement speed. *IEEE Wireless Communication* 27(2): 218–228.
6. Nayak, S. and Patgiri, R. (2020). "6G: Envisioning the Key Issues and Challenges," CoRR, vol. abs/2004.040244, [Online]. Available: https://arxiv.org/abs/2004.04024
7. Chiuchisan, I., Costin, H., and Geman, O. (2014). Adopting the internet of things technologies in healthcare systems. In: 2014 international conference and exposition on electrical and power engineering (EPE), pp. 532–535.
8. Rao, B.P., Saluia, P., Sharma, N., Mittal, A., and Sharma, S.V. (2012). Cloud computing for internet of things & sensing based applications. In: 2012 sixth international conference on sensing technology (ICST). IEEE, pp. 374–380.
9. Datta, S.K., Bonnet, C., Gyrard, A., Da Costa, R.P.F., and Boudaoud, K. (2015). Applying internet of things for personalized healthcare in smart homes. In: 2015 24thWireless and optical communication conference (WOCC). IEEE, pp. 164–169.
10. Azimi, I., Rahmani, A.M., Liljeberg, P., and Tenhunen, H. (2017). Internet of things for remote elderly monitoring: A study from user-centered perspective. *Journal of Ambient Intelligent Humanized Computer* 8(2): 273–289.
11. Darwish, A., Hassanien, A.E., Elhoseny, M., Sangaiah, A.K., and Muhammad, K. (2017). The impact of the hybrid platform of internet of things and cloud computing on healthcare systems: Opportunities, challenges, and open problems. *Journal of Ambient Intelligent Humanized Computer* 75: 1–16.
12. Tyagi, S., Agarwal, A., and Maheshwari, P. (2016) A conceptual framework for IoT-based healthcare system using cloud computing. In: 2016 6th international conference-cloud system and big data engineering (Confluence). IEEE, pp. 503–507.
13. Kim, S. and Kim, S. (2018). User preference for an IoT healthcare application for lifestyle disease management. *Telecommunication Policy* 42(4): 304–314.

14. Gubbi, J., Buyya, R., Marusic, S., and Palaniswami, M. (2013). Internet of things (IoT): A vision, architectural elements, and future directions. *Future Generation Computer System* 29(7): 1645–1660.

15. Fox, A., Griffth, R., Joseph, A., Katz, R., Konwinski, A., Lee, G., Patterson, D., Rabkin, A., and Stoica, I. (2009). Above the clouds: a Berkeley view of cloud computing. Department of Electrical Engineering and Computer Sciences, University of California, Berkeley, Rep. UCB/EECS, 28(13).

16. Alasmari, S. and Anwar, M. (2016). Security & privacy challenges in IoT-based health cloud. In: 2016 international conference on computational science and computational intelligence (CSCI). IEEE, pp. 198–201.

17. Owasp.org (n.d.). Code Injection Software Attack | OWASP Foundation. [online] Available at: https://owasp.org/www-community/attacks/Code_Injection. Accessed 9 December 2020.

18. Zhang, Z., Xiao, Y., Ma, Z., Xiao, M., Ding, Z., Lei, X., Karagiannidis, G.K., and Fan, P. (2019). 6G wireless networks: vision, requirements, architecture, and key technologies. *IEEE Vehicular Technology Magazine* 14(3): 28–41.

19. Chinmay, C. (2020). Joel JPC Rodrigues, a comprehensive review on device-to-device communication paradigm: Trends, challenges and applications. *Springer International Journal of Wireless Personal Communication* 114: 185–207. https://doi.org/10.1007/s11277-020-07358-3

20. Chinmay, C. (2019). Advanced classification techniques for healthcare analysis. IGI global book series – advances in medical technologies and clinical practice (AMTCP), pp. 1–405. https://doi.org/10.4018/978-1-5225-7796-6

21. Open Mind: The Internet of Everything (IoE) | Openmind. [online] Available at: https://www.bbvaopenmind.com/en/technology/digital-world/the-internet-of-everything-ioe/. Accessed 9 December 2020.

22. Mucchi, L., Jayousi, S., Caputo, S., Paoletti, E., Zoppi, P., Geli, S., and Dioniso, P. (2020). How 6G technology can change the future wireless healthcare. In: 2020 2nd 6G Wireless Summit (6G SUMMIT).

23. Ullah, K., Shah, M.A., and Zhang, S. (2016). Effective ways to use internet of things in the field of medical and smart health care. In: 2016 international conference on intelligent systems engineering (ICISE). IEEE, pp. 372–379.

24. Qi, J., Yang, P., Min, G., Amft, O., Dong, F., and Xu, L. (2017). Advanced internet of things for personalized healthcare systems: A survey. *Pervasive Mobile Computing* 41: 132–149.

25. Han, C. and Chen, Y. (2018). Propagation modeling for wireless communications in the terahertz band. *IEEE Communication Magazine* 56(6): 96–101.

26. Sharad, E.N., Kaur, I.K., and Aulakh, K.S. (2020). Evaluation and implementation of cluster head selection in WSN using Contiki/Cooja simulator. *Journal of Statistics and Management Systems* 23(2): 407–418. https://doi.org/10.1080/09720510.2020.1736324

27. Chauhan, S., Arora, R., and Arora, N. (2021). "Researcher issues and future directions in healthcare using IoT and machine learning," In G. C. Meenu Gupta and V. H. C. de Albuquerque (eds), *Smart Healthcare Monitoring Using IoT with 5G*, 1st edition. Boca Raton, London, New York: CRC Press, Taylor and Francis Group, pp. 177–196.

28. Chauhan, S., Pahwa, K., and Ahmed, S. (2023). Telemedical and remote healthcare monitoring using IoT and machine learning. In: Gupta M, Ahmed S, Kumar R, Altrjman C (eds), *Computational Intelligence in Healthcare*. Boca Raton: CRC Press, pp. 47–66.

29. Han, C. and Chen, Y. (2018). Propagation modeling for wireless communications in the terahertz band. *IEEE Communication Magazine* 56(6): 96–101.

30. Who.int. (2020). WHO | Bangladesh. [online] Available at: https://www.who.int/workforcealliance/countries/bgd/en/. Accessed 14 December 2020.

31. Aazam, M., Huh, E.N., St-Hilaire, M., Lung, C.H., and Lambadaris, I. (2016). Cloud of things: Integration of IoT with cloud computing. In: Koubaa A, Shakshuki E (eds), *Robots and sensor clouds*. Switzerland: Springer, pp 77–94.

32. Shah, J.L. and Bhat, H.F. (2020). Cloud IoT for smart healthcare: Architecture, issues, and challenges. In: Raj P, Chatterjee J, Kumar A, Balamurugan B (eds), *Internet of things use cases for the healthcare industry*. Switzerland: Springer. https://doi.org/10.1007/978-3-030-37526-3_5

33. Mahmoud, M.M.E. et al. (2018). Enabling technologies on cloud of things for smart healthcare. *IEEE Access* 6(24): 31950–31967.

34. Gupta, P., Agrawal, D., Chhabra, J., and Dhir, P.K. (2016). IoT based smart healthcare kit. In: 2016 international conference on computational techniques in information and communication technologies (ICCTICT). IEEE, pp. 237–242.

35. Yogesh, S. and Chinmay, C. (2020). Augmented reality and virtual reality transform for spinal imaging landscape. *IEEE Computation Graph Appl*, 1–13. https://doi.org/10.1109/MCG.2020.3000359

36. Catalyst.nejm.org. (n.d.). Healthcare big data and the promise of value-based care. [online] Available at: https://catalyst.nejm.org/doi/full/10.1056/CAT.18.0290. Accessed 13 December 2020.

37. Anwar, S., Nasrullah, M., and Hosen, M.J. (2020). COVID-19 and Bangladesh: Challenges and how to address them. *Front Public Health* 8: 154. https://doi.org/10.3389/fpubh.2020.00154.

9 6G-Based Smart Healthcare Solutions

Beyond Industry 4.0 Trends and Products

Chander Prabha and Deepak Kumar Jain

CONTENTS

9.1 Introduction: Background and Driving Forces.. 171
9.2 Requirement of 6G in Smart/Intelligent Healthcare System........................ 173
9.3 6G Technologies in Healthcare... 175
9.4 6G Healthcare Applications and Challenges... 176
9.5 Use Cases in 6G.. 178
9.6 Conclusion 180
References.. 181

9.1 INTRODUCTION: BACKGROUND AND DRIVING FORCES

Present healthcare systems depend mainly on 4G and 5G communication technologies to support healthcare solutions. However, these technologies due to limited bandwidth can't facilitate the accelerated surge of healthcare solutions in the long term. When comparing 4G and 5G, the 5G networks support improved services in terms of reliability, bandwidth, data rate, and latency [1]. 5G services from the smart healthcare perspective provide:

- better connectivity of the internet to the IoMT (Internet of Medical Things) via mMTC (massive Machine Type Communication)
- for telemedicine, high-quality video calling [2]
- improved visualization in treatment and diagnosis via eMBB (enhanced Mobile Broad Band)
- use of Augmented Reality (AR) and Virtual Reality (VR) techniques
- for monitoring emergency situations, support drones, and autonomous vehicles via URLLC [3]

However, the use of 5G is not sufficient for the evolution of smart healthcare and for handling healthcare in disaster-like situations. Major reasons for this are security and privacy in remote areas, providing pervasive communication for telemedicine,

DOI: 10.1201/9781003321668-9

and connectivity issues for ultra-dense IoMT devices during remote surgery using AR/VR, etc.

Next-generation healthcare solutions will use hybrid technology comprising the Internet of Things (IoT), 5G, 6G, fog computing, and cloud computing [3]. It, thus, solves security problems and improves performance and network coverage. 6G is the latest technology in the field of wireless cellular communication. It provides a sustainable healthcare system even in remote areas for the citizens. The key motivation for 6G technology development is to benefit society and humanity by improving their quality of life [4–6]. Table 9.1 shows the differentiation between 5G, B5G, and 6G.

6G promises many deliverables and services; yet, a lot of challenges to overcome like core network – IoE, truly AI-driven integration, 1 THz operational frequency, 1 Tbps data rate, 3D spectral requirements, less than 1 ns end-to-end delay, less than 10 ns radio delay, and many more. Many technologies and services are being proposed keeping 6G vision in mind like tactile internet, teleoperated vehicles, holographic presence, IoBNT (Internet of Bio-Nano Things), aerial networks, visible light communication, radio frequency coexistence, and Terahertz (THz), etc. [7]. A powerful communication infrastructure can be developed using the mentioned technologies for smart healthcare solutions. It would provide extreme reliability, unbreakable connection, scalability,

---

TABLE 9.1
Differences between 6G, B5G, and 5G Healthcare Requirements

Requirements	5G	B5G	6G
Type of applications	eMBB, URLCC, mMTC	Relible eMBB, mMTC, URLLC, Hybrid (eMBB+URLLC)	MBRLLC, HCS, MPS, mURLLC, mLLMT, mBBMT, MBBLL
Type of devices	Smartphones, Drones, Sensors	Drones, Sensors, Smartphones, XR requirements	DLT devices and Sensors, BCI and XR equipment, CRAS, smart implants
Operational frequency	3–300 MHz	500 MHz	1 THz
Spectral efficiency	10* in bps/Hz/joules	100* in bps/Hz/joules	1000* in bps/Hz/joules
Data rate	1Gbps	100Gbps	1Tbps
End-to-end delay	5 ms	1 ms	< 1 ms
Radio delay	100 ns	< 100 ns	< = 10 ns
Processing delay	100 ns	50 ns	< = 10 ns
Wavelength	3 mm	1 mm	300 μm
Architecture	Massive MIMO	Massive MIMO	Intelligent Surface
Core network	IoT	IoT	Internet of Everything (IoE)
Integration of AI	Partially	Fully	AI-driven truly
Integration of XR	Partially	Fully	Fully
Integration of satellite	Partially	Fully	Fully
Integration of haptic communication	Partially	Fully	Fully
Features	Extremely high-streaming rate	Extremely high-streaming rate	More secrecy, privacy, and security

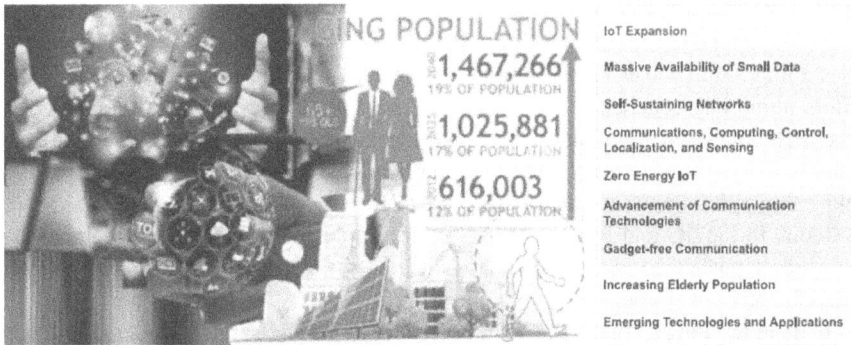

FIGURE 9.1 Driving force behind 6G [8, 9].

ultra-massive connectivity, frequent rapid response, continuous monitoring without any hindrance, and quick preventive actions in emergency situations.

Figure 9.1 shows the driving force behind 6G. The present system of smart health-care provides basic amenities, and the major drawback is time and space. However, in near future, with the evolution of 6G, this will not be a barrier. In smart healthcare monitoring, ambulances equipped with IoT devices and technologies serve only as a transporter of patients in emergencies. Presently, the services provided to elders are very unsatisfactory requiring extensive care from expert medical staff. A system like the detection of accidents in ambulances is unavailable in present health systems. It requires detection in real time to serve medical services on the spot and on time.

In this chapter, the categorization of healthcare is done into remote healthcare, hospital, and emergency response unit. Further, the investigation of the problem along with possible solutions is done in each area with regard to smart healthcare systems. The next section describes the requirements of 6G in smart healthcare systems. The 6G usage could help in handling emergency situations in smart healthcare more effec-tively. The next section represents the requirements of 6G in smart healthcare systems. Further, it explores 6G technologies in the third section. Smart healthcare system challenges and applications have been discussed in the fourth section. The fifth sec-tion presents the use cases of 6G and solutions pertaining to healthcare beyond indus-try 4.0 and beyond. The chapter ends with a conclusion in the last section.

9.2 REQUIREMENT OF 6G IN SMART/INTELLIGENT HEALTHCARE SYSTEM

The IoT has played a crucial part in relaxing the burden by means of an in-home care approach on healthcare professionals. Especially for the elderly population, during the pandemics and epidemics like COVID-19, IoT, and IoMT for healthcare have proven to be in their highest demand. However, to cope with this increase in demand, the question here is, "whether the current technology would be capable or not." The solution lies in the 6th generation networks. The basic requirements of 6G healthcare services are mentioned in Table 9.1. 6G is truly AI-driven and is also abbreviated as the 6th sense [9]. Prices are expected to be 1,000 times cheaper in the 6G era. It uses XR (extended radio) instead of NR-Lite of 5G. To achieve 1 THz frequency, it uses a maximum wavelength of 300 μm. The use of such a high frequency (1 THz) offers numerous benefits, thus making it more appropriate for 6G communication like high data rates, high bandwidth, high throughput, and capacity [10]. Real-time communications are required in some applications of healthcare like telesurgery, and holographic communication using AR/VR, etc. to boost intelligent healthcare systems. In the 5G and B5G eras, these were implemented partially, which can be boosted or pushed forward many steps ahead with 6G. Figure 9.2 shows an intelligent healthcare system.

It includes IoMT comprised of a BSR sensor (blood sample reader) via IWD (intelligent wearable device), MRI, prescription online, and CT scan. H2H service is implemented via mobile hospitals, remote doctors, pathology, and data scientists. To implement smart healthcare systems effectively and without any interruption, 6G will be an added advantage. The healthcare sector will fully lean on this 6G

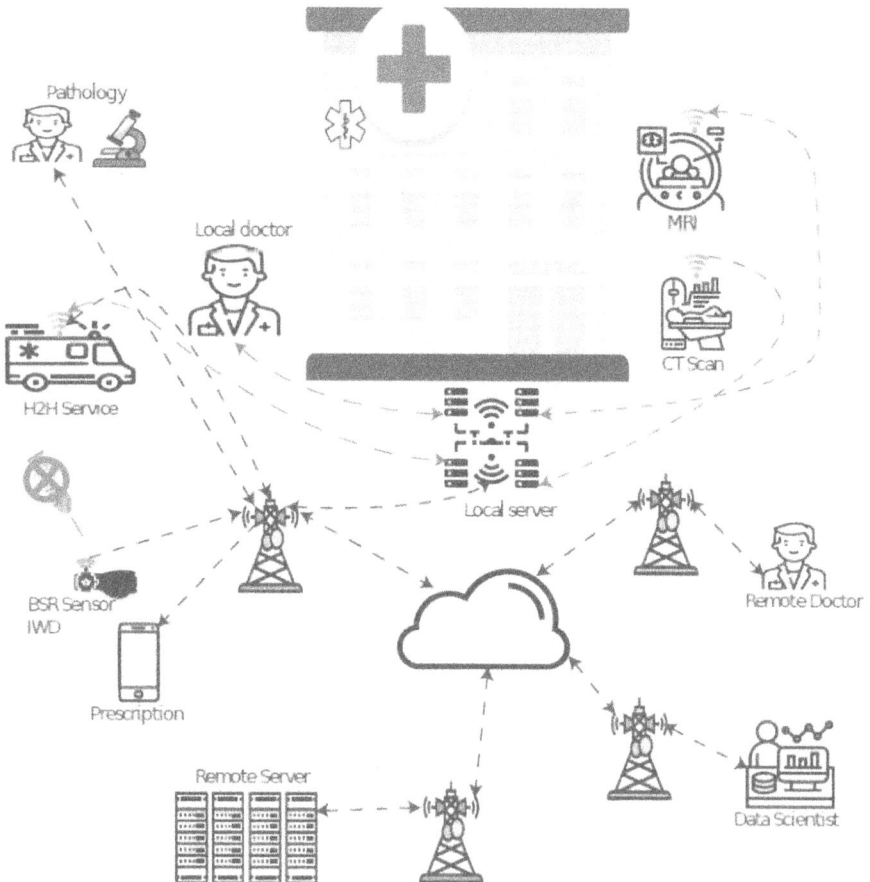

FIGURE 9.2   Intelligent healthcare system.

communication technology as it will reform the healthcare sector completely by providing alternative solutions to current challenges faced in healthcare [10].

The aim of 6G is to provide QoS (Quality of Services), QoL (Quality of Life), and QoE (Quality of Experiences). The requirements like H2H (Hospital-to-Home) services may tend to increase with the use of edge technology along with AI (Artificial Intelligence). Smart healthcare will transition to intelligent healthcare in 6G. From 2030 onward, IoE will replace IoT, intelligent phones would take over smartphones, and all intelligent devices (AI-driven) would have the capability to connect to the network. Thus, more accurate predictions, decisions, and experiences would be shared by intelligent devices while connected to healthcare systems.

The QoS parameters of 6G are superior to 5G and B5G due to the type of applications it supports. The AR/VR, holographic communications, and tactile internet are part of QoE that requires an extremely high-data rate that is expected to be nil or low latency. In the healthcare sector, there is a need for high QoE for H2H service, critical operations, and intelligent hospitals. The QoL represents an enhanced lifestyle in healthcare along with QoS and QoE. The QoL is basically a core parameter of intelligent healthcare and 6G communication technology is capable of providing the same. The QoL includes health monitoring of patients remotely, IWD connection management, telesurgery, accident detection, precision medicine prescription, etc. One of the attractive features of QoL is H2H services implemented in an intelligent vehicle via a mobile hospital.

9.3   6G TECHNOLOGIES IN HEALTHCARE

AI-incorporated algorithms featuring 6G will help in the accurate tracking of a patient's condition with the support of automated warnings at regular intervals. It involves relevant engagement with health providers in real time. This will reduce the overall medical costs and duration of stay of patients in hospitals, further reducing morbidity and mortality rates. Some of the 6G technologies in the upcoming healthcare sector that can be applied are:

- *In-on-off body communications*: In this, the body layer is categorized as in, on, and off-body communication. ICT tools will be used in this technique for remotely monitoring the health of people. Sensors in the form of molecules and nanostructure are represented in in-body communication to build biological communication networks [11]. Figure 9.3 shows an in-body scenario of communication.

The in-body communication networks help in removing limitations of the present healthcare system, i.e., closed-loop monitoring and predictive therapy system. By the 2030s, the sensors will be more precise, accurate, and reliable for diagnostic purposes. Such sensors being a part of in-body sub-networks will provide updates and interact with distributed cloud repositories in future.

- *Intelligent nanoscale inner body communications*: 6G technology is very significant in linking IoBNT (Internet of Bio-Nano Things) and IoNT

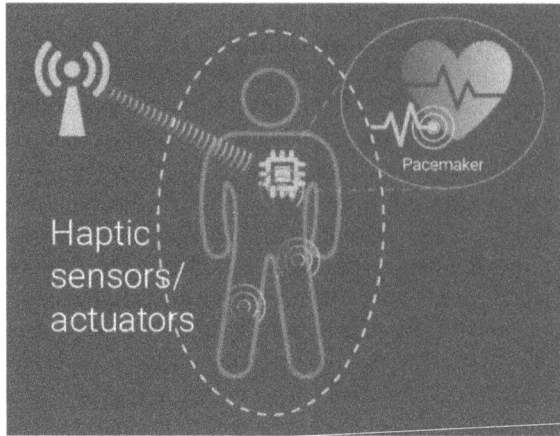

FIGURE 9.3   In-body scenario.

(Internet of Nano-Things) together [12, 13]. This will bring a new revolution as medical information is gathered for taking appropriate actions remotely by doctors or nurses. In IoBNT, a critical study can be investigated within the body by examining intrabody.

- *Human bond communications*: The detection and transmission of data like thoughts or experiences will soon become reality with the use of human senses in 6G. Information saved in the emotion sensors serves as a perception of information. Numerous actions, feelings, and behaviors of a person can be recorded at a given moment. It also includes monitoring and examining behavioral patterns, noting facial expressions, measuring actions, voice intonation, etc. The AI techniques would be able to recognize the meaning behind any type of emotion and can respond quickly. Emotion-based sensors have numerous applications. Many health wearables and smart watches help in managing daily tasks along with avoiding health issues by tracking and evaluating a person's physical condition and dealing with stress and anxiety reactions.
- *Visible light communication (VLC)*: It is a type of optical wireless technology that transmits data via light rays. The data is gathered from the body and to provide efficient, interrupted transmission and enhanced connectivity for extensive communication among users, 6G would offer benefits by providing a downlink channel [14, 15].

9.4   6G HEALTHCARE APPLICATIONS AND CHALLENGES

The major application fields of 6G in the healthcare sector are within the hospital environment, providing remote healthcare, and in emergency/disaster situations. These are depicted in Figure 9.4. The basic human need from the diagnosis of disease to its treatment is getting better healthcare. In the hospital environment, numerous smart medical equipment and trained staff are there to provide the

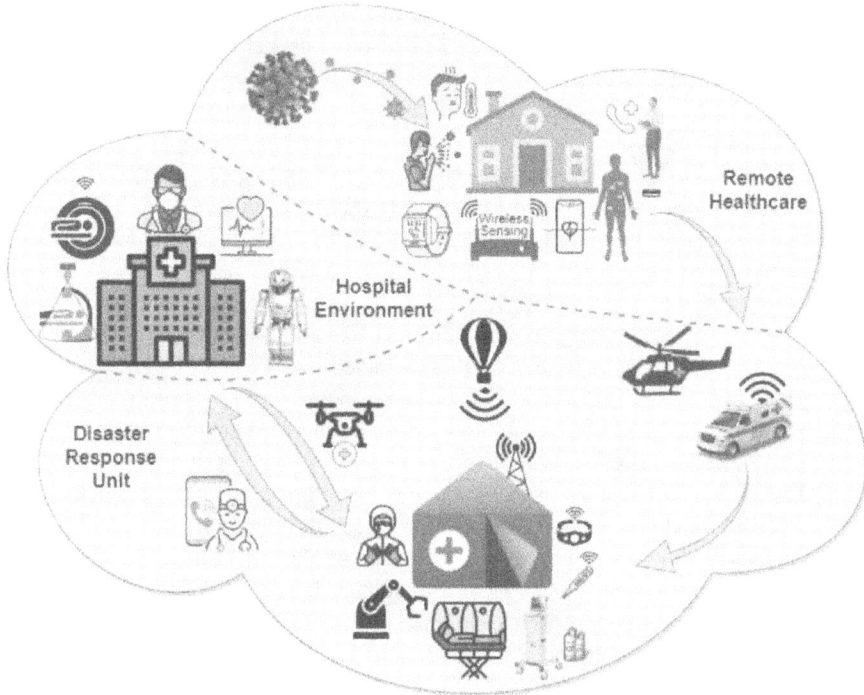

FIGURE 9.4   Application areas of 6G in healthcare.

best medical services. For inter-disciplinary communication among the staff and patients, the preferably used technologies are email, two-way radios, mobile phones, pagers, etc. However, presently, improved methods have been introduced based on AI in healthcare services to maintain the patient's health records electronically. It reduces time, human errors, and improves communication among patients and doctors resulting in better decisions during the diagnosis of a disease. High-precision robots are being used in surgeries to support medical doctors. The data can be sent directly to the repository (server) by using IWD and sensors through IoMT more precisely without any loss in 6G [16, 17].

During a disaster or emergency scenario, the hospital environment becomes over-powered too quickly due to a large number of casualties. Sometimes situations are uncontrollable in a pandemic due to an increase in the chances of spreading infection from patient to medical staff. Another reason may be limited patient capacity, shortage of equipment, and medical staff in hospitals. One of the biggest challenges during the pandemic is about ensuring the safety of medical staff involved in treating infected patients. The solutions to the aforementioned challenges presented are:

- interaction between clinicians and patients should be minimized;
- use of IoMT; and
- use of intelligent robots in the hospital environment.

The sensors and IWD can monitor and transmit patient records to doctors over the internet. Robots can be used to deliver medical supplies, help in medical check-ups, disinfect the patient's area, etc. In the hospital or H2H, the massive-scale implementation of these in improving the smart healthcare sector is expected with 6G in the future, thus providing more security to patients, doctors, and medical staff [18].

The 6G is still in the development phase and several aspects related to healthcare challenges are discussed before. However, various challenges may occur while implementation [19–21]. Numerous challenges while employing 6G communication technologies in healthcare are:

- One important challenge is to make 6G compatible with earlier technologies due to its use of higher frequency bands like VLC and THz (require new network architecture and transceiver design, have high-propagation losses, and low coverage area issue). So, making 6G backward compatible with the previous one is a challenging task.
- The next challenge is associated with the high cost and complexities involved due to the dense configuration of cell development.
- Further higher frequency usage raises major health issues like damaging skin or eye cell tissues. So, health standards need to be chased for the healthcare and safety of users while developing these 6G technologies.
- 6G technologies must be energy-efficient. In disaster situations, the longevity of devices supporting 6G must be maintained due to the scarcity of energy resources.
- Security and privacy: A lot of cryptographic algorithms with powerful authentication mechanisms having shorter key length helps in the transmission of encrypted health-related information on and within the body. Numerous tools are required to study the reactivity in biomolecules and sudden catastrophic symptoms.
- Technological aspects: Retrieval of data from the body to the cloud as a result of communication among body layers is feasible with 6G. However, continuous monitoring and correlating data may possess a challenge due to the use of numerous sensors lying between micro to macro.
- Ethical aspects: The users of smart or intelligent healthcare must have higher health literacy. They must participate in driving processes being the data owners of their health records. A framework needed to employ unified regulatory procedures to maintain the integrity and ethical aspects of healthcare records and the making of it still possess challenges.

9.5   USE CASES IN 6G

The goals of 6G in healthcare include digital world experience and ensuring security, trust, and resilience. Privacy in 6G can be ensured by including AI/ML. One of the challenges in healthcare is the aging population, which should be taken up diligently. To provide them with major healthcare facilities at home itself as daily life support, there is a need to incorporate intelligent systems and technologies into our daily lives. Some of the service scenarios of healthcare are:

Scenario A: For diagnostic purposes, monitoring of patient's health like blood pressure, heart rate, etc. There is a growth of virtual and augmented reality (VR/AR) in the healthcare sector due to an increase in the elderly population globally. The usage of AR in the healthcare field would be more reliable with 6G, and it allows doctors to utilize clinical devices and examine the state of new drugs interaction within the patient's body.

Scenario B: The treatment would be using in-body sensors and actuators (e.g., a wireless insulin pump and a wireless pacemaker controlling heartbeat, etc.) in diabetic patients to ensure the right glucose level. Patients having motor disabilities can do movement via a muscle controller.

In-body appliances and applications are life critical, and it is, naturally, important to ensure the required safety and service to the patients of the healthcare provider. In addition, operations performed to ensure the quality of life are battery-driven, leading to constraints of major energy consumption. For supporting in-body networks consisting of ingestible devices and micro-sized implants, there is a need to support reliable and extreme connectivity for consistency, conciseness, and improved efficiency. Figure 9.5 shows the practical usage of 6G in healthcare.

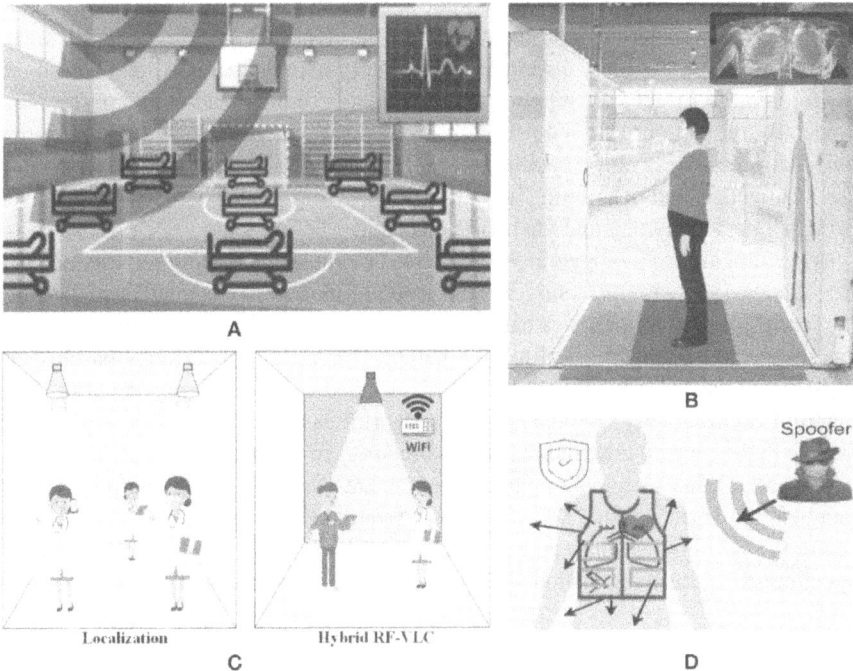

FIGURE 9.5 6G usage in healthcare (A) wireless-sensing scenario in hospital, (B) lung screening via THz, (C) VLC use for capacity enhancement and localization, (D) wireless body area network security via a smart vest.

During the COVID-19 pandemic, many nations have faced crowding and long queues outside hospitals, the reason being a lack of resources and medical facilities to handle such situations. One possible solution was the use of IoMT devices. However, due to a shortage of these devices and connectivity issues, the results of monitoring were not too accurate. Wi-Fi sensing via 6G can be advantageous in such situations for patient monitoring and tracking [22]. The same strategies can be applied in hospitals, where no existing medical solutions and facilities are feasible for tracking and monitoring (Figure 9.5 [A]).

Numerous sensing technologies can be employed for the identification of various critical diseases. One such technique is terahertz imaging (Figure 9.5 [B]). In this, the beams of terahertz frequency are directed over the specified area of disease detection (e.g., the chest of the person) [23]. Advanced AI and deep-learning algorithms are used to segregate these images for the identification of healthy and infected cells. The THz screening has no adverse effects on living cells [24].

The global positioning system (GPS) is useful for localization and outdoor positioning. However, it can't provide precise indoor positions owing to the complex electro-magnetic (EM) propagation environment [25]. In pandemic situations, when hospitals become overcrowded with patients, it turns more troublesome to spot the medical staff, doctors, and patients. In this situation, the Wi-Fi real-time positioning system will be helpful to spot the patients as well as the medical staff and also for providing prompt responses to critical patients, and for real-time coordination. But again, in sensitive areas, Wi-Fi would not help so VLC points can be used (Figure 9.5 [C]). Precise positions and locations can be identified of doctors and patients via VLC due to their small coverage area. Elderly people activities, medical robotics, and remote surgery are a few other applications of localization and positioning. Especially remote surgery requires very high positioning and precise localization and such preciseness can be achieved via THz. Especially in remote surgery, precise localization and positioning are required. The said preciseness can be achieved through THz technology and via hybrid THz and VLC systems.

6G healthcare technologies are expected to be robust against any security and privacy attacks. Say, in remote surgery, end-to-end link security is mandatory because any sort of link failure or attack can revamp the instructions forwarded to the robotic apparatus and endangers the life of a patient. Initially, cryptography-based techniques (high complexity) were being used for handling privacy and security. Now quantum cryptography (low complexity) algorithms have been introduced, which provide highly secure communication and security in healthcare.

Presently, edge technologies based on AI are used for differentiating medical data before it is transmitted and storing its private information in the local memory. Figure 9.5 (D) shows a smart vest employing a radiology technique capable of refining and eliminating the manipulation of signals against spoofing and jamming attacks.

9.6   CONCLUSION

There is a need for advancements in communication technology due to the increase in disaster and pandemic situations to manage existing and future health crises. Keeping this viewpoint, from a communication perspective, various weaknesses and challenges of healthcare are discussed. The solutions are provided via 6G in all environments. The healthcare standards are to be followed while implementing the 6G in healthcare systems while minimizing the adverse effects and providing a quick response in any kind of emergency scenario. The use of IoMT, VLC, PLS, wireless sensing, and automated vehicles may revolutionize healthcare. However, in reality, the precise integration of 6G with healthcare is still an open challenge while maintaining standards.

REFERENCES

1. Dong Li. 5G, and intelligence medicine–how the next generation of wireless technology will reconstruct healthcare? *Precis. Clin. Med.*, vol. 2, no. 4, pp. 205–208, December (2019).
2. G. Cisotto, E. Casarin, and S. Tomasin. Requirements and enablers of advanced healthcare services over future cellular systems. *IEEE Communication Mag.*, vol. 58, pp. 76–81 (2020).
3. A. Ahad, M. Tahir, and K. Yau. 5G-based smart healthcare network: Architecture, taxonomy, challenges, and future research directions. *IEEE Access*, vol. 7, pp. 100747–100762 (2019).
4. M.A. Rahman, M.S. Hossain, N.A. Alrajeh, and N. Guizani. B5G and explainable deep learning assisted healthcare vertical at the edge: COVID-19 perspective. *IEEE Networks*, vol. 34, pp. 98–105 (2020).
5. S. Dang and O. Amin et.al. What should 6G be? *Nat. Electron.*, vol. 3, pp. 20–29 (2020).
6. Transforma Insights Research. (May 2020). Global IoT Market, Will Grow to 24.1 Billion Devices in 2030, Generating $1.5 Trillion Annual Revenue.
7. S. Nayak and R. Patgiri. 6G communication technology: A vision on intelligent healthcare (2020). [Online]. Available: arXiv:2005.07532.
8. L. Mucchi et al. "How 6G technology can change the future wireless healthcare." In Proc. 2nd 6G Wireless Summit (6G SUMMIT), pp. 1–6 (2020).
9. W. He, D. Goodkind, and P. Kowal. "An aging world: 2015." U.S. Census Bureau, International Population Reports, P95/16-1 (2016). Available at https://www.census.gov/content/dam/Census/library/publications/2016/demo/p95-16-1.pdf
10. C. Hsu and R. Hristov et al. Enabling identification and behavioral sensing in homes using radio reflections. In CHI '19 New York, NY: Association for Computing Machinery, pp. 1–13 (2019).
11. C. Liu, W. Feng, Y. Chen, C.-X. Wang, and N. Ge Cell-free satellite-UAV networks for 6G wide-area internet of things. *IEEE J. Sel. Areas Commun.*, vol. 39, no. 4, pp. 1116–1131, April (2021).
12. N.A. Abbasi and O.B. Akan. An information theoretical analysis of human insulin-glucose system toward the internet of bio-nano things. *IEEE Trans. Nanobiosci.*, vol. 16, no. 8, pp. 783–791 (2017).
13. J. Wang, M. Peng, Y. Liu, X. Liu, and M. Daneshmand. Performance analysis of signal detection for amplify-and-forward relay in diffusion-based molecular communication systems. *IEEE Internet Things J.*, vol. 7, no. 2, pp. 1401–1412 (2020).
14. S. Ariyanti and M. Suryanegara. "Visible light communication (VLC) for 6G technology: The potency and research challenges." In Proc. IEEE 4th World Conf. Smart Trends Syst. Security Sustain. (WorldS4), pp. 490–493 (2020).
15. J. Chen and Z. Wang. Topology control in hybrid VLC/RF vehicular ad-hoc network. *IEEE Trans. Wireless Commun.*, vol. 19, no. 3, pp. 1965–1976 (2020).
16. W. Taylor and Q.H. Abbasi et al. A review of the state of the art in non-contact sensing for COVID-19. *Sensors*, vol. 20, p. 5665 (2020).

17. M. Giordani, M. Polese, M. Mezzavilla, S. Rangan, and M. Zorzi. Toward 6G networks: Use cases and technologies. *IEEE Commun. Mag.*, vol. 58, no. 3, pp. 55–61 (2020).
18. A. Rahman, S. Dash, A.K. Luhach, N. Chilamkurti, S. Baek, and Y. Nam, A. Neuro-fuzzy approach for user behavior classification and prediction. *J. Cloud Comput.*, vol. 8, no. 17, pp. 1–15 (2019).
19. M. Z. Chowdhury, M. Shahjalal, M. Hasan, and Y.M. Jang. The role of optical wireless communication technologies in 5G/6G and IoT solutions: Prospects, directions, and challenges. *Appl. Sci.*, vol. 9, no. 20, p. 4367 (2019).
20. M. Katz and I. Ahmed. "Opportunities and challenges for visible light communications in 6G." In Proc. IEEE 2nd 6G Wireless Summit (6G SUMMIT), pp. 1–5 (2020).
21. M. Giordani and M. Zorzi. Non-terrestrial networks in the 6G era: Challenges and opportunities. *IEEE Netw.*, vol. 35, no. 2, pp. 244–251, March/April (2021).
22. S. Chen, Y. Liang, S. Sun, S. Kang, W. Cheng, and M. Peng. "Vision, requirements, and technology trend of 6G: How to tackle the challenges of system coverage, capacity, user data-rate and movement speed. *IEEE Wirel. Commun.*, pp. 1–11 (2020). https://doi.org/10.48550/arXiv.2002.04929
23. S. Tian and W. Yang. Smart healthcare: Making medical care more intelligent. *Glob. Health J.*, vol. 3, pp. 62–65 (2019).
24. N. Rothbart, O. Holz, and R. Koczulla et al. Analysis of human breath by millimeter-wave/terahertz spectroscopy. *Sensors*, vol. 19, pp. 2719 (2019).
25. S. Dang, O. Amin, B. Shihada, and M. Alouini. What should 6G be? *Nat. Electron.*, vol. 3, pp. 20–29 (2020).

10 Influence of AI and 6G-Enabled IoT in Smart Healthcare
Challenges and Solutions

Kritika Upadhyay and Manisha Bharti

CONTENTS

10.1 Introduction 184
10.2 Literature Review 184
10.3 Medical Advancement in Recent Years.. 185
10.4 Integration of Wireless Technology... 186
    10.4.1 Artificial Intelligence-Enabled Medical Services 186
    10.4.2 Next Generation Wireless Network 6G 188
    10.4.3 IoT-Embedded Systems in Monitoring Devices 188
10.5 Implementation of Technology 189
    10.5.1 Systematic Allocation of Wheelchair 191
    10.5.2 Medical Integrated System 191
    10.5.3 Effective Healthcare Solutions 191
        10.5.3.1 Confidential.. 191
        10.5.3.2 Privacy 191
        10.5.3.3 Accessibility.. 191
        10.5.3.4 Integrity... 191
        10.5.3.5 Recent Data Collection 191
        10.5.3.6 Secure.. 192
        10.5.3.7 Optimization 192
        10.5.3.8 Configuration 192
        10.5.3.9 Protection 192
        10.5.3.10 In-Depth Analysis.. 192
10.6 Smart Healthcare Challenges and Applications 192
    10.6.1 Maintaining Protection Mechanisms 193
    10.6.2 Adoption of New Models... 193
    10.6.3 Complex Design for Carrier Wave.. 193
    10.6.4 Availability of Semiconductor 193
10.7 Potential Solutions to Smart Healthcare and Emerging
Technologies 194
    10.7.1 Edge Level 194

DOI: 10.1201/9781003321668-10

10.7.2 Fog Level 194
10.7.3 Cloud Level 194
10.8 Summary of Research Guidelines for Smart Healthcare 194
       10.8.1 Collection of Facts and Figures 195
10.9 Conclusion 196
References 196

10.1 INTRODUCTION

6G is one of the prominent features of wireless technology attracting the attention of many researchers in this area. It has the power to revolutionize every domain of technological development including healthcare, defense application, education sector and many more areas involving the use of latest technology. This provides the right opportunity to dwell into the various aspects of 6G in future. It will extend the performance of existing communication standards by improving latency and capacity of data transmission. To advance the development of sensing technology, it uses sub-mm waves (wavelength less than 1 mm) and frequency selection. This approach has potential advantages to make 6G operational in the coming years.

6G provides various methodologies [1] for defining its role in health sector even in case of a pandemic. To address the status of patient's health in new healthcare system, cognitive data analytics [2] can be used which is having low latency. The role of new technology in medical field and its impact on patient's health plays a vital role in implementing such phenomenon [3] in healthcare systems. Factors such as human error, virtual existence of technology and medical diagnosis affect decides the future of AI-enabled IoT in medical science. Smart healthcare is composed of many components of wireless technologies including edge computing, cloud computing and thus detailed analysis [4] provides answers related to medical signal security, computing process and shows the upcoming challenges related to this research domain. The major challenges in this field of medical science includes end-to-end communication between systems, systematic management, effective sensors, and security policies of the organization.

10.2 LITERATURE REVIEW

Transmission of large amount of medical data possesses high risk and serious leakage issues; thus, various models have been designed for analyzing privacy performance in real time. Combination of AI, IoT and 6G infrastructure will be able to provide the platform for computations including random decisions about processing, exchanging and storage. Xu et al. proposed conventional neural network design of four-layered architecture [5] and thus improved the security of data by 20% with adaptability to nonlinear data as well. IoMT (Internet of Medical Things) overcomes critical issues of advanced medical system in terms of response time, availability of cloud storage thus provides effective methodology for reliable architectures. Figure 10.1 illustrates the components of smart medical healthcare systems.

Fog computing follows the latest trend in sensor-based monitoring systems which gain more interest of researchers in exploiting its features [6]. Another challenge for

AI 6G

IoT

Smart Healthcare

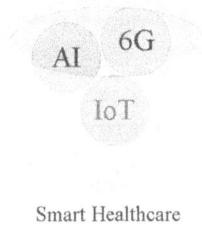

FIGURE 10.1   Components of smart medical healthcare systems.

mankind in nearby future is the detection of diseases by analyzing health state of human body as observed in COVID-19 pandemic that despite having latest medical equipment detection of symptoms itself consumed a lot of time in its prevention. Choyon et al. [7] proposed effective monitoring system as a solution to aid future virus attacks by detecting biological data of patient's health and thus can provide immediate medical support. Guo researched on improving the trust on sophisticated modern technology by optimizing features of PHY (physical) and MAC layer [8] in data-dependent learning model. Vulnerability to suspicious data, less effective network design arouses the need to explain the trade-offs between performance and algorithms. In recent years, shift in design paradigm of entire healthcare landscape has brought revolution in reshaping human–technology symbiosis. Pang et al. in his research reviewed the convergence of engineering and automation [9] in biomedi-cal field to bridge the gap between research and present demand. Vision of bio-medical engineering has shifted from illness treatment to fitness management and has become more analytic in terms of patient orientation. In [10], various aspects of healthcare treatment are observed following 7P features of personalized patient-friendly healthcare systems.

The organization structure of this chapter is as follows – the next section con-tains literature review carried out for smart healthcare systems, the second section describes recent medical advancement carried out in biomedical sector and the impact of culmination of tri-technology (AI, IoT and 6G) is illustrated in the third section. Implementation of technological models is shown in the fourth section and the fifth section describes the challenges posed by integration of smart technology with healthcare. Finally, the sixth section includes potential solutions to overcome challenges, followed by summary and conclusion in the last sections.

10.3   MEDICAL ADVANCEMENT IN RECENT YEARS

Rapid advancement in technology and innovation have become keystones of the healthcare and medical sector. The power of recent advancement and development in medical field is illimitable. This progress will allow medical healthcare profes-sionals to gather information, diagnose, cure and handle medical operations more effectively.

Nowadays, there are various medical technologies emerging with full pace which includes effective diagnosis of disease, patient monitoring, personalized medicines

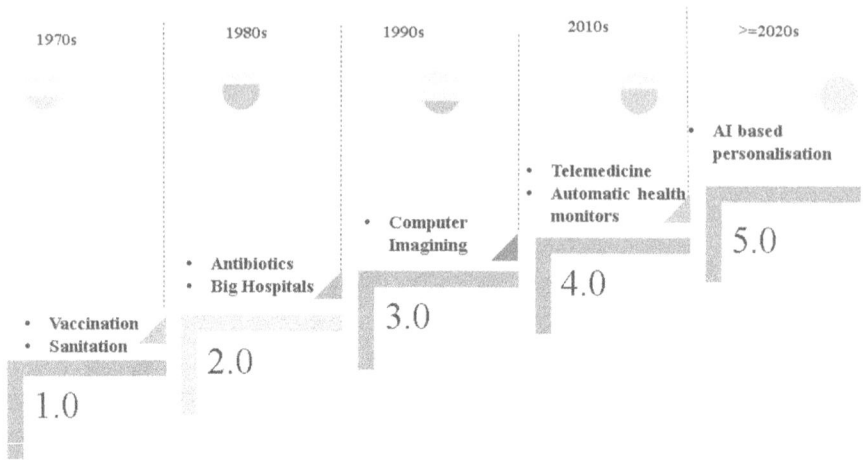

FIGURE 10.2   Timeline of advancement in medical healthcare systems.

using AI technology and IoT. Timeline of advancement in medical healthcare systems is shown in Figure 10.2.

Many tech giants (Google, Microsoft) have started investing in emerging digital medical development as the demand for robotic assistance [11] is rapidly increasing. Technology will advance day by day and there will be new discoveries and inventions. In the field of medical technology, use of robotic surgeries and intelligent diagnosing aids are common nowadays that are responsible for taking intelligent decisions.

10.4   INTEGRATION OF WIRELESS TECHNOLOGY

As the number of users using internet are increasing exponentially in today's world, demand for wireless technology is also growing rapidly. The benefits associated with wireless are manyfold – users can access real-time information and installation of this technology is easy to handle. With such advancement in this area of research, integration of these technologies could bring revolution in future and can open pathways for new inventions.

10.4.1   ARTIFICIAL INTELLIGENCE-ENABLED MEDICAL SERVICES

AI is the simulation of human intelligence in machine that defines the ability of computer systems to think like human brain. The basic idea behind AI is data analysis and algorithms in which huge amount of data is fed into machines and thereby learning takes place. AI holds advantages in medical sector as well but detail impact of using this technology needs to be analyzed.

AI involves investigating data, training data, analyzing correlation patterns to predict the future outcome. It has its focus on three domains of cognitive

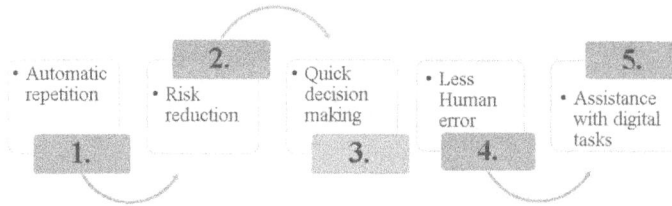

FIGURE 10.3   Benefits of artificial intelligence in processing big medical data.

intelligence – learning, reasoning and self-correction. Learning process involves conversion of data into useful information by creating suitable algorithms in a step-by-step manner. Reasoning process decides the most suitable path to get the desired outcome and self-correction process ensures that accurate results are produced by the algorithm.

AI has gained more importance in recent years as it can perform task better than humans since processing large data can bury a human researcher while AI can quickly turn it into actionable information. Some of the advantages associated with AI is listed in Figure 10.3. AI can be classified into four different types, namely reactive, limited memory, theory of mind and self-awareness as shown in Figure 10.4.

Reactive AI is designed for a specific task and acts on the received input. There is no effect of past decisions on the task performed. Limited memory AI takes input and adds a certain piece of it to programmed representation and thus changes the way AI makes new decisions.

Theory of mind AI includes updatable representation of the world that specifies an understanding toward other entities also. Self-awareness AI extends the theory of mind to predict the internal state of another task as well. Various application of

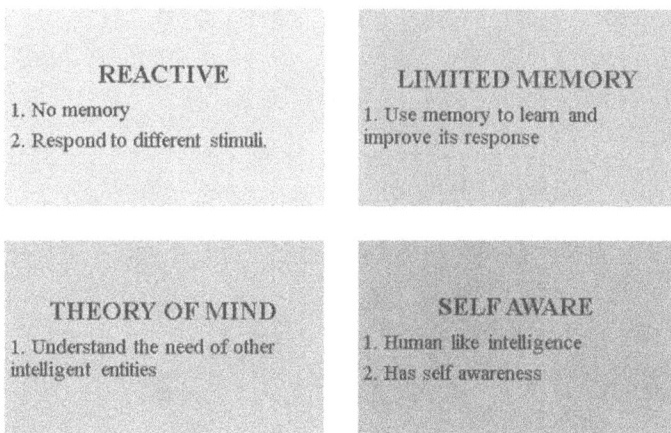

FIGURE 10.4   Classification of artificial intelligence.

AI can be found in healthcare such as online virtual health assistants and chatbots to help the customers in finding medical information like schedule appointments and billing process. The concept of smart healthcare in smart cities [12] requires special services to manage utilities and transportation to community using sensors integrated with machine learning.

10.4.2 NEXT GENERATION WIRELESS NETWORK 6G

6G is said to be 50 times faster than 5G and expected to be commercially available before 2030. It will be able to use higher frequency and thus provide higher capacity and much lower delay. Such technologies involving massive parallel-computing architectures will help to solve scheduling operations and research problem in more efficient way. This will limit the need for on-site presence of medical staff and doctors in remote areas.

Application of 6G in various spheres of technology is depicted in Figure 10.5. Several reasons support the need for using 6G includes technology convergence, high-performance computing, IoT-supporting machine-to-machine communication and edge computing.

10.4.3 IoT-EMBEDDED SYSTEMS IN MONITORING DEVICES

IoT is a combination of interrelated computing systems having unique identifiers that can transfer information without human-to-computer or human-to-human

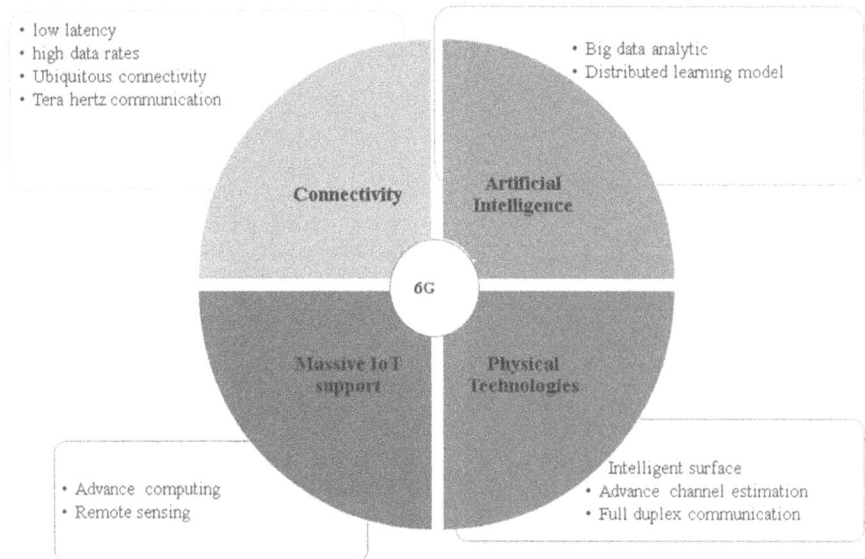

FIGURE 10.5   Applications of 6G technology.

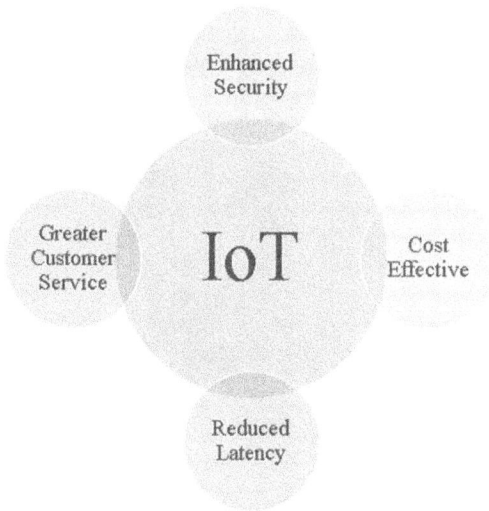

FIGURE 10.6 Benefits of internet of things (IoT) in healthcare systems.

interaction. It has an ecosystem which consists of many smart systems with web-enabled applications. These devices have in-built sensors that collect the information through a common gateway and send it to cloud for analyzing and further processing. It has the property to work irrespective of human intervention; however, human can interact with these devices to install them, giving commands or accessing data.

The applications deployed in IoT provide specific protocols for their connectivity, networking and communication. It offers several benefits to industry-specific applications and some of them are listed in Figure 10.6. Some of the common advantages include improved customer experience, save time as well as money, also enhance employee productivity by integrating different business models.

Enabling IoT in smart healthcare systems would help in providing information anytime from anywhere on any device thus saving time consumed in the administration process, and improvising the communication between connected devices. Automation of task involved in medical process will improve its quality as well as reduce the need of human intervention, especially in remote areas. BSN (body sensor network) [13] has emerged as one of the core developments of miniaturized wireless sensor units to monitor basic activities of patient like temperature, respiration rate, etc.

10.5 IMPLEMENTATION OF TECHNOLOGY

Smart healthcare-based systems focus on integrated technology of AI, IoT and 6G to provide advanced medical facilities. Failure and recovery of software and hardware

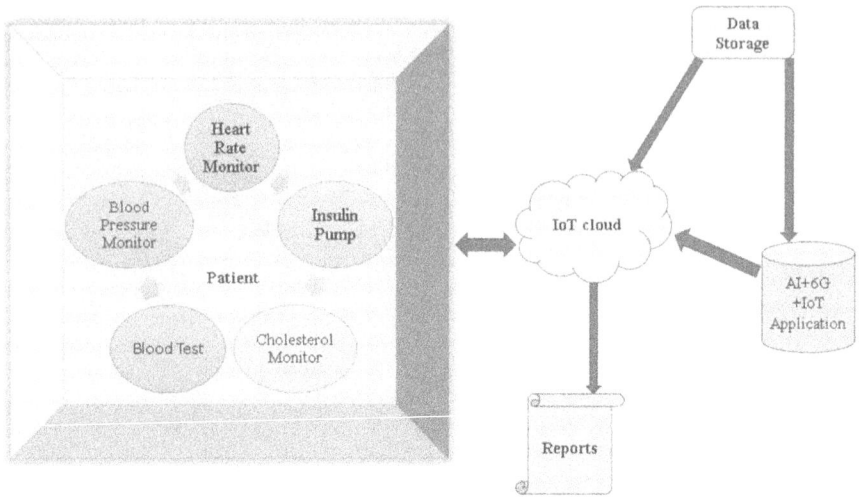

FIGURE 10.7 Workflow of process in healthcare systems.

of medical devices play a vital role in deciding performance associated with patient health condition.

As shown in Figure 10.7, different medical devices are dedicated to performing function such as blood pressure device to give details regarding heart condition. It aims at providing a comprehensive report of patient's health (as shown in Figure 10.8) by analyzing inter-dependency of biological and mechanical functionality of healthcare.

Following examples give the illustration of processes carried out in smart health-care model.

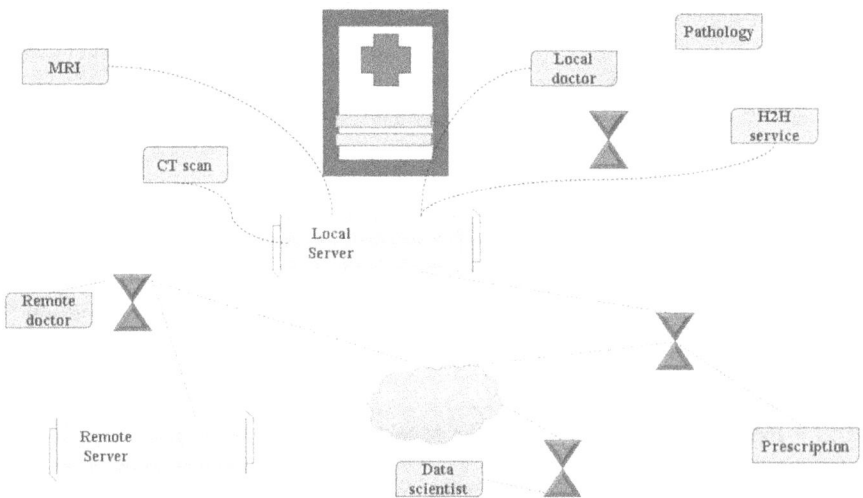

FIGURE 10.8 Illustration of smart healthcare model.

10.5.1 Systematic Allocation of Wheelchair

In accordance with the health condition of physically disabled and senior citizens, researchers have created fully automated smart wheelchairs that have various sensors and new-fangled technology.

These sensors help in monitoring and identifying the movement of wheelchair and provide information related to current health status of the patient. Wireless technology has played a very crucial role in accelerating this work.

10.5.2 Medical Integrated System

IoT focus on the development of two entities which include problems related to population growth and a lack of health competence. It can improve the working capabilities of physically disabled people and senior citizens. Body sensor network is introduced to escalate integration of the system.

The design of medical system determines that wireless technology can create fruitful environment in providing real-time accurate data. There are various IoT-based medical-integrated system that includes language training system for teens, smart medical system in cities and advanced system for prisons.

10.5.3 Effective Healthcare Solutions

Nowadays, electronic devices and instruments can be operated with the help of smartphones using sensors and AI. Different apps in smartphones provide assistance to the patient, enhance medical education and provide necessary training in healthcare field. The development of various software products proves that smartphones are helpful gadget in healthcare sector.

The key requirements essential for effective implementation of smart healthcare systems are shown in Figure 10.9.

10.5.3.1 Confidential
It maintains the authorization of only signed users for gathering medical information.

10.5.3.2 Privacy
It allows users to strictly follow privacy policy and avoid disclosure of any sensitive information outside the organization without consent.

10.5.3.3 Accessibility
It ensures the use of medical services without any further delay in times of need.

10.5.3.4 Integrity
It provides accuracy in describing prescription and diagnosis with complete authorized data and end-to-end communication.

10.5.3.5 Recent Data Collection
It needs to ensure that only recent medical data is analyzed and used for diagnosis with real-time communication.

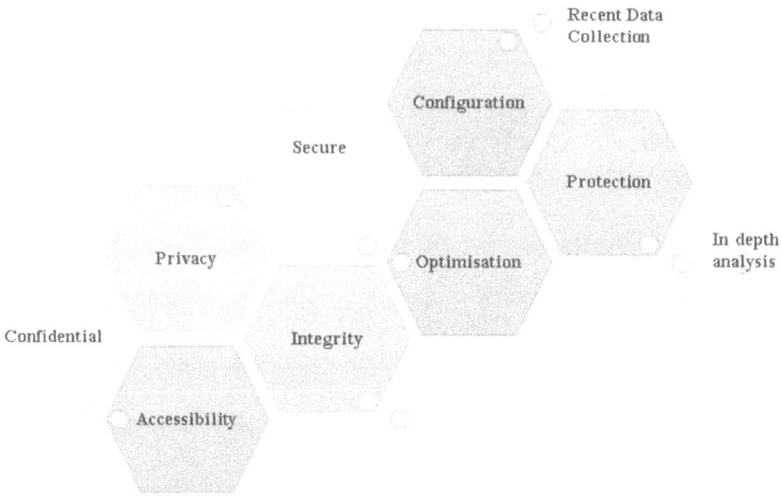

FIGURE 10.9   Key requirements of healthcare systems.

10.5.3.6   Secure

It follows coordination of accessibility, integrity and privacy of data to prescribe medicine to patient.

10.5.3.7   Optimization

Smart healthcare-based systems need to optimize resources such as data, power and maintain its quality of performance.

10.5.3.8   Configuration

Smart systems should be able to automatically configure any downloads and any latest update of software.

10.5.3.9   Protection

System should be able to protect itself from any virus attack and suspicious activity and report against them.

10.5.3.10   In-Depth Analysis

Various factors need to be analyzed before determining the condition of patient such as past medical history, allergies and immunity of body, etc. so that different monitoring devices can be configured.

10.6   SMART HEALTHCARE CHALLENGES AND APPLICATIONS

Wireless network devices can be consolidated into the healthcare environment. Advanced healthcare diagnosis for patients and various medical facility functions are performed by using IEEE802.15.4 wireless network and CDMA cellular network [14].

It also helps in collecting real-time information and provide optimum aids to the patient at hospital as well as at home environment. However, few challenges are encountered in the process of implementation of such systems which are listed next.

10.6.1   MAINTAINING PROTECTION MECHANISMS

The key technical challenges involved in implementation of smart healthcare system are energy efficiency and avoidance of signal attenuation due to water droplets present in surrounding air and obstruction due to buildings. Another dimension to protection mechanism includes end-to-end robust security and data protection mechanism to handle large amount of patient data.

10.6.2   ADOPTION OF NEW MODELS

Implementation of new models include innovation in the design of antenna, its miniaturization and combination of edge cloud – distributed AI models.

10.6.3   COMPLEX DESIGN FOR CARRIER WAVE

Complex models need to be designed to route the data through complex paths to destination as water vapors present in the atmosphere block the THz waves and reflect it.

10.6.4   AVAILABILITY OF SEMICONDUCTOR

Semiconductor material using multi-THz frequencies need to be designed by aligning enormous arrays of extremely tiny antennas to get a particular frequency range.

One of the vital applications [15] of smart healthcare systems includes treatment of chronic patients as shown in Figure 10.10. Such patients are affected by issues governing their quality of life and in most of the cases environmental factors are not considered in treatment due to their dynamic nature. However, with the concept of smart health, the scenario is changing, and the dynamics of healthcare are also shifting.

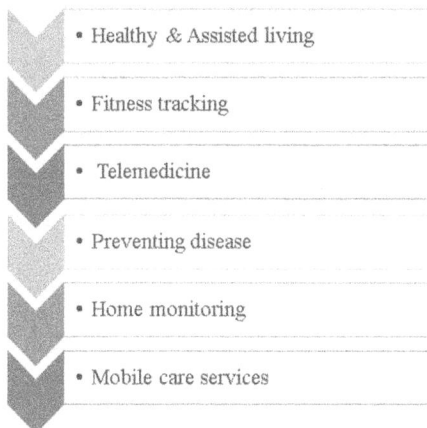

- Healthy & Assisted living
- Fitness tracking
- Telemedicine
- Preventing disease
- Home monitoring
- Mobile care services

FIGURE 10.10   Applications of smart healthcare systems.

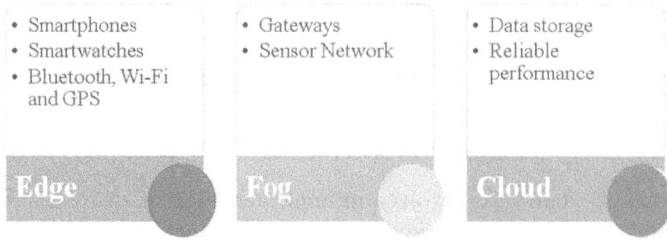

• Smartphones	• Gateways	• Data storage
• Smartwatches	• Sensor Network	• Reliable
• Bluetooth, Wi-Fi		performance
and GPS		

| Edge | Fog | Cloud |

FIGURE 10.11   Architecture level IoMT-integrated systems.

10.7   POTENTIAL SOLUTIONS TO SMART HEALTHCARE AND EMERGING TECHNOLOGIES

One of the practical solutions for effective utilization of smart healthcare facilities include concern over medical data fusion which will allow more accurate analysis of real-time diagnosis to curb diseases more efficiently. Multi-layered architecture (as shown in Figure 10.11) employs another general solution in more elaborative way which comprises of:

10.7.1   EDGE LEVEL

It includes embedded systems in compact portable devices such as smartwatches and ensures processing based on wireless sensors.

10.7.2   FOG LEVEL

Information gathered from edge-level devices is processed for storage.

10.7.3   CLOUD LEVEL

It is responsible for remote storage and reliability for high performance.

The main aim of such advanced techniques is to inaugurate fast computing systems for settling down the challenging issue of quality in medical market. NIB (Industrial Network in Box) [16] provides a highly mobile management tool for systematic medical applications.

10.8   SUMMARY OF RESEARCH GUIDELINES FOR SMART HEALTHCARE

Smart healthcare has knowledge influence from diverse fields as a result, there is a need to explore respective domains to identify its paradigm. The main aim is to rectify the latest trends in research guidelines [17] that will need attention in the coming years. To set a common ground to address the challenges, a systematic approach is needed starting from data assembling to the implementation part. Since this industry incorporates various technologies together for serving better quality, its functioning involves a dynamic approach in terms of the transformation of data into intelligence

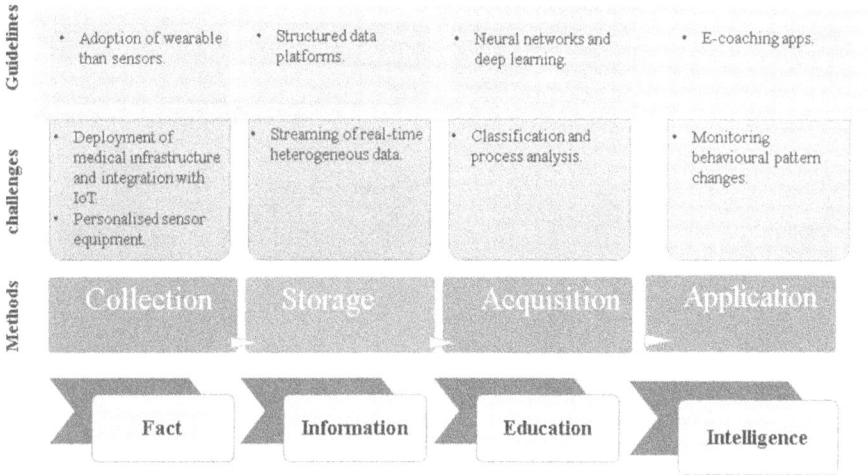

FIGURE 10.12 Architecture of smart healthcare systems.

which is difficult in the medical sector. In this, the data management system is a sensitive matter that could place life at stake. The smart healthcare paradigm follows a context-dependent approach where similar data set for specific parameter could have different interpretations depending on the age of the patient, geographical location, and so on. Hence, there is a need to put together various platforms concerning the healthcare system to have a well-structured environment that could deal with the generation of huge heterogeneous medical data, facilitation of sensors, etc.

The concept of collaboration of mobile devices with healthcare (m-health), acquisition of ICT with medical science (e-health), and networking infrastructure in smart facilities (s-health) pave the way to overcome the challenges and grasp the opportunities that will shape the healthcare field in the future. The architecture of smart healthcare systems is shown in Figure 10.12.

10.8.1 COLLECTION OF FACTS AND FIGURES

To extract the useful information from facts, it is necessary to gather them. Since there is an exponential increase in the data being transferred in medical system, it is difficult to estimate its real aggregate. Figure 10.13 discusses the steps involved in collection of facts and figures for medical data analysis. Moreover, extracting the personalized information requires deep processing that possesses many challenges including cost and reliability. In conventional medical infrastructure, network is formed by sensors which communicate data to central unit. The process looks to be simple but communication in dense environments requires radio planning. Another phase of data collections holds difficulties in passage followed by wearables and sensors that impact platforms like IoMT.

Sensors are known to be a well-known research area of e-health that are mostly found in healthcare facility. Collection of data by sensors is personalized and

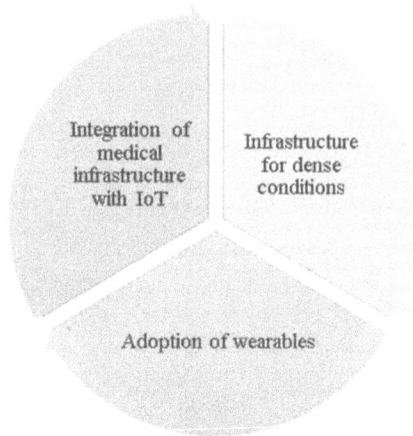

FIGURE 10.13 Steps involved in collection of facts and figures for medical data analysis.

contextual, according to the needs of patients. The significance of sensors is worth emphasizing for its integration in wearable technology like designing costumes equipped with sensors (to track patient's health), inserting sensors inside human body is also a fascinating research area to tackle new viruses.

10.9 CONCLUSION

This book chapter focuses on the upgradation of healthcare industry by collaboration of advanced technologies and biomedical industry. With the growing population, it is important to renovate health surveillance monitoring system based on AI-enabled IoT and 6G network. Smart healthcare solutions provide a unique framework to channelize medical services in effective manner by overcoming barriers of geographical topology and man–machine interaction. It aims to collaborate the concept of sustainable future with wireless mechanics. Deployment of AI in medical sector would provide quick data analysis and high degree of remote monitoring, thus making it viable to a large community. IoT provides various safeguard mechanisms to preserve data integrity and confidentiality. Combination of the aforementioned three technologies will improve working efficiency of surveillance system by automation, training and learning of big medical data. Despite several benefits of embedded technology, it suffers from data privacy issues and ethical judgment also needs to be addressed in running algorithms-based treatment. Thus, personalized health-tracking systems pave the way for patient-oriented systems.

REFERENCES

1. Sabuzima Nayak and Ripon Patgiri. 6G Communication Technology: A Vision on Intelligent Healthcare. *Studies in Computational Intelligence Journal*, 1–18 (2020).
2. P. K. Padhi and F. Charrua-Santos. 6G Enabled Tactile Internet and Cognitive Internet of Healthcare Everything: Towards a Theoretical Framework. *Applied System Innovation*, 4, 66 (2021).

3. S. Yeasmin. Benefits of Artificial Intelligence in Medicine. 2nd International Conference on Computer Applications & Information Security (ICCAIS), 1–6 (2019).
4. F. Alshehri and G. Muhammad. A Comprehensive Survey of the Internet of Things (IoT) and AI-Based Smart Healthcare. *IEEE Access*, 9, 3660–3678 (2021).
5. L. Xu, X. Zhou, Y. Tao, L. Liu, X. Yu and N. Kumar. Intelligent Security Performance Prediction for IoT-Enabled Healthcare Networks Using an Improved CNN. *IEEE Transactions on Industrial Informatics*, 18, 3, 2063–2074 (2022).
6. Luca Greco, Gennaro Percannella, Pierluigi Ritrovato, Francesco Tortorella and Mario Vento. Trends in IoT-Based Solutions for Health Care: Moving AI to the Edge. *Pattern Recognition Letters*, 135, 346–353 (2020).
7. M. M. S. Choyon, M. Rahman, M. M. Kabir and M. F. Mridha. IoT Based Health Monitoring & Automated Predictive System to Confront COVID-19. IEEE 17th International Conference on Smart Communities: Improving Quality of Life Using ICT, IoT and AI (HONET), 189–193 (2020).
8. W. Guo. Explainable Artificial Intelligence for 6G: Improving Trust between Human and Machine. *IEEE Communications Magazine*, 58, 6, 39–45 (2020).
9. Z. Pang, G. Yang, R. Khedri and Y. -T. Zhang. Introduction to the Special Section: Convergence of Automation Technology, Biomedical Engineering, and Health Informatics Toward the Healthcare 4.0. *IEEE Reviews in Biomedical Engineering*, 11, 249–259 (2018).
10. H. Zhu et al. Smart Healthcare in the Era of Internet-of-Things. *IEEE Consumer Electronics Magazine*, 8, 5, 26–30 (2019).
11. J. H. Han and J. Y. Lee. Digital Healthcare Industry and Technology Trends. IEEE International Conference on Big Data and Smart Computing (BigComp), 375–377 (2021).
12. D. J. Cook, G. Duncan, G. Sprint and R. L. Fritz. Using Smart City Technology to Make Healthcare Smarter. *Proceedings of the IEEE*, 106, 4, 708–722 (2018).
13. P. Gope and T. Hwang. BSN-Care: A Secure IoT-Based Modern Healthcare System Using Body Sensor Network. *IEEE Sensors Journal*, 16, 5, 1368–1376 (2016).
14. C. Yan and W. Chung. IEEE 802.15.4 Wireless Mobile Application for Healthcare System. International Conference on Convergence Information Technology (ICCIT), 1433–1438 (2007).
15. Shuo Tian, Wenbo Yang, Le Grange, Jehane Michael, Peng Wang, Wei Huang and Zhewei Ye. Smart Healthcare: Making Medical Care More Intelligent. *Global Health Journal*, 3, 62–65 (2019).
16. A. H. Sodhro et al. Toward ML-Based Energy-Efficient Mechanism for 6G Enabled Industrial Network in Box Systems. *IEEE Transactions on Industrial Informatics*, 17, 10, 7185–7192 (2021).
17. A. Solanas, F. Casino, E. Batista and R. Rallo. Trends and challenges in smart healthcare research: A journey from data to wisdom. IEEE 3rd International Forum on Research and Technologies for Society and Industry (RTSI), 1–6 (2017).

11 Success Stories for IoT-Enabled 6G for Prediction and Monitoring of Infectious Diseases with Artificial Intelligence

S. Chandrakala and G. Revathy

CONTENTS

11.1 Introduction 200
11.2 Diseases Introduction 200
    11.2.1 COVID-19..200
    11.2.2 Infectious Diseases Caused after COVID-19 200
    11.2.3 Other Diseases Symptoms 201
    11.2.4 Heart Failure...201
    11.2.5 Heart Attack Symptoms 201
11.3 Machine Learning Models 202
    11.3.1 Random Forest (RF)...202
    11.3.2 Support Vector Machine (SVM)...202
    11.3.3 K-Nearest Neighbour (KNN) 203
    11.3.4 Logistic Regression..203
    11.3.5 Naïve Bayes 203
11.4 6G Fusion with ML 203
    11.4.1 Need of Fusion of IoT, ML and 6G..204
    11.4.2 Impact of 6G in Healthcare 204
11.5 Literature Survey 205
11.6 Dataset 208
11.7 Proposed Work System...208
    11.7.1 ML Connectivity Flow Diagram 208
    11.7.2 Implementation 209
11.8 Conclusion 212
References...213

DOI: 10.1201/9781003321668-11

11.1 INTRODUCTION

The chapter forecasts the importance of IoT, ML and the fusion for 6G in various infectious diseases and their immediate alert and other medical assistance for post-Covid recovered patients. Out of many diseases, we have taken case studies of various post-Covid patients affected by heart attacks and other issues after the immediate recovery from COVID-19. Many people are suffering from heart attacks these days, and doctors are in short supply due to the pandemic crisis. To lower the number of deaths, we must be able to predict heart attacks. In this chapter, ML plays a significant part in addressing this issue. This prophecy saves a person's life. The random forest algorithm is utilized in this chapter to forecast heart attacks ahead of time. This chapter describes the architecture for checking heart rate and other data monitoring approaches, as well as how to leverage ML techniques; one example of it is heart attacks can be predicted using the collected heart rate data and other health-related information using the random forest classification technique.

11.2 DISEASES INTRODUCTION

The various diseases after post-Covid situations, the symptoms and the case study of heart failures have been discussed.

11.2.1 COVID-19

SARS-CoV-2 are among the different forms of corona viruses with high pathogen city. Corona virus disease 2019 is the result of the subsequent Spartan acute respiratory syndrome coronavirus (SARS-CoV-2) (COVID-19). COVID-19 is initially thought to be a respiratory infection [1]. Furthermore, COVID-19-affected patients with prevailing cardiac problems had worse respiratory symptoms; nonetheless, new onset of cardiac dysfunction is common in this group [2].

11.2.2 INFECTIOUS DISEASES CAUSED AFTER COVID-19

It's possible with the intention of social limitations premeditated to stop the blowout of SARS-CoV-2 were also linked with a decline in incidence of other infectious diseases. Evidence implies that as societal limitations were relaxed, infection incidence rates (IRs) began to increase (e.g., mask mandates). The resurgence of infectious disease makes it more challenging to control the ongoing COVID-19 pandemic. The 386,711 patients who made a total of 1,221,568 visits to hamlet clinics had an average age of 27.29 (23.93) years. Nearly 184,217 of these patients were female and 202,494 (52.3 percent) were male. Brood with ages 0–3 years had significantly more diagnoses of respiratory and gastrointestinal contagion (IR ratio, 2.64; 95 percent CI, 2:30–2.91; P.001). Additionally, SARS-CoV-2 was not the only respiratory infection to see a significant increase in prevalence across all age groups (IR ratio, 1.74; 95 percent CI, 1.56–1.94; P.001).

11.2.3 OTHER DISEASES SYMPTOMS

When we are in good health, we take breathing for granted and rarely give our lungs the credit they deserve for keeping us alive. We realize that breathing is the only thing that really matters, when our lung condition deteriorates. A sign of chronic obstructive pulmonary disease (COPD), a chronic inflammatory lung disease, is a restriction of airflow from the lungs. Symptoms include wheezing, coughing, production of mucus (sputum) and difficulty in breathing.

- Breathing difficulties, particularly when engaging in physical activity.
- A wheezing sound.
- Tightness in the chest.
- Persistent cough that occasionally results in the production of sputum, which can be clear, white, yellow or greenish.
- Respiratory infections that happen regularly.
- There is not enough vigour.
- Loss of weight that wasn't intended to happen.
- Ankle, foot or leg swelling.

11.2.4 HEART FAILURE

Patients who have pneumonia are more likely to develop heart failure. Furthermore, numerous investigations have found a link between heart failure and COVID-19. Twenty-three percent of heart issues were treated out of 191 COVID-19 patients from Wuhan [3]. Heart failure was present in 52 percent of the 54 individuals who died. Another study from Wuhan indicated that 24 percent of COVID-19 patients who died had heart failure [4–6].

According to several studies, the heart condition that happens after COVID-19 is due to stress. As a result, emotional discomfort and anxiety performance are a critical part in aggravating heart failure in COVID-19 patients. When people are infected with COVID-19, they are promptly isolated from their homes and a home quarantine is implemented [7, 8]. This home quarantine in and of itself is stressful for them. Due to age and other health circumstances such as diabetes, hypertension, hyperlipidemia, coronary artery disease, and so on, a lack of boldness also contributes to heart failure.

11.2.5 HEART ATTACK SYMPTOMS

The following are some of the signs and symptoms of a quick or irregular heartbeat: When a person gets up, they feel light-headed or dizzy. After getting infected with COVID-19, the menace of cardiopulmonary events may increase. One observational study based on data from National Veteran Health Administration database found an augmented menace of cardiovascular trial in COVID-19 patients compared to two sets of controls (contemporary [during the COVID-19 pandemic] and historical [pre-COVID-19 pandemic]) in one year (an extra 45.29 incidents/1,000 people) [8–12].

Stroke, dysrhythmias, myocardial infarction, pericarditis, myocarditis, heart failure and thromboembolic illness were all linked to an elevated risk. The things that the COVID-19 patients can do are:

- Hand washing can be performed frequently and distancing among people can be maintained.
- Home routines can be restructured.
- Emphasis can be given for the healthy weight.
- Good eating habits can be maintained.
- Exercises can be performed moderately.
- Alcohol can be avoided.
- Smoking or tobacco products can be avoided.
- Self-medication can be avoided.
- Telemedicine contacts can be arranged.
- Arrange for vaccination after three months post-recovery if not vaccinated before.
- HT, DM and dyslipidaemia can be controlled.
- Meditation, yoga can be practiced within the tolerance limits.

The things that the COVID-19 patients should avoid doing are:

- Continuous symptoms such as cough, weariness, fever, and dyspnoea should be limited to 60 percent of maximal heart rate, even if symptoms appear two to three weeks later.
- Cardiovascular exercises in known cardiac patients should be avoided for three months.
- Any medication should be taken only after consulting a cardiologist.
- Any warning signs such as heavy temperature, oxygen saturation level below 93 percent, chest pain, and dizziness should not be ignored.

11.3   MACHINE LEARNING MODELS

11.3.1   RANDOM FOREST (RF)

"RF is a classifier that uses the average of a number of decision trees on diverse subsets of a given dataset to improve the projected accuracy of that dataset." The projected correctness of a dataset is increased by a classifier called random forest by averaging the results of several decision trees on various subsets of the dataset [1, 2, 13].

11.3.2   SUPPORT VECTOR MACHINE (SVM)

Support vector machines are high-dimensional feature space popular among the neural information processing systems (NIPS) community, but they have since become a major fragment of ML explore everywhere in the world [14]. Using pixel maps as input, SVM completes a handwriting detection task with accuracy comparable to advanced neural networks with expanded features. With an emphasis on pattern classification and regression, it is also used for a variety of tasks, including handwriting analysis, facial analysis and other things. The foundation for SVM have become more and more popular due to a number of promising qualities, like improved pragmatic recital. The formula makes use of the structural risk minimization (SRM) principle, which is praised for being superior to the empirical risk minimization (ERM) theory used in traditional neural networks. The superior guarantee on the projected risk is minimized by SRM, whereas the accuracy of the training data is minimized by ERM. SVM has a stronger capacity for generalization as a result of this distinction, which is what statistical learning is all about. SVMs were originally designed to tackle classification problems; however, they have lately been extended to solve regression issues.

11.3.3   K-Nearest Neighbour (KNN)

The K-nearest neighbour (KNN) algorithm stays as a powerful ML technique that is simple to implement and administer [15]. It may be cast-off to address cataloging and deterioration problems. Close proximity is connected with comparable objects, and dissimilar things exist far apart from one other, according to the KNN algorithm. In other words, things that are comparable are close together.

11.3.4   Logistic Regression

Logistic regression, also known as the logistic model or logit model, examines the association amid several autonomous factors and a categorical reliance on variable by appropriate facts to a logistic curve and determining the chance of an event occurring [16]. When the dependent variable isn't binary or has added more than two groupings, a multinomial logistic regression can be utilized.

11.3.5   Naïve Bayes

Naïve Bayes is a probabilistic contraption erudition technique that can be practical to a multiplicity of categorization problems. That is, changing the value of one feature has no impact on the value of any other feature in the algorithm. Each characteristic in the Naïve Bayes method is assumed to be unrelated to the others [17, 18]. The technique is simple to code, and the predictions are made quickly, because it is a probabilistic model. As a result, it is scalable, and it has long been the preferred solution for real-world applications (apps) that must respond to user requests immediately. Forecasting the session of the trial dataset is modest and swift. It can also anticipate many classes. When the postulation of unconventionality is met, a Naïve Bayes classifier beats other models like logistic regression while using less training data.

11.4   6G FUSION WITH ML

According to current research, 6G is anticipated to have improved capacity, coverage, dependability, energy efficiency, decreased latency and, most outstandingly, a unified "human-centric" network system motorized by artificial intelligence (AI).

The 6G network is, therefore, capable of making a large number of automated judgments each second [19]. Simple network resource allocation is one option among many. It can indicate that the patient has to get to a hospital right away. But if AI decision-making becomes more rapid and data-intensive, it may become more dangerous without the knowledge of designers and consumers. The possible explainable AI (XAI) solutions reduce such worries by making the black box AI decision-making process more transparent.

11.4.1 NEED OF FUSION OF IoT, ML AND 6G

Wireless communications and networks of the sixth generation (6G) will continue to expand in frequency and bandwidth, and their data rates and spectral efficiency will increase significantly. It may be necessary to expand the 6G wireless network in order to support contemporary random access (RA) for IoT and ML assumed the assortment and compression of the IoT. Modern communications and signal-processing technologies, as well as clever protocol design, can accomplish this. The IoT and ML are strong candidates for 6G-enabled RA technologies like massive multiple-input-multiple-output (MIMO), OFDMA, non-orthogonal multiple access (NOMA), sparse signal processing, or novel orthogonal design techniques. For dispersed IoT and ML applications, grant-free transmission in 6G should be planned. IoT and ML applications frequently take part in self-organizing decision-making [20].

IoT powered by 6G will benefit from the most recent advancements in AI technology. It will increase IoT innovation and discovery while producing new knowledge and understanding. Each of these initiatives aims to highlight the inherent multidisciplinary aspect of the developing IoT with ML area. IoT will face various obstacles thanks to the hypothetical, scientific and decent frameworks that resolves the established 6G-enabled IoT and ML, improving technology for humanity.

11.4.2 IMPACT OF 6G IN HEALTHCARE

The rise in the number of chronic patients makes prevention essential. Prevention is a means of maintaining a healthy lifestyle (physical activity, food, routine health checks, etc.), as well as a means of preventing the deterioration of chronic illnesses. Actively promoting the well-being of post-Covid patients is one of the goals of the healthcare system [21].

6G is viewed as a complete and omnipresent connectivity fabric that enables the collection of many/all the required data from individuals (healthy and not), ranging from the activation of on-demand health check-ups to how much water a person has consumed daily (using sensors on the bottle, for example) to how many calories they have consumed daily (using sensors on/into the body).

Five use cases that 6G communication technologies can support:

Initial, eMBB-Plus assuming the role of eMBB in the 5G standard; it is anticipated to improve mobile communications in terms of interference, handover, data transfer, data processing and interoperability while also offering a high level of security and privacy.

BigCom is the next. By guaranteeing network coverage and a sufficient level of service everywhere, it helps to bring communication services to rural areas.

SURLLC. It should give 5G mMTC less latency and more security reliability than 5G URLLC.

3D-InteCom. It is primarily concerned with full-dimensional MIMO topologies, unmanned aircraft, underwater communications, and 3D network analysis, planning and optimization that take network node heights into account.

UCDCs or uCDCs as they are frequently abbreviated. It contains cutting-edge communication paradigms and prototypes, including holographic and tactile internet and human-bond communications, among others.

Pathology, local doctors, remote doctors and data scientist are all a part of the hospital-to-home (H2H) services, which implement mobile hospitals, and the Intelligent Internet of Medical Things (blood sample reader [BSR] sensor, intelligent wearable devices [IWD], online prescription, MRI, and CT Scan).

In order to usher in the intelligent future, it is likely that 6G will be a communication technology that is entirely controlled by AI. Because all smart devices will transition to being intelligent in the 6G era, we will see a number of changes from smart things to intelligent things as a result of the development of AI and mobile schmoozing. After 2030, when IoE becomes intelligent, it will replace IoT as the dominant technology. Intelligent phones will gradually replace smart phones in the marketplace. Internet-connected gadgets that use AI will be seen as intelligent. As a result, the intelligent device, which could be small, will be able to communicate with other intelligent devices and predict events.

11.5   LITERATURE SURVEY

Heart disease is the most prevalent long-term post-COVID-19 consequence among COVID-19 survivors, according to a research. The availability of the post-COVID-19 dataset, which is limited in scope, is the driving force for this study. Data on post-COVID problems is gathered in this research [1] by personally contacting COVID-19 patients who had previously been impacted. After pre-processing to deal with missing values, the dataset is oversampled to generate many examples, and the model is trained. For the purpose of predicting heart disorders after COVID-19 infection, deep neural networks are used in the aforementioned work to expand a binary classifier based on a mounding assembly.

Corona viruses mostly damage the cardiovascular system among the numerous components of the human body. The foundations of corona viruses, with an emphasis on COVID-19, are discussed in this work [2], as well as their effects on the cardiovascular system. Corona virus infection in 2019 can result in viral pneumonia, as well as other pulmonary symptoms and consequences. A high percentage of affected role have original cardiovascular disease or jeopardy factors for heart disease. Age, as well as other health-related issues such as hypertension, sugar levels, heart disease, and cerebrovascular illness, are the key determinants that dictate a person's mortality.

Patients with underlying cardiovascular illness and/or cardiac risk factors make up a high percentage of the population. Elevated high-sensitivity troponin levels indicate very serious cardiac damage, which is recurrently realized in a variation of conditions and is linked to mortality. According to the findings of this study, corona virus disease 2019 is accompanying with a high-seditious cargo that can root vascular inflammation, myocarditis and cardiac arrhythmias.

More research is being done to find specific vaccinations and anti-vaccines for SARS-CoV-2. In addition, evidence-based guidelines should be followed to control cardiovascular risk factors and diseases. Corona virus illness 2019 (COVID-19) continues to cause widespread distress and missed deadlines around the world. COVID-19 primarily affects the cardiovascular system, according to accounts from hospitalized patients, although the global impact is unknown.

Using ML algorithms, Naresh Kumar and colleagues created an effective automated disease diagnosis model. The death rate from these disorders could be reduced if disease was diagnosed early. Diabetes, heart disease, and the coronavirus are three of the major illnesses covered in this work. The analysis of the data is carried out in a real-time database using a ML model that has already been deployed in Firebase and pretrained using the same dataset. The results of the illness detection are then displayed in the android applications. Logistic regression is used to perform prediction calculations. Diabetes, heart disease, and the corona virus can all be identified early. A comparative investigation findings indicate that the suggested strategy can help doctors give patients timely treatment and drugs.

According to Muhammad Nabeel and colleagues, the most dangerous issue facing today's society is the heart's incapability to ticker adequate blood to change that needs in the body. This problem is particularly prevalent among the elderly. Exercise boosts blood flow, and if you don't do it, you'll start to experience the signs of heart failure. Every year, cardiovascular diseases claim millions of lives. When a blood clot prevents enough blood from flowing, a heart attack happens. The heart muscle starts to deteriorate due to a lack of blood when blood flow is blocked. A heart attack usually happens between the ages of 40 and 50, claims scientific research. As a result, this study's objective is to analyze the illness of heart attack in terms of a variety of traits. Dietary restrictions are essential for heart attack patients to keep their blood pressure and cholesterol levels within healthy ranges [22]. This benefits in maintaining strong cardiac muscles and excellent health.

Discussing the Health Internet of Things is Hemantha Krishna Bharadwaj et al. (H-IoT). Data gathering and processing are the two main elements of this. Here, the H-IoT and ML algorithms are cast-off to handle the vast amount of data involved in healthcare, where precise prediction is necessary to save many lives [23]. Many serious illnesses, including heart disease, lung cancer, and kidney disease, are covered together with the various ML techniques. Applications of various healthcare systems, such as those for monitoring infants, emotion recognition, and cognitive monitoring systems, are also described.

Amani Alhahiri et al. provided an explanation of how the health prediction system uses a hybrid of IoT and ML. In this learning, ML algorithms are swotted in relation to their application to IoT medical data. They've also come to the conclusion that every ML algorithm has flaws of its own. Additionally, it is stated that in order to predict the crucial healthcare data, the best method must be found based on the type of IoT dataset selected [24].

Yogesh Kumar and colleagues presented their work on the use of a dataset with 14 attributes to detect heart failure using quantum-enhanced ML. After the heart failure data has been standardized using techniques like min-max, PCA and standard scalar, the data is then optimized using the pipeline technique [25]. It demonstrates how cutting-edge quantum machine learning methods, including quantum random forest (QRF), quantum K-nearest neighbour (QKNN), quantum decision tree (QDT) and quantum Gaussian Naïve Bayes (QGNB), outperform traditional ML methods in the detection of heart failure. Quantum random forest was the algorithm with the best accuracy rate (0.89), F1 score (0.88), precision (0.89) and recall (0.89), among quantum-based ML algorithms. Additionally, the processing speeds of classical and quantum-enhanced approaches are contrasted. By 150 microseconds, QRF has the quickest execution time.

Muhammed Golec et al. developed the IFaasBus architecture, a lightweight security and privacy system based on data collected from numerous IoT devices, in order to safeguard the lives of many people. It relies on a number of technologies, such as serverless computing, the IoT, ML, and function as a service, to help those with Covid-19 disorders. To protect the confidentiality of the patient's medical records, IFaaSBus employs the OAuth-2.0 authorization protocol, JSON Web Tokens, and transport layer socket protocol. In comparison to using non-serverless computing, IFaaSBus' response time is slower when dealing with up to 1,100 concurrent requests. The accuracy rate of the k-closest neighbour model, which achieved a 97.51 percent accuracy rate, is the highest of all ML techniques when compared [26].

Jimin Liu et al. used a variety of classifiers, such as SVM, KNN, logistic regression (LR), RF, Extra Tree (ET), gradient boosting decision tree (GBDT), XGBoost, LightGBM, CatBoost, and multilayer perceptron, to determine the best base learners. The LR simple linear classifier is used as the meta learner in order to circumvent the overfitting issue caused by the base learners. The proposed approach was compared to ten single classifier models using a combined heart dataset derived from various UCI ML sources as well as a different publicly available heart attack dataset [27].

Without the use of human feature engineering, Muhammed Umer et al. proposed a smart healthcare framework that makes use of cloud and IoT technologies to improve heart failure patient survival prediction. The intelligent IoT-based system keeps track of patients using real-time data and gives heart failure patients prompt, efficient and high-quality therapy. The suggested system uses deep-learning techniques as well to classify heart catastrophe affected role as alive or dead. The context collects data from IoT-based sensors and transfers it to a cloud web server so that it may be processed. To evaluate a patient's status, deep-learning algorithms further process these information. A medical professional who is qualified to provide emergency aid is given access to patients' medical data and processing findings [28].

According to Liang Tan et al., patients who pass away from COVID-19 typically have a co-morbid cardiovascular disease. By adopting wearable medical equipment to identify cardiovascular illness in real time, COVID-19 death rates could be decreased. Technical limitations are also mentioned in this chapter. To begin with, wearable medical equipment's standard wireless communication technology struggles to keep up with the demands of real-time connectivity. Second, the enormous volume of real-time cardiovascular data cannot be handled by current monitoring platforms due to the lack of efficient streaming data-processing tools. Third, it can be challenging to ensure that there are enough doctors on hand to make a prompt, efficient and accurate diagnosis because manual diagnosis on monitoring platforms is the norm. This study suggests a real-time, 5G-enabled cardiovascular monitoring system for COVID-19 patients that is deep learning-based. Initial transmission and reception of wearable medical device data occurs over 5G. Data about the electrocardiogram is gathered using the Flink streaming data-processing framework. The patient with COVID-19's cardiovascular condition is predicted using convolutional neural networks and long short-term memory network models [29].

11.6 DATASET

PSG polysomnography (ECG and EEG), blood pressure and airflow are all noted along with the date and time. According to a study, theta frequencies appear when blood flow drops below 17–18 ml/100 g/min and alpha frequencies disappear when blood flow falls below 25–35 ml/100 g/min. A blood flow range of 17–18 ml/100 g/min is crucial because as neurons twitch, transmembrane gradients collapse and brain cells die. Blood flows of 12–18 ml/100 g/min make the delta frequencies visible. At blood flow rates lower than 10–12 ml/100 g/min, EEG activity decreases and cellular damage becomes irreversible. Even when a patient is sleeping, it is still possible to predict their outcome.

11.7 PROPOSED WORK SYSTEM

Blood flow, blood pressure and air flow are connected to a Wi-Fi module on an Arduino board, which sends the data to a Naïve Bayes Classifier. The IoT sensor's data is divided into two groups by the RF: safe and unsafe. RF is used to identify people who are at risk of cardiac arrest, and the doctor or his family are immediately notified and instructed to take the appropriate precautions. The circumstances surrounding non-cardiac arrest patients are regularly confirmed, and their values are routinely assessed. The 6G role immediately helps the family with the nearby hospital facilities' assistance for patients in need of treatment emergencies.

11.7.1 ML CONNECTIVITY FLOW DIAGRAM

Figure 11.1 shows a simple sample diagram for random forest.

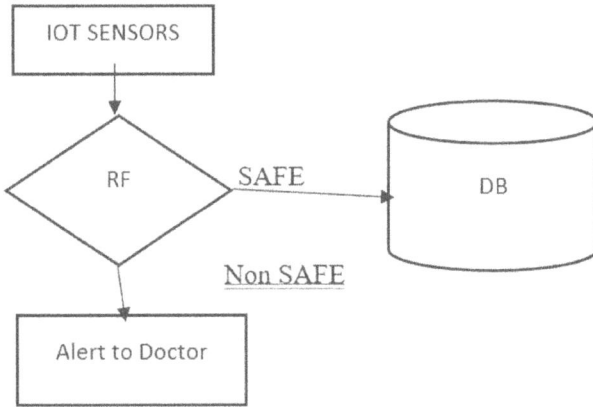

FIGURE 11.1   Block diagram of the proposed system.

11.7.2 Implementation

Using an Arduino board and a GSM module, IoT devices are connected. Circuit diagram for Figure 11.2 is shown with examples of sensors [30]. A brief output sample is taken after the sensors are connected.

The IoT sensor data along with the normal records of patient age, gender, past attack history, blood sugar level and cholestral level is passed to the ML

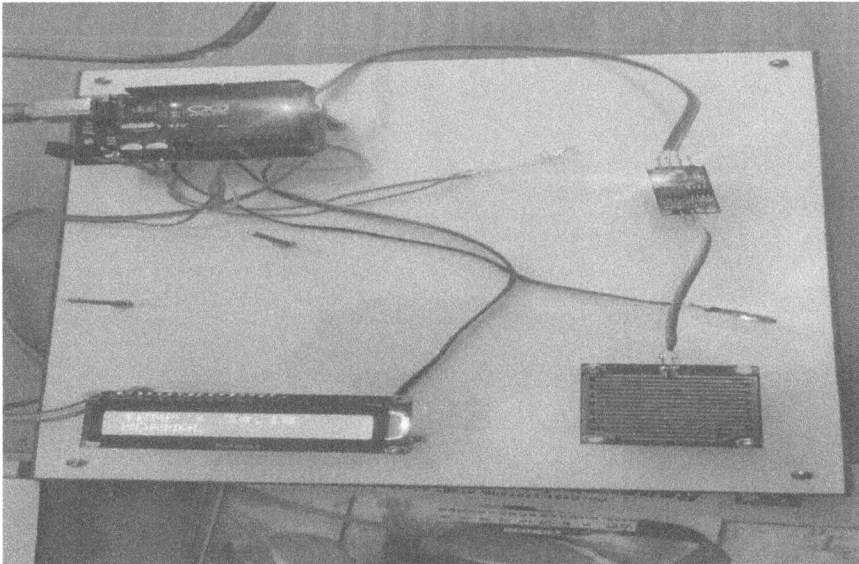

FIGURE 11.2   Circuit diagram.

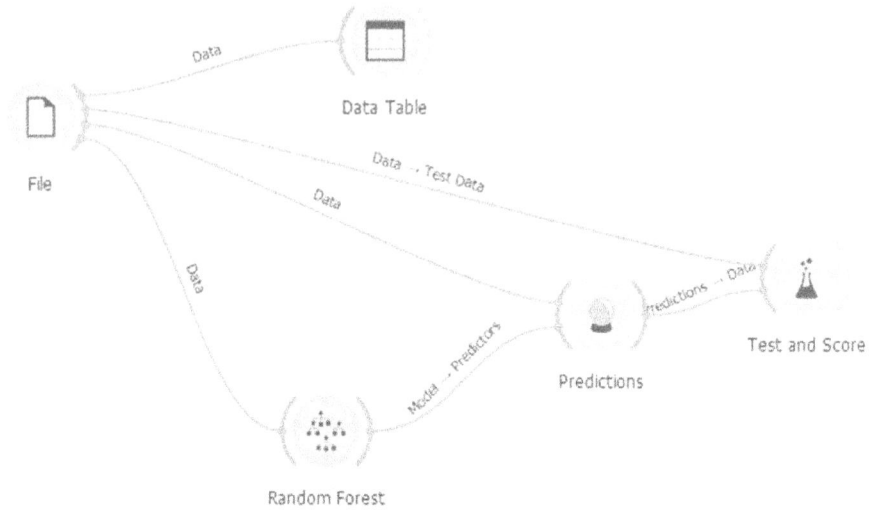

FIGURE 11.3   Random forest implementation in Orange tool.

algorithms [31, 32]. The implementation is performed with Orange tool and the results are recorded.

Figure 11.3 shows the implementation of random forest (data passed to RF, predictions and final test and score) in Orange tool. Figure 11.4 shows KNN (data passed to KNN, predictions and final test and score) implementation in Orange tool. Figure 11.5 shows SVM (data passed to SVM, predictions and final test and score)

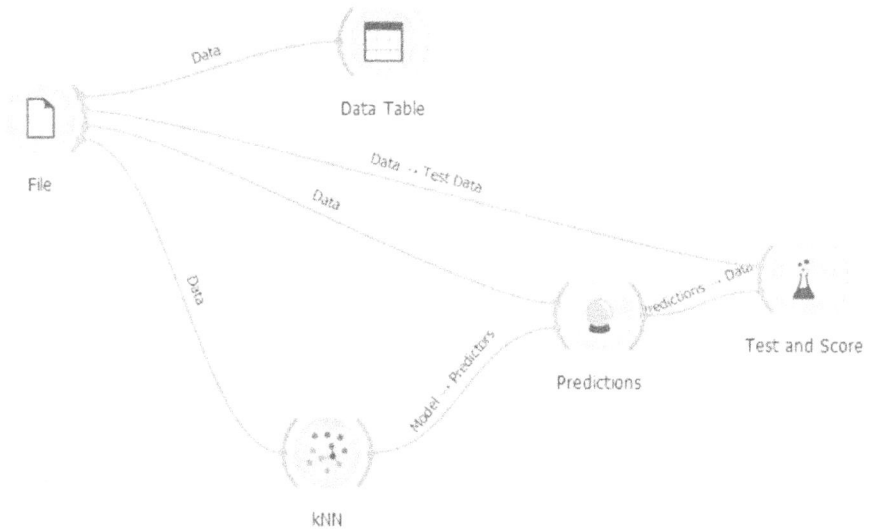

FIGURE 11.4   KNN implementation in Orange tool.

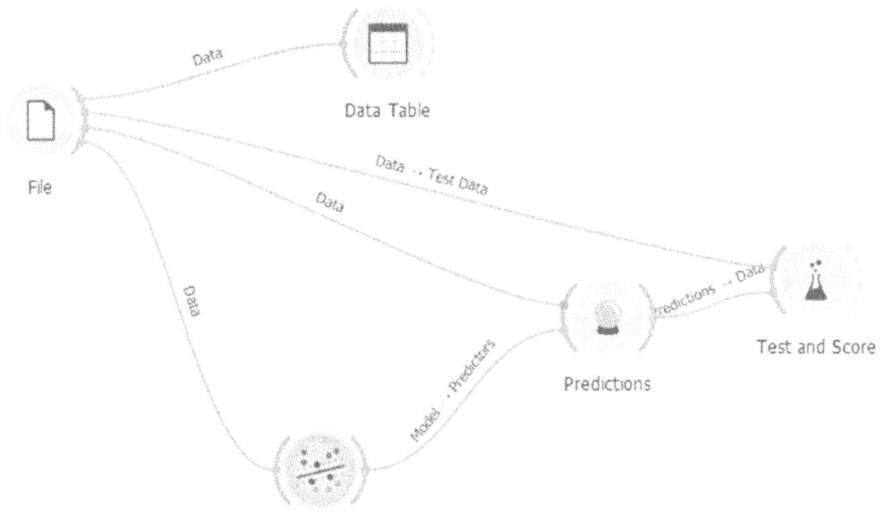

FIGURE 11.5   SVM implementation in Orange tool.

implemetation in Orange tool. Figure 11.6 shows Naïve Bayes (data passed to NB, predictions and final test and score) implementation in Orange tool. Figure 11.7 shows logistic regression (data passed to LR, predictions and final test and score) in Orange tool.

Figure 11.8 gives overall comparison of all ML algorithms. The comparisons of RF, SVM, NB, LR and KNN are compared and the result showed RF displays more accurate results than all other algorithms.

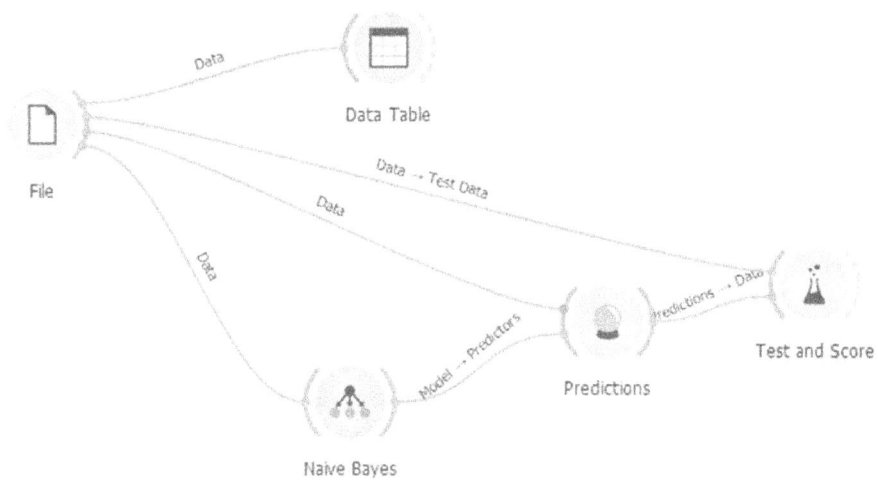

FIGURE 11.6   Naïve Bayes implementation in Orange tool.

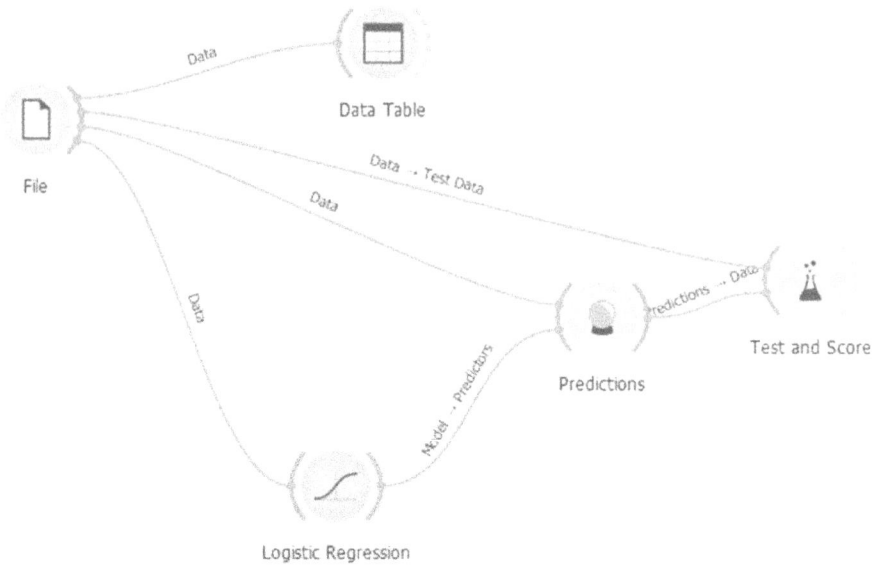

FIGURE 11.7   Logistic regression in Orange tool.

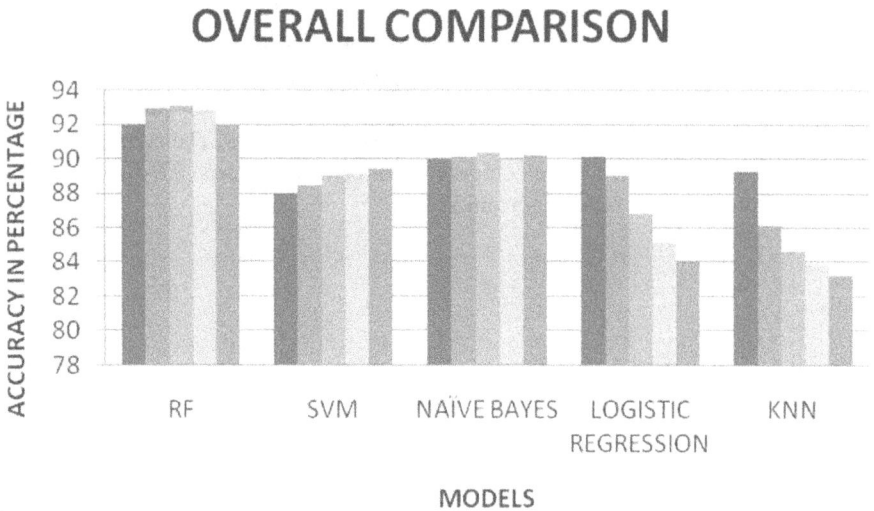

FIGURE 11.8   Overall comparison of ML algorithms.

11.8   CONCLUSION

Fedyor expressed his gratitude by saying, "It's a fantastic honour." "In order to preserve a life. You helped a lot of people," expressed Leigh Bardugo in *Shadow and Bone* It's a fantastic quote. During a pandemic, such as COVID-19, it is extremely difficult to admit every patient to a hospital and examine their results. As a result of our proposed strategy, many lives have been spared, and people who are in good health do not need to attend a hospital or learn about new ailments. As far as our proposed work is concerned, test centres for COVID-19 patients can be setup using the various IoT sensors. If any person suspects that they have COVID-19, they can come to this test centres and can verify whether they are ok or not related to their health. The need of nearest hospital assistance and the nearest medical assistance can be easily obtained with the fusion of 6G. Since the patients with an abnormal condition alone will be given medical emergency, they can easily find the specialization doctor based on the disease and hence 6G assists in finding the nearest medical partner to sort out their issue. If they are declared ok suggests they need not go to the hospital and the chances of getting infected from other disease from any other person from the hospital is negligible. If they are not ok suggests they can verify the seriousness of their health issue. If immediate attention has to be given to their health issue signifies they can go to the hospital with all the health-related parameter from the test centres. The various parameters from the test centre can be temperature, pulse rate, pressure level, heart beat rate, sugar level, and any other health-related issue. A patient can be admitted to the hospital and receive treatment if they need care or if they are experiencing an emergency. They can carry out their treatments as necessary. We can guarantee that a patient's life is preserved because our method yields 90 percent accurate results.

REFERENCES

1. Karthick, D. and Priyadharshini, B. "Predicting the chances of occurrence of Cardio Vascular Disease (CVD) in people using classification techniques within fifty years of age." Second International Conference on Inventive Systems and Control (ICISC). Coimbatore, 2018, pp. 1182–1186.
2. Article on premature heart disease, available at https://www.health.harvard.edu/heart-health/premature-heartdisease.
3. Jabbar, M.A., and Samreen, S. "Heart disease prediction system based on hidden naïve bayes classifier." International Conference on Circuits, Controls, Communications and Computing (I4C). Bangalore, 2016, pp. 1–5.
4. Singh, J., Kamra, A., and Singh, H. "Prediction of heart diseases using associative classification." Fifth International Conference on Wireless Networks and Embedded Systems (WECON). Rajpura, 2016, pp. 1–7.
5. Wu, Z., and McGoogan, J.M. "Characteristics of and important lessons from the coronavirus disease 2019 (COVID-19) outbreak in China: Summary of a report of 72 314 cases from the Chinese center for disease control and prevention." *JAMA* 323(13): 1239–1242 (2020).
6. Heng, Y., Luo, R., Wang, K., Zhang, M., Wang, Z., and Dong, L. et al. "Kidney disease is associated with in-hospital death of patients with COVID-19." *Kidney International* 97(5): 829–838 (May 2020).
7. Klok, F.A., Kruip, M.J.H.A., van der Meer, N.J.M., Arbous, M.S., Gommers, D., Kant, K.M. et al. "Confirmation of high cumulative incidence of thrombotic complications in critically ill ICU patients with COVID-19: An updated Analysis." *Thromb Research* 191: 148–150 (2020).
8. Martínez-Martínez, J.M. et al. "Prediction of the hemoglobin level in hemodialysis patients using machine learning techniques." *Computer Methods and Programs in Biomedicine* 117(2): 208–217 (2014).
9. Decaro, C. et al. "Machine learning approach for prediction of hematic parameters in hemodialysis patients." *IEEE Journal of Translational Engineering in Health and Medicine* 7: 1–8 (2019).
10. Radović, N. et al. "Machine learning approach in mortality rate prediction for hemodialysis patients." *Computer Methods in Biomechanics and Biomedical Engineering* 7: 1–12 (2021).

11. Mansor, H., Shukor, M.H.A., Meskam, S.S., Rusli, N.Q.A. Mohd, and Zamery, N.S. "Body Temperature Measurement for Remote Health Monitoring System." *IEEE Xplore* (2014).

12. Dang, S., Amin, O., and Shihada, B. et al. "What should 6G be?" *Nature Electronics* 3: 20–29 (2020). https://doi.org/10.1038/s41928-019-0355-6.

13. Nayak, S., Patgiri, R., and Singh, T.D. "Big computing: Where are weheading?" *EAI Endorsed Transactions on Scalable Information Systems* 4: 283–300 (2020).

14. Lin, C.-H., Chen, W.-L., Li, C.-M. et al. "Assistive technology using integrated flexible sensor and virtual alarm unit for blood leakage detection during dialysis therapy." *Healthcare Technology Letters* 3(4): 290–296 (2016).

15. Tekale, S., Shingavi, P., Wandhekar, S., Chatorikar, K.A. Vidya Pratishthan's "Prediction of Chronic Kidney Disease Using Machine Learning Algorithm." *IJARCCE* 7(10): 92–96 (2015).

16. Zhang, Z., Ho, K.M., and Hong, Y. "Machine learning for the prediction of volume responsiveness in patients with oliguric acute kidney injury in critical care." *Critical Care* 23: 112 (2019).

17. Tomašev, N., Glorot, X., Rae, J.W., Zielinski, M., Askham, H., and Saraiva, A. et al. "A clinically applicable approach to continuous prediction of future acute kidney injury." *Nature* 2019.

18. Thakur, N., and Han, C.Y. "A study of fall detection in assisted living: Identifying and improving the optimal machine learning method." *Journal of Sensor and Actuator Networks* 2021.

19. Wang, S. et al. "Explainable AI for B5G/6G: Technical Aspects, UseCases, and Research Challenges." *Networking and Internet Architecture* December 2021.

20. Liang, Q, Durrani, T.S., Liang, J., Koh, J., Wang X. "Guest editorial special issue on 6G-enabled internet of things." *IEEE Internet of Things Journal* 8(20): 15037–15040 (October 15, 2021).

21. How 6G Technology Can Change the Future Wireless Healthcare, 978-1-7281-6047-4/20/$31.00 ©2020 IEEE.

22. Nabeel, M. et al. "Heart Attack Disease Data Analytics and Machine Learning." International Conference on Innovative Computing (ICIC), 2021.

23. Bharadwaj, H. et al. "A Review on the Role of Machine Learning in Enabling IoT Based Healthcare Applications." IEEE Access 2021.

24. Aldahiri, A. et al. "Trends in Using IoT with Machine Learning in Health Prediction System." *Forecasting* 2021.

25. Kumar, Y. et al. "Heart Failure Detection Using Quantum-Enhanced Machine Learning and Traditional Machine Learning Techniques for Internet of Artificially Intelligent Medical Things." *Wireless Communications and Mobile Computing* 2021.

26. Golec, M. et al. "iFaaSBus: A Security- and Privacy-Based Lightweight Framework for Serverless Computing Using IoT and Machine Learning." *IEEE Transactions on Industrial Informatics*, May 2022.

27. Liu, J. et al. "Predictive Classifier for Cardiovascular Disease Based on Stacking Model Fusion." *Processes* 2021.

28. Umer, M. et al. "IoT Based Smart Monitoring of Patients' with Acute Heart Failure." *Sensors* 2021.

29. Tan, L. Toward real-time and efficient cardiovascular monitoring for COVID-19 patients by 5G-enabled wearable medical devices: A deep learning approach." *Neural Computing and Application*, 2021.

30. https://dias.library.tuc.gr

31. Chuang, H.-C., Shih, C.-Y., Chou, C.-H. et al. "The development of a blood leakage monitoring system for the applications in hemodialysis therapy." *IEEE Sensors Journal* 2009.

32. https://orange3.readthedocs.io

12 Emerging Internet of Things (IoTs) Scenarios Using Machine Learning for 6G Over 5G-Based Communications

Raghav Dangey, Arjun Tandon, and Amit Kumar Tyagi

CONTENTS

12.1 Introduction 216
12.2 Background Work 217
12.3 Problem Statement and Motivation 217
    12.3.1 Motivation 217
        12.3.1.1 IoT as a Catalyst for 5G 218
        12.3.1.2 Role of IoT in the Future with Blockchain 218
        12.3.1.3 Vision of IoT 218
    12.3.2 Foundation of IoT Architecture 219
12.4 Existing Solutions – IoT Opportunities and Prospects 219
    12.4.1 Implementation of AI-Cases for 5G-IoT Networks 220
        12.4.1.1 Big Data Processing Enhancement 220
        12.4.1.2 Expanding the Horizon of Healthcare 220
        12.4.1.3 Intelligent Networking 221
        12.4.1.4 Smart Transportation Systems 221
        12.4.1.5 Utilizing Abundant Data of Inter-connected
                IoT Devices 221
    12.4.2 How IoT Has Enabled a Smart Environment? 222
12.5 Discussion on 5G-Enabled IoT from 5G Cellular Technologies 223
    12.5.1 5G-Empowered IoT – GlobaL Ingenuities 223
    12.5.2 Spectrum Necessities of 5G-IoT 224
    12.5.3 Structures Active in 5G PHY Layer to Support 5G-IoT 225
    12.5.4 Structures Active in 5G Networking Layer to Support 5G-IoT 227
    12.5.5 Architectural View of 5G-IoT 228
    12.5.6 QoS in 5G-IoT 228

DOI: 10.1201/9781003321668-12

        12.5.7 Standardization in 5G-IoT 228
        12.5.8 Proposed Model 229
    12.6 Emergence of 6G 230
        12.6.1 6G vs 5G: A Comparative Study 231
    12.7 Trending Research Issues and Challenges of 5G-IoT.................................232
        12.7.1 Can 5G Achieve a Blend between Connectivity Ease and Security?........232
        12.7.2 Is 5G Sufficiently Flexible to Allow for Various Types of
                Network Configuration?..234
        12.7.3 How Will 5G Take Account of a Higher Density of Connected
                Devices?...234
        12.7.4 Is 5G Future-Proof?..234
    12.8 Conclusion 235
    References..235

12.1   INTRODUCTION

Technology has become one of the fastest growing areas in communication, and the largest digital carrier of data worldwide. It is clear that device mixing has become increasingly advanced through diverse multimedia competencies with at least third generation connectivity. As a result, this has seen the demand for the increased production of smart devices with better network connectivity and computing capabilities. It has also led to the share of smart connections and devices percentage growing significantly from 45% in 2015 to 86% in 2022, an increment of more than twofolds during the figured time frames; it is projected that more than 74 billion devices are to be connected by the year 2026. The rollout of the 5G networks around the globe by the service providers is growing significantly due to ensuring that the end consumers demand higher safety, great bandwidth, and fast connectivity.

Significant advances in wireless sensing devices, communications, and informatics have enabled ubiquitous intelligence, predicting the future IoT. People are increasingly looking forward to the IoT on a personal and business level. Via health, smart homes, and smart learning, the IoT greatly raises a person's quality of life. Note that for a professional approach, the IoT has applications in logistics, smart supply chains, smart transportation, and remote monitoring.

In addition, the various developments in wireless network informatics and telecommunications have paved the realization of universal intelligence and the ideology of global computing in which the objectives were geared to embedding technology in day-to-day life. Smart homes, smart learning, and e-health are just a few examples of how IoT is significantly improving living standards at the individual level. For professionals, the IoT uses a smart supply chain, logistics, transportation, automation, and remote monitoring. Recent trends show the blend of diverse technologies such as embedded systems and integration of sensors with the device to device, cyber-physical systems, and fifth-generation communications with IoT as the center. Since new business models have been put in place due to technological advancements, many have been set for IoT implementations that require high privacy, complete security coverage, ultra-low latency, and massive data connectivity.

The involvement in the diversified environments and devices brings a vast variety of expectations and requirements, thus focusing more on the IoT due to its vast range of applicability from human-centric to industry 5.0/4.0. Since IoT introduces significant protection measures for significant protection challenges and due to the wide variety of demanding situations and functionality, there is always a significant dependency of the IoT on the cellular network coverages since the long-term evolutions of LTE were introduced [1].

12.2   BACKGROUND WORK

The 5G-based IoT was created due to anticipated changes in consumer preferences and user demand for a new IoT experience. To ensure they overcame current IoT effects like communication issues and slow data transmission, the developers had to put in significantly more effort. This improved effective data sharing. The 5G-based IoT has been shown to have high-data rates, highly scalable and fine-grained networks, extremely low latency, stability, resilience, and security. It also has a high-connection density and is mobile. IoT apps will, therefore, be able to offer improved services thanks to 5G by capturing more data through a faster and more secure connection. Since the qualities of the 5G network are related to the communication requirements, they may be resolved under 5G. As long as the trend is maintained, the communication requirements will be easy to meet. As a result of reducing latency and increasing data transmission speed, the 5G network was created. Between devices, the 5G networks also use communication technology to increase spectral efficiency and enable users to connect nearby without interruptions or destructions. The 5G network developed the integration of edge computing-enhanced IoT to improve the quality of user experience.

12.3   PROBLEM STATEMENT AND MOTIVATION

The advancements in ML have led to a new approach to solving this issue. In this chapter, we will study the trends, prospects, and challenges in the world of 5G IoT using ML techniques to deliver effective IoT connections.

12.3.1   MOTIVATION

The secret to managing all that data without hiccups and with less power use is machine learning. The 5G network can evaluate data trends and employ learned models to transfer data more effectively thanks to ML. Due to the discussion's application to the bulk of modern inventions, readers may be inspired to devote time to IoT research and development.

Note that IoT as a key player in smart cities.

The IoT can rightfully be considered to be the foundation for building a realistic smart city because it unites trillions of nodes in a single network that allows remote monitoring and management [2]. IoT may aid in diagnosing and monitoring distributed processes with the added potential of predicting future events by using learning technologies like ML and DL. Additionally, thanks to reduction and optimization, controlling complex systems becomes realistically feasible because of the cheap cost of IoT. The implementation of IoT can go beyond problems with modern cities including a lack of fresh water, monitoring of rubbish dumps, traffic jams, and air pollution. Traffic management, city air management tools, smart infrastructure, smart parking, and smart waste management are examples of facilities.

12.3.1.1 IoT as a Catalyst for 5G

IoT and 5G might change how we communicate in the future. Today, every business wants to gain access to the related client base that these two technologies may enable. With its abundant bandwidth, 5G supports IoT and, shortly, may improve virtual and augmented reality experiences. Although 5G networks have the ability to serve a wide range of IoT-based services, they are unable to fully satisfy the needs of the newest smart applications. As a result, there is a growing need to imagine 6G wireless communication technologies to get beyond the primary drawbacks of the current 5G networks. Additionally, the use of AI in 6G will offer answers for extremely difficult issues pertaining to network efficiency. Future 6G wireless communications has to accommodate large amounts of data-driven applications as well as a growing number of users. In contrast to other studies, this one focuses on recent developments and trends in 6G technology, network requirements, key enabling technologies for 6G networks, and a thorough comparison of 5G and 6G use cases.

12.3.1.2 Role of IoT in the Future with Blockchain

Blockchain provides a modern, safe data format. Information is organized into chronologically ordered blocks. When a data block's capacity is achieved and it is connected to the previous filled block, a chain of data blocks, or "blockchain," is generated. Since there is a record of each transaction in a dispersed environment, the records are resistant to manipulation and hacking, offering a high level of security. Recent years have seen a rise in IoT research. However, this study has mostly been domain-specific because its discussion was narrowed to particular subtopics. The forces behind this, however, are constrained in that they can only talk generally about their areas of specialization without delving deeper into other related topics. With its vast capacity, 5G supports the IoT and may soon improve virtual and augmented reality experiences.

12.3.1.3 Vision of IoT

IoT has been described by Atzori et al. in terms of three visions. The three visions are things-oriented, which focuses on general things, knowledge-oriented, which focuses on how to represent, store, and organize knowledge, and internet-oriented, which focuses on connectivity between the objects [3].

These ideas opened the way for the IoT as it is defined by the International Telecommunication Union (ITU): "from anytime, anyplace connectivity for anyone; we will now have the connectivity for anything." The main aim is to "plug and play smart items," to put it briefly.

12.3.2 FOUNDATION OF IoT ARCHITECTURE

The foundation of IoT architecture consists of three elements:

- **Hardware:** The sensor nodes, embedded communication, and interface circuitry are included.
- **Middleware:** This consists of tools for processing, analyzing, and storing data.
- **Presentation layer**: It is made of powerful visualization tools that provide user-facing data in an understandable style across a range of platforms and applications.

The IoT architecture is influenced by a variety of factors. Therefore, efforts are being made in current research to provide the most optimum design that addresses network challenges including scalability, security, addressability, and effective energy consumption. Every time a node joins the network or when the software operating on those nodes has to be installed or updated, an IoT network's security and privacy are also put to the test. The remote wireless reprogramming methodology is suggested in this situation. This protocol enables the node to check each piece of code and scan the installation process for any malicious intrusions.

The information is subsequently translated into a human-readable format by the information converter that relies on the application and stored on the storage medium. The AL provides services to customers using visualization technology. So, by using eGNs and BS at the sensing and control layers to control the SNs' sleep time interval, energy efficiency is accomplished. It can be done by properly allocating hardware resources utilizing the IPL's robust and methodical (with respect to energy) resource allocator. The hierarchal architecture is contrasted with the index tree which is efficient in energy, self-organized things (SoT), hierarchical clustering index tree which consumes optimum amounts of energy, and the object group localization designs (OGL). After careful evaluation, it is determined that the suggested architecture has a functional advantage over rivals. There should be room for adjusting to changes during the initial deployment period. IoT hardware- and open-source software-based solutions should be suggested for this. In this context, using cell phones as IoT nodes is one method of cost-cutting serving as IoT nodes.

12.4 EXISTING SOLUTIONS – IoT OPPORTUNITIES AND PROSPECTS

Due to the great interest in the IoT field, many countries including UAE, Brazil, China, and Canada have supplied different models for intelligent cities, smart cranes and urban devices, innovative warning systems against floods, and the smart-grid. Thirty-three IoT projects are now being funded by the European Research Cluster, which is an institution of the European Union. The organization's main goal is to create IoT architectures that are interoperable in terms of technology and knowledge while maintaining security, dependability, and scalability. As a result, the benefits listed were favorable for the nation's economy, growth, urbanization, infrastructure, employment rate, and inhabitants' access to healthcare and other services. Enterprises were also able to achieve their business demands thanks to IoT implementations. The cloud gateway uses the data obtained from the nodes for analysis in a Microsoft cloud-based architecture. Additionally, enabling security and marketing effectiveness is the intended solution. Daimler launched Car2go, using IoT architecture and IBM services.

12.4.1 Implementation of AI-Cases for 5G-IoT Networks

One of the key reasons for the installation of numerically demanding and empowering AI-based algorithms is the extremely high-data rates. Because of the network's high-data transmission capacity, efficient algorithms using deep learning for wireless 5G-IoT nodes, such as simulated speech recognition and video classification, are possible [4]. Adding and incorporating the intelligence factor on IoT nodes or a fog-based node toward the edge locations would help reduce time latency, increases link capacity, and boosts the security of the network. 5G-IoT networks might potentially leverage AI-based methodologies to more effectively manage their efficiency at the physical, application, and network levels in order to increase data rates by anticipating network traffic patterns, making it simpler to offer users AI-based apps [5]. To make the network self-organized, configurable, and adaptive, AI techniques might be used to study network traffic and capacity trend analysis, for example. AI-based optimization techniques might help with dynamic spectrum management, organizing massive data, IoT node interoperability, integrating incorporating various gadgets devices, ultra-densifying devices, even an extended battery life at the physical and network levels [6]. The following is a list of some present-day and potential future AI-based applications that might be enabled by 5G-IoT:

12.4.1.1 Big Data Processing Enhancement

Massive data processing and crowded communication channels may be addressed by 5G intelligent IoT. The purpose of the 5G intelligent IoT, which blends AI algorithms with 5G technology, is to intelligently analyze massive volumes of data while enhancing channel use and optimizing communication channels [7]. The most up-to-date IoT practices and the 5G network's dependable and quick speed foster an environment for developing Big Data applications with the highest potential, such as facial recognition and natural language processing. The constant connectivity offered by 5G generates a massive volume of data. In 5G IoT-based networks, this data collection may also be used as a channel for communication and decision-making. Additionally, it will support the integration of massive IoT devices and the management of the large volume of data, which is probably measured in TBs [8].

12.4.1.2 Expanding the Horizon of Healthcare

The utilization of AI and 5G in the medical sector can be upgraded to save lives of millions of people by bringing about modifications to the existing system. A tailored, emotion-aware healthcare system with a focus on emotional care has been developed by Chen et al. utilizing 5G, notably for children, the mentally ill, and the elderly [1]. A genetic algorithm was used to trace the apt point for 5G-based drone stations within the constraints of energy, cost, and coverage. From 2030 onward, the whole health business will be dominated by the promised 6G communication technology. It will rule a variety of industries in addition to the health industry. The future of healthcare may be entirely AI-driven and reliant on 6G connectivity technologies, which will alter how we see lifestyle. In light of this, we imagine a healthcare system for the 6G future of communication technologies. Aspects of quality of life (QoL), intelligent wearable devices (IWD), the intelligent internet of medical things (IIoMT), hospital-to-home (H2H) services, and new business models are also addressed in this perspective as necessary innovations to improve our way of life. We also discuss how 6G communication technology is used in telesurgery, epidemics, and pandemics.

12.4.1.3 Intelligent Networking

One major use case of AI is its application in 5G networks including those of the design descriptions in automated networks which make use of ML-based techniques for decision-making. The goal of implementing a more adaptive regulating mechanism alongside the core NFV functions is to lower system costs while maintaining a competitively high level of QoS. By the time 6G networks are implemented, edge and core computing will be considerably more smoothly linked as a part of a combined communications/computation infrastructure framework. As 6G technology is put into use, this might result in a number of benefits, including easier access to artificial intelligence (AI) capabilities.

12.4.1.4 Smart Transportation Systems

One of the biggest innovations that seems to be taking a foreground in real-time world is consistent connectivity through combination of 5G and IoT. Because of this integration, it is now able to access the internet more rapidly. Automakers are looking at additional ways to introduce this technology into the realm of transportation systems now that their interest has risen. An internet connection was used in the investigation of self-driving cars. A smart transportation system allows passengers' cellphones and the automobile itself to connect. A smart transportation system, like other IoT devices, can provide extra possibilities for improved control. The placement of sensors at traffic signals offers the information needed to decide on effective traffic routes and decrease vehicle propagation times. The total traffic system has been enhanced by the combination of IoT and 5G. IoT has assisted in eliminating human labor in sectors like traffic management, which can help to lower expenses.

12.4.1.5 Utilizing Abundant Data of Inter-connected IoT Devices

By correlating the massive amounts of data already available, it is possible to predict accidents and criminal activity using the massive amounts of data created by IoT-based devices connected continuously to 5G. As a result, it aids in the generation of enormous amounts of data (massive data sets may then be utilized to uncover parallels, correlations, and patterns), the development of novel ideas that can become projects for large corporations, and the provision of numerous communication channels. With the use of IoT, real-time data extraction is feasible. The new infrastructure for handling everyday traffic has been made possible by

IoT devices. Environment detection has been made possible via wireless network technologies. Additionally, it shows that IoT has been adopted as a surveillance method. Creating large data from IoT devices has helped plan and enhance urban environments. IoT Big Data analytics have also demonstrated their benefit to society. The highly demanding IoT application often tend to have their interaction needs satisfied by increased data rates. Reduced time delays, upgraded coverage, and backing for several devices. The idea of a genuinely global IoT is made possible by its support for a huge number of devices. 5G may serve as a single interconnection framework, enabling seamless communication of "things" with the internet, due to its concentration on the integration of diverse access methods [9]. Curating predictions with the data available and making decisions for updating technology to enhance life of quality.

The combination of 5G along with AI and IoT seems to improve and empower businesses by forecasting with the help of data available and curating suitable control decisions [10].

12.4.2 How IoT Has Enabled a Smart Environment?

The idea of a "smart environment" has gained enormous popularity in the last ten years. The concept is vast, encompassing home/office, utilities, healthcare, transportation/logistics, and many other areas. Augmented reality maps, self-driving cars, smartphone ticketing, and passenger counts have all been effectively deployed in the transportation and logistics industry. Additionally, these technologies are presently being continually enhanced. IoT-enabled robot taxis are being developed for prospective use. Similar benefits accrued to society through telemedicine, wearable technology, smart biosensors, smart ambulances, and remote patient monitoring in the IoT-enabled healthcare arena [11], has been depicted in Figure 12.1.

The idea of practical, cost-effective smart homes and cities has improved not just the infrastructure and framework of the country but also the lives of the end users. Smart healthcare successfully manages consumer health. To keep a track of the training routines and to verify them, the smart gym concept is highly beneficial to end users.

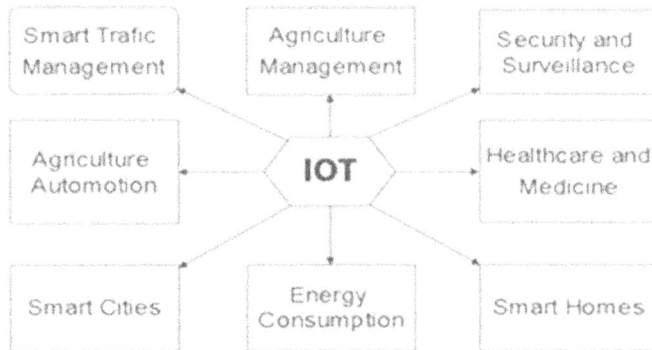

FIGURE 12.1   Domains representing IoT.

TABLE 12.1
How IoT Has Enabled a Smart Environment?

Applications	Communication Enablers	Network Types	Modules
Smart Cities	Wi-Fi, 3G, 4G, Satellite	MAN, WRANs	Urban IoT architectures, protocols, and supporting technologies.
			Information hub for the smart city that is integrated.
Smart Homes	Wi-Fi	WLAN	Software-defined networks (SDNs) are used in a cloud-based home solution for location identification of defective locations.
Smart-Grid	3G, 4G, Satellite	WLAN, WANs	A method for monitoring transmission lines in real time to prevent disasters.
Smart-Schools	Wi-Fi	WLAN	Controls student reports, assignments, and information.
Smart Buildings	Wi-Fi	WLAN	Controlling access to services within a typical smart building.
Smart Transport	Wi-Fi, Satellite	WAN, WLANs, MANs	Smart passenger counting and smart ticketing.
Smart Health	Wi-Fi, 3G, 4G, Satellite	WLAN, WPANs, WANs	Distant medical care.
Smart Industry	Wi-Fi, Satellite	WLAN, WPANs, WANs	Remote monitoring uses less energy, and improved decision-making.

Because modern humans are increasingly socially involved, there is a need for time to automatically update one's social occurrences immediately on social media. As a consequence, while dealing with privacy and security concerns, the benefits of IoT were also apparent at the end user level [12]. In a summary, Table 12.1 summarizes the technological specifications that are currently being included in published literature on IoT-enabling smart environments.

12.5 DISCUSSION ON 5G-ENABLED IoT FROM 5G CELLULAR TECHNOLOGIES

12.5.1 5G-Empowered IoT – Global Ingenuities

Around the world, several activities are being conducted to implement and standardize 5G-enabled IoT. Beyond 4G, many European initiatives are also available [1]. The research and technological practices were also started by International Mobile Telecommunications (IMT) in 2013 and the standardization was completed in 2016. It was determined in 2015 that the group and committee in charge of technical specifications, which would be in charge of creating 5G RAN, will be formed by the Third Generation Partnership Project (3GPP) [13]. The International Telecommunication Union-Radio Communication (ITU-R) has been tasked with designing and defining 5G technology by 2020 throughout the same period.

TABLE 12.2
Spectrum Types, Their Characteristics, and Uses

Spectrum Type	Characteristics	Use Cases
Low-frequency band (below 1 GHz)	• Higher coverage and mobility • Wider channels availability	1. Massive machine-type communications 2. Indoor applications
Higher frequency millimeter waves (mmWave) bands	• Short-range with low latency • High capacity due to wider channelization	1. Enhanced mobile broadband communications 2. Urban and sub-urban applications
Mid-frequency bands	• Short range with low latency and high-capacity transmission for a few macro-based stations	1. 5G implementation in uncrowded/ open areas 2. Urban deployment

12.5.2 Spectrum Necessities of 5G-IoT

To suffice the growing needs and requirements of consistently rising traffic, new generation concepts and innovations, wireless domain innovation, and the development of 5G-enabled IoT to require cutting-edge services and solutions. According to 5G Americas, a mixture of low-, mid-, and high-band spectrums is preferable in order to acknowledge the utilizations of 5G that enable IoT. Some use cases are better served by mixing many bands than others. Each band is compared under different usage scenarios [13]. In addition to conventional spectrum requirements, the 3GPP has designed a new 5G air interface known as New Radio (NR) [1, 14].

There is still a disconnect between the assurances and guarantees put forth by 5G network and its actual deployment of 5G technology when examining the abovementioned frequency features and needs in Table 12.2 and Figure 12.2. Therefore, the establishment of 5G requires the use of certain technology. For instance, mmWave transmission and reception have a high-route loss and a high rate of absorption from atmospheric factors like rain and vegetation. To increase coverage and reduce path-loss at mmWaves, there's a high chance that it is a micro version cellular design. This created the foundation for the novel idea of a compact, low-power cellular base station (BS).

Currently, a 4G BS uses hundreds of antenna ports to effectively manage its traffic. M-MIMO technology, which aims to integrate several antennas on a single BS, is used to resolve this. The installation of the IoT was the goal of the 5G technology, which attempted to integrate numerous heterogeneous access methods. Beam division

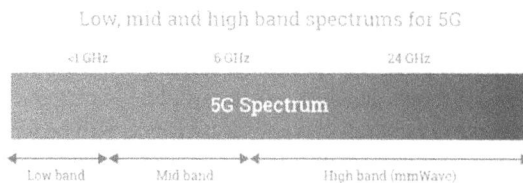

FIGURE 12.2 Spectrum types graphic.

multiple access (BDMA), a cutting-edge technology utilized by the 5G network, splits the beam based on the location of the mobile devices, whereas BS allows each device to receive an orthogonal beam. This allows for repeated access to the devices, greatly boosting capacity with little disturbance. To maximize spectrum efficiency, mmWaves, M-MIMO, and beamforming are also used in 5G technology, which likewise needs high throughput and low latency. By incorporating the full-duplex technology, which focuses on the transceiving mechanism of antennas, this need is addressed [13]. A 5G transceiver must be able to operate in both Time Division Duplexing (TDD) and Frequency Division Duplexing (FDD) modes to be able to transmit and receive data at the same time and on the same frequency. This is acquired by using transistors made from silicon which takes up the role of switches and ensure transmission at the same frequency [1]. Even though the aforementioned techniques are in the infant stages, research is carried out to acknowledge the inadequacies and curate an efficient 5G system.

12.5.3 STRUCTURES ACTIVE IN 5G PHY LAYER TO SUPPORT 5G-IoT

Some of the elements that have been normalized for the LTE or advanced LTE concepts are MIMO, CoMP, and HetNets [1]. These technologies provide huge connections and fast data rates, which is exciting. Therefore, these ideas are used in 5G technology. These ideas are first explored to provide context for the next subsections [13].

- **Carrier aggregation/accumulation:** Carrier aggregation is a method that improves network performance in the uplink, downlink, or both by increasing data capacity, throughput, and rates. It improves spectrum use by merging two or more carriers from the same or different frequency bands into a single aggregated channel. Based on 3GPP Release 10, carrier aggregation was implemented in 4G LTE-A. It combines up to five LTE-A component carriers (CCs), each with 20 MHz of capacity, bringing the total available bandwidth to 100 MHz. There are high chances of mobile devices getting multiple CC when utilizing carrier aggregation [13]. One CC is chosen as a major component carrier (PCC) in uplink and downlink while the others must be chosen as subsidiary component carriers (SCC). Different 3GPP versions now contain a much larger number of CCs [15]. Even though carrier aggregation is extremely strong and powerful, the product of intermodulation may hinder with the signal due to the inter- and intra-band carrier aggregation [1].
- **Massive-MIMO (M-MIMO):** A mix of antenna expansion and sophisticated algorithms is needed for MIMO systems. Although it has many facets, MIMO has been utilized in wireless communications for a while now. Both mobile devices and network frequently include multiple antennas to improve connectivity, provide faster speeds, and improve user experiences. Massive MIMO, a variation of MIMO, increases the number of antennas on the base station to outperform outdated systems. In addition to having additional antennas, the network and mobile devices need more intricate architecture to coordinate MIMO operations. These developments are achieving the performance enhancements required to support the 5G consumer experiences [13]. To increase the capacity of tiny cells, this approach

makes it possible to deploy high-order multi-user MIMO (MU MIMO) [16]. An omnidirectional antenna is used in the macro cell to supply control-plane communication at lower band frequencies, while a highly directed M-MIMO beam is used to send user-data traffic at mmWave band frequencies [1]. As a result, more MIMO technologies are being used. The benefits of M-MIMO have proven to be advantageous especially since it can boost the radiation up to 100 times [16].

- **Coordinated Multipoint Processing (CoMP):** CoMP uses distributed MIMO to transmit and receive from various antennas, some of which may not be in the same cell, in order to lessen received spatial interference and improve the quality of the received signal. Along with physical layer security (PLS) development, CoMP has shown to be a fantastic interference mitigation solution. With appropriate base station synchronization, it offers great secrecy coverage probability and interference performance (BSs). CoMP-based resource allocation methods provide a significant increase in capacity and, thus, less interference [13, 17]. When combined with MU-MIMO, CoMP is a particularly successful strategy for boosting cell-edge coverage and lowering outages brought on by blocking and channel issues. The CoMP is a transceiver technology that reduces interference problems [1]. This is accomplished by leveraging channel state information to coordinate transmission and reception among the widely dispersed BSs [17].

- **Heterogeneous Networks (HetNets):** The pico base station need to coordinate hinderance for the control and traffic channels with major macro-interferers to offer services to the user terminals [18]. Each wireless access network in the HetNet ecosystem has unique properties, including capacity, access technology, security, power consumption, latency, coverage, and access cost. HetNets have the intriguing property that certain wireless access networks are layered over others in a way that naturally creates a multilayer structure or hierarchical cellular mobile network. A mobile user must be equipped with a multi-interface device that can identify and connect with the access network that fits personal expectations and the requirements of apps to fully utilize HetNets and benefit from what these networks have to offer [1, 18, and 19].

- **D2D communications:** It is regarded as a typical way to use the method of transferring data from the base point to each device. As a result, device-to-device communication was selected as a method for data transfer on a 5G network since it is thought to be more advanced and effective. D2D communication also has a lot of benefits because it doesn't rely on a base station to provide data. For instance, improving spectral efficiency and system capacity, lowering latency on the network and energy consumption in the EU, disassembling the 5G mobile network, and extending network coverage. D2D is a potential technology for 5G; in addition to enhancing connection in the next networks, D2D offers greater data rates, more capacity, and better QoS [20] In the context of 5G, "D2D communication" refers to a paradigm in which devices speak with one another directly rather than sending data over the network infrastructure [1].

- **Centralized Radio Access Network (CRAN):** A 5G design called the cloud radio access network (CRAN) makes use of cloud computing to accomplish its goals. The possibilities of CRAN are also diminished by problems with security, fronthaul, and a centralized baseband unit (BBU) pool restriction. For the centralized BBU processing to function properly, fronthaul links in CRAN must have very low latency and large bandwidth. In real-time applications, a link's capacity is typically constrained and time-delayed, decreasing the CRAN's spectrum and energy efficiency as a result [1, 21]. To address the CRAN fronthaul concerns, a heterogeneous CRAN (HCRAN) that isolates the user plane from the control plane was proposed.

12.5.4 STRUCTURES ACTIVE IN 5G NETWORKING LAYER TO SUPPORT 5G-IoT

- **Software-defined wireless sensor networking (SD-WSN):** A combination of SDN and WSNs is the SD-WSN. The logical plane for control from the networking device in the decentralized segment is the main aim of using the approach for constructing 5G networks [22]. A centralized software-based paradigm like SDN is required to ensure a constant QoS due to the growing needs of the many linked devices. The deployment of additional connections and nodes, resource allocation, and other network management challenges will all be much simplified by the SDN [23, 24].
- **Virtualization of Network Function (NFV):** Network slicing, a feature of virtual network architecture that enables the construction of many virtual networks on top of a single physical infrastructure, will be made possible by NFV in 5G. The demands of applications, services, devices, consumers, or operators may then be accommodated through the customization of virtual networks [25]. These standards serve as the foundation for each element of the architecture, enhancing stability and interoperability. The components of NFV architecture are software programs called virtualized network functions (VNFs) that provide network services including file sharing, directory services, and IP setup [13, 25].
- **Cognitive radios (CRS):** There is a shortage of spectrum due to the existing IoT applications, which range from crucial to huge in terms of connection and network resource overload. Therefore, it is imperative to make effective and wise use of the spectrum to meet the rising demand. In a radio set, the first part relates to recording the spatial and temporal fluctuations with less interference. An optimum spectrum can then be recorded for transmission. Typically, this is a region of the spectrum known as a "spectrum hole" or "white space" [26]. Interference is lessened in three different ways if it is being utilized by any authorized user. First, jump over to the other spectrum hole. Second, by limiting its power level, and third, by switching the modulation method that is being employed. Depending on its hardware, a CR can broadcast and receive utilizing a variety of frequencies, modulation techniques, transmission powers, communication techniques, protocol specifications, and transmission access techniques. The RF front end of cognitive radio contains a wideband antenna, power amplifier, and adaptive filter, to set

its conventional counterparts apart. Wideband sensing is made possible by an RF front end with these features. A CR should also be able to pick up weak signals across a broad range. The cognitive radio cycle is followed by the CR as it attempts to adapt to the requirements of a radio environment [26, 27].

The cycle has three fundamental steps:

1. Sensing spectrum
2. Spectrum evaluation
3. Decision on the spectrum

Depending on the quality of each use case, several spectrum choice criteria might be explored [1]. All these structures make the CR effective for successful deployment in 5G [13].

12.5.5   ARCHITECTURAL VIEW OF 5G-IoT

For the base of massive IoT data analysis, a 5G framework should be capable of providing a scalable network, virtualization, cloud services, etc. In essence, a 5G-IoT-based architecture needs to offer an independent HetNet that is self-configurable under the application requirement. The primary components of a cellular 5G architecture are the front-haul, mid-haul, and back-haul networks. The remote radio-head (RRH) is connected to the BBU through the front-haul network. Back-haul describes the coaxial cable and/or optical fiber link that connects the BBU to the main wired network. The link between RRH and the next link is referred to as the mid-haul. The radio network and network cloud are the two logical layers included in the 5G cellular network architecture. It may be explained that a high-data rate can be attained by employing steerable antennas at the BS and the mobile station with cutting-edge CMOS technology and the mmWave spectrum [1]. Owing to the mmWave spectrum's unsuitability for mobile communications – specifically due to propagation problems such as path losses, blocking, air, and rain absorption, etc. By deploying big antenna arrays, directing up the beam energy, and coherently collecting it, these problems are now mostly handled [13].

12.5.6   QoS IN 5G-IoT

The spectral efficiency and latency of a 5G cellular network may be utilized to understand its QoS. Although the latency requirements for user and control plane data differ, non-orthogonal signals and radio access methods can be employed to improve the spectrum efficiency of a 5G network [28]. In the case of a 5G network, there is a significant improvement in cell spectral efficiency as well as a 50% reduction in control plane latency [29, 30].

12.5.7   STANDARDIZATION IN 5G-IoT

There are primarily two types of standards involved in the 5G-IoT standardization process. One set of standards deals with network technology, protocols, standards for wireless communication, and standards for data aggregation. The second is a regulatory requirement that covers data security and privacy [1].

12.5.8 PROPOSED MODEL

The proposed models for researching the threats to emerging trends and prospects on 5G-IoT are summarized in Table 12.3 [31]. Along with references of models, their techniques, and specifications are summarized in Table 12.4.

TABLE 12.3
Proposed Models on Threats Research with Descriptions Summarized

S. No	Year	References	Description	Security Aspect Affected
1	2018	Xin Zhang and Fengtong Wen [21]	The USD and UDS are two algorithmic models proposed for a new user who is anonymous in the IoT segment.	Authentication
2	2018	Mohammad Dahman Alshehri and Farookh Khadeer Hussain [22]	Proposes a secure communications paradigm between IoT nodes utilizing hexadecimal values combined with a cluster-based fuzzy logic implementation approach.	Confidentiality and trust management
3	2019	Priyanka Anurag Urla, Girish Mohan, Sourabh Tyagi, and Smitha N. Pai [23]	The model presented here is a multi-stage security paradigm that uses fully homomorphic encryption (FHE) and elliptical curve cryptography (ECC) to mitigate cryptographic threats.	Integrity
4	2019	Hongsong Chen, Caixia Meng, Zhiguang Shan, Zhongchuan Fu and Bharat K. Bhargava [24]	Proposes a unique method for detecting low-scale DoS attacks that includes trust assessment using the Hilbert-Huang transformation in Zigbee WSN.	Availability and trust management
5	2019	Michail Sidorov, Ming Tze Ong, Ravivarma Vikneswaran, Junya Nakamura, Ren Ohmura and Jing Huey Khor [20]	Offers a radical safety and security framework curated for a lightweight and simple RFID protocol that highlights the supply chain management through blockchain.	Authentication
6	2019	Munkenyi Mukhandi, David Portugal, Samuel Pereira, and Micael S. Couceiro [26]	Presents a basic security architecture that includes MQTT and robot operating system for robotic communication in industrial IoT. The two main techniques are data encryption and authentication.	Authentication and integrity
7	2019	Pooja Shree Singh, Vineet Khanna [27]	Provides a speech recognition prog built on Mel-frequency cepstral coefficients (MFCC) for user identification and authentication that may be used in an IoT context to protect the privacy, confidentiality, and integrity of data.	Confidentiality, integrity, and privacy

TABLE 12.4

References of Models, Their Techniques, and Specifications [31]

References	Technique Used	Confidentiality (C)	Integrity (I)	Availability (A)	Trust (T)	Authenticity (Ay)
Xin Zhang and Fengtong Wen [21]	Data encryption method				✓	✓
Mohammad Dahman Alshehri and Farookh Khadeer Hussain [22]	Fuzzy-logic-based ram algorithmic method	✓			✓	
Priyanka Anurag Urla, Girish Mohan, Sourabh Tyagi, and Smitha N. Pai [23]	A multi-level data encryption method	✓	✓			
Hongsong Chen, Caixia Meng, Zhiguang Shan, Zhongchuan Fu and Bharat K. Bhargava [24]	Mathematical evaluation method			✓	✓	
Michail Sidorov, Ming Tze Ong, Ravivarma Vikneswaran, Junya Nakamura, Ren Ohmura and Jing Huey Khor [20]	Block chain-based authentication method					✓
Munkenyi Mukhandi, David Portugal, Samuel Pereira, and Micael S. Couceiro [26]	A cryptographic-based data encryption method		✓			✓
Pooja Shree Singh, Vineet Khanna [27]	Socket programming	✓	✓			✓

12.6 EMERGENCE OF 6G

Wireless communication has been more important over the last few decades. The global deployment of fifth-generation (5G) communications, which have many more capabilities than fourth-generation communications, is expected to begin soon. Between 2027 and 2030, the sixth-generation (6G) system, a new wireless communication paradigm with full AI support, is expected to be in operation. Faster system capacity, higher data rate, lower latency, higher security, and enhanced quality of service (QoS) compared to the 5G system are some of the fundamental issues that must be solved after 5G.

Throughput, latency, energy efficiency, rollout costs, reliability, and hardware complexity are all trade-offs in 5G technology. After 2030, 5G is unlikely to be able to keep up with demand. Following that, 6G will bridge the demand gap between the market and 5G. The main goals of 6G systems are (i) massive data rates per device, (ii) huge number of connected devices, (iii) global connectivity, (iv) reduced delays, (v) decreasing consumption of energy by battery free devices and nodes in IoT, (vi) extremely reliable connectivity, and (vii) connected intelligence with ML capability. These goals are based on historical trends and predictions of future needs.

The simultaneous wireless connection of the 6G system is predicted to be 1,000 times greater than that of the 5G system. In contrast to the enhanced mobile broadband (eMBB) in 5G, it is anticipated that ubiquity services will also be a major part of 6G. A crucial component of 5G, ultra-reliable low-latency communications will be a key driving force in 6G communication, with capabilities including end-to-end (E2E) latencies lower than one millisecond, nearly 99.99% dependability, and 1 Tbps peak data throughput. The 6G communication system will be capable of supporting numerous linked devices. The major use cases of this revolutionizing technology would be along the lines of a super smart society, connected robotics and autonomous systems, wireless human–computer interactions, industrial automation, haptic advancements and communications, IoE, and so on [30].

12.6.1   6G vs 5G: A Comparative Study

The following table gives a detailed survey highlighting the similarities and contradictories of 5G and 6G technologies respectively (refer Table 12.5).

TABLE 12.5
Comparison of 5G and 6G

Features	5G	6G
Frequency bandwidth	It is allocated for loa and high-band frequencies: sub 6 GHz and more than 224.25 GHz	This is mainly allocated for higher band frequencies ranging between 95 GHz to 3 THz
Data rate	One of the fastest connections currently available with approximately 20 Gigabits being transmitted per second.	Predicted to have almost five times the data rate of that of 5G, transmitting around 100 Gigabits per second.
E2E delay	Approximately 1 millisecond	Approximately 0.1 millisecond
Architecture and framework	Heavy and dense sub 6 GHz with smaller cells of millimeter waves.	Cell free smart surfaces at high frequencies
Device types	It can be deployed in smartphones, sensors, drones, etc.	It can be used in distributed ledger technologies, smart implants, and so on.
Traffic capability	Around 10 Mbps/m^2	Ranges between 1 and 10 Gbps/m^2

12.7 TRENDING RESEARCH ISSUES AND CHALLENGES OF 5G-IoT

One may witness a drift from different wireless technologies including 1G, 2G, 2.5G, 3G, 3.5G, and 4G toward 5G. It is acknowledged because 5G technology exceeds its predecessors in addressing the major challenges of cellular networks.

The following issues are annexed:

- Increased bandwidth
- Massive data rate
- High connectivity
- Reduced end-to-end latency
- Cost-effectiveness
- Accordant quality of service
- Device computational capabilities
- Device intelligence services

Some summarized challenges in the 5G-IoT network and their solutions are described in Table 12.6 [1].

The 5G-IoT network of the future should be able to handle the huge connection of devices by offering high and reliable QoS, according to current trends. A 5G network must support both critical and large-scale IoT [1, 32].

12.7.1 CAN 5G ACHIEVE A BLEND BETWEEN CONNECTIVITY EASE AND SECURITY?

Unauthorized codes can be inserted into mobile phone devices to control network services and collect data traveling via networks, among other security-related problems, as a result of their uncontrolled access to networks. The transmission of data through various devices and nodes using synchronized and coexisting technologies require security at each node so as to maintain the safety of network services [33]. As a consequence, manufacturers may design systems that have the intelligence required to understand, validate, and allocate a session and authority with certain values. Because of this, end users may simply do their work without difficulties or disruptions in connectivity. It is hard to ensure the security and safety of connected IoT-based 5G networks just through software improvement. Cooperation, affiliation, and coordination are all necessary for increased security. The adoption of a secure boot and a reliable execution environment improves the security of intelligent devices and prevents illegal usage of other devices. The combination of intelligent systems and software security will increase the safe communication of networked IoT devices while also inspiring new concepts for future wireless communication networks [34, 35].

With the deployment of more and more 5G networks, the limits of 5G networks have been revealed, which undoubtedly supports the exploratory research of 6G networks as the next generation solutions. These studies address the fundamental privacy and security concerns raised by 6G technology. As a result, we developed a survey on the current status of 6G security and privacy in order to synthesize and develop this essential study as a basis for future research.

TABLE 12.6
Challenges in the Industry of 5G IoT and Their Solutions

S.No.	Challenges	Solutions
1	Flexibility in the 5G physical layer radio architecture to meet the various IoT requirements.	A random-access channel is used in the design of appropriate radio numerology to enable high-connection densities and to handle transceiver flaws and channel degradation.
2	Radio access technologies (RATs) and significant signaling overhead in network control systems for network edge devices.	An extensive overview of client-controlled HetNets for 5G networks is given, along with distributed and hybrid control techniques.
3	It is introduced that several businesses, like Tata Communications, Dell IoT Services, and Sierra Wireless, are creating IoT technologies globally.	
4	Effective LPWAN (low power wide area network) enabling technologies.	The newest and most promising technology is described as LoRa.
5	Spectrum resources are insufficient to support IoT devices and enable 5G technologies. The radio access channel also has several restrictions for handling 5G devices with IoT capabilities.	Spectrum resources are insufficient to support IoT devices and enable 5G technologies. The radio access channel also has several restrictions for handling 5G devices with IoT capabilities.
6	The effective recharging of widely used IoT devices is a laborious operation when considering 5G-IoT situations.	It is possible to charge IoT devices wirelessly using both near- and far-field methods. Additionally, a brand-new networking concept known as wireless power communication network is presented that unifies wireless power transfer and communication.
7	To meet the demands of the 5G-enabled IoT, which include higher data rates, lower latency, constant quality of service, and vast amounts of spectrum resources.	The architecture of the 5G cellular network is given together with its supporting technologies, such as M-MIMO and D2D communication. These include ultra-dense networks, cognitive radios, millimeter-wave (mm-wave) solutions for 5G networks, cloud technologies, and other related upcoming technologies.
8	Backhaul is a bottleneck that must be overcome to maintain the high quality of service in a 5G paradigm. Since backhaul connects the very busy, dense cells to the core, its requirements must be taken into consideration.	The presentation of a combination radio access and backhaul framework effectively handles the QoS challenges. Backhaul as a Service (BHaaS), an SDN architecture with RAN intelligence, Self-Optimizing Network (SON), and caching capabilities, offers a comprehensive view of the end-to-end network and also allows for optimization.
9	Mobile tasks are frequently delegated to remote infrastructures, such as cloud platforms, due to the limited computational power and battery life of mobile devices (MDs), which results in an inevitable offloading transmission delay.	A crucial method for the deep learning edge services in 5G networks is computation offloading. A heuristic offloading technique is developed and shown to reduce the transmission latency of deep-learning tasks.

12.7.2   Is 5G Sufficiently Flexible to Allow for Various Types of Network Configuration?

The traffic produced by the nodes in IoT differs from the ones generated in cellular systems. In fact, majority of the traffic in IoT occurs in the uplink.

Furthermore, messages conducted through IoT networks are usually quick and of little size. IoT devices have limited energy and computing resources as well. In terms of how they connect to 5G networks, these IoT devices differ from traditional cellular devices. It may be challenging to establish the best system parameter configuration for a certain IoT use case [36].

12.7.3   How Will 5G Take Account of a Higher Density of Connected Devices?

The rapid proliferation of mobile devices necessitates an extensible and energy-efficient communication infrastructure. One million devices might be connected across $0.38 \ mi^2$ using 5G technology, compared to just 2,000 using 4G. This extensive coverage will significantly diminish the battery life of electronics.

The slim band of IoT, also called narrow band IoT, is a major part of the intelligent 5G IoT network which is essential for ideal energy consumption. An intelligent 5G-IoT ecosystem will, therefore, provide the ability to process massive amounts of data with minimum ping, network stability, and continued service availability [37, 38].

Intelligence for IoT-based devices is necessary for appropriate device administration and management, especially when all linked elements generate substantial traffic over the internet [37].

12.7.4   Is 5G Future-Proof?

One of the main and difficult physical layer goals of coverage improvement (CE), among the numerous difficulties stated for IoT access technologies, is to increase the maximum coupling necessary to enable tactile internet and multimedia applications. Other significant issues include security/privacy, energy efficiency, and widespread networking. Major research developments have been carried out with respect to this area due to high expectations of IoT networks that incorporate 5G-enabled techniques with several use cases [39]. In addition to these activities, academics are working to address issues with the physical and architecture layer, energy efficiency, channel access, and spectrum efficiency of 5G-enabled IoT technologies.

High-data rates are needed for applications like high-definition video streaming, augmented reality (AR), and virtual reality (VR); these applications often ask for speeds of up to 25 Mbps. Now due to a lack of communication or data flow among systems, the 5G-IoT-based network may completely disintegrate [40, 41, and 42]. Deep learning is used enormously in IoT as well as mobile applications in order to execute real-time operation on processing of data. Sending massive volumes of data to the cloud for deep learning would consume a lot of energy and cause a lot of transmission delay, which reduces the efficacy of deep-learning activities. This is due to the poor performance of data transfer speeds. By minimizing human participation while boosting network performance, the main aim of SON's is to surge the quality of service and reduce the expenses related to the operations in the network. The main goal of incorporating AI-related technologies into 5G-IoT infrastructures is to provide the network the ability to intelligently adapt its configurations in response to shifting environmental conditions or requirements. The new 5G network should be able to offer efficient strategies for radio resource management (RRM), mobility management (MM), management and orchestration (MANO), and service provisioning management in order to replace special utility networks with complex network reconfigurations [39, 40, and 41].

12.8 CONCLUSION

This chapter provided a thorough analysis of the 5G wireless technologies, which have emerged as essential facilitators for the wide adoption of IoT technology. It reviewed the development of cellular wireless technologies and made the argument for how 5G wireless technology improves upon its forerunner technologies, enabling widespread IoT implementation. In this research, we have also covered the various architectural elements of 5G networks, with a focus on the significant advancements made over 4G networks at the physical and network layers.

The chapter also goes into great detail about the difficulties in implementing QoS requirements in contemporary 5G-IoT, whose traffic characteristics differ significantly from another legacy 5G network applications because it is primarily in the uplink rather than the downlink direction. For the cloud-based application layer programs running cutting-edge artificial intelligence, machine- and deep-learning algorithms for effective real-time data processing and prediction, high-data transfer rates with minimal latency from the 5G-IoT nodes are essential. These contemporary applications, such as smart transportation, smart healthcare, smart school, smart industry, etc., that operate on top of 5G-IoT are also explored. Additionally, key performance indicators (KPIs) and criteria for acceptable performance are provided. The difficulties with standardization caused by the numerous nodes utilizing the 5G-IoT network are another subject covered in this study (HetNets). The thorough analysis provided in this study will aid in better-coordinated efforts from both businesses and academics to advance 5G-IoT technology.

REFERENCES

1. Shafique, Kinza, Khawaja, Bilal, Sabir, Farah, Qazi, Sameer & Mustaqim, Muhammed. "Internet of Things (IoT) For Next-Generation Smart Systems: A Review of Current Challenges, Future Trends, and Prospects for Emerging 5G-IoT Scenarios." *IEEE Access*, 2020, pp. 23022–23040. doi: 10.1109/ACCESS.2020.2970118.
2. Deshmukh, A., Sreenath, N., Tyagi, A. K. & Jathar, S. "Internet of Things Based Smart Environment: Threat Analysis, Open Issues, and a Way Forward to Future," 2022 International Conference on Computer Communication and Informatics (ICCCI), 2022, pp. 1–6, doi: 10.1109/ICCCI54379.2022.9740741.
3. Harrison, Luke. "The Internet of Things (IoT) Vision." Interconnections – the Equinix Blog, Equinix, 12 March 2015. Accessed 3 Aug. 2022.
4. Madhav, A. V. S., Tyagi, A. K. 2023. Explainable Artificial Intelligence (XAI): Connecting Artificial Decision-Making and Human Trust in Autonomous Vehicles. In: Singh, P.K., Wierzchoń, S.T., Tanwar, S., Rodrigues, J.J.P.C., Ganzha, M. (eds)

Proceedings of Third International Conference on Computing, Communications, and Cyber-Security. Lecture Notes in Networks and Systems, vol. 421. Singapore: Springer. https://doi.org/10.1007/978-981-19-1142-2_10

5. Nair, M. M., Kumari, S., Tyagi, A. K. (2001). Internet of Things, Cyber Physical System, and Data Analytics: Open Questions, Future Perspectives, and Research Areas, 2021. In: Goyal D., Gupta A. K., Piuri V., Ganzha M., Paprzycki M. (eds) Proceedings of the Second International Conference on Information Management and Machine Intelligence. Lecture Notes in Networks and Systems, vol. 166. Singapore: Springer. https://doi.org/10.1007/978-981-15-9689-6_36

6. Kumar Tyagi, A., Abraham, A., Kaklauskas, A., Sreenath, N., Rekha, G., & Malik, S. (Eds.). 2022. Security and Privacy-Preserving Techniques in Wireless Robotics (1st ed.). CRC Press. https://doi.org/10.1201/9781003156406

7. Rashid, Salman & Razak, Shukor. Big Data Challenges in 5G Networks, 2019, 152–157, Accessed 3 August 2022. doi: 10.1109/ICUFN.2019.8806076.

8. Chen, M., Yang, J., Hao, Y., Mao, S. & Hwang, K., "A 5G Cognitive System for Healthcare." *Big Data and Cognitive Computing*, vol. 1, no. 1, March 2017, p. 2.

9. Ribeiro, Jair. "Introduction to the Future with 5G, AI, and IoT." The Startup, 12 December 2020.

10. Kiss, P., Reale, A., Ferrari, C. J. & Istenes, Z. "Deployment of IoT applications on 5G edge." In 2018 IEEE International Conference on Future IoT Technologies (Future IoT), Eger, 2018, pp. 1–9.

11. Gomez, Carles, et al. "Internet of Things for Enabling Smart Environments: A Technology-Centric Perspective." *Journal of Ambient Intelligence and Smart Environments*, vol. 11, no. 1, 30 January 2019, pp. 23–43.

12. Ammad, Muhammad, Shah, Munam, Islam, Saif, Maple, Carsten, Alaulamie, Abdullah, Rodrigues, Joel, Mussadiq, Shafaq & Tariq, Usman. "A Novel Fog-Based Multi-Level Energy-Efficient Framework for IoT-Enabled Smart Environments." *IEEE Access*, 2020, pp. 150010–150026.

13. THALES. "5G and the IoT (What Is IoT in 5G?) – Thales." Accessed 3 August 2022.

14. "5G Spectrum Explained | Blog." Carritech Telecommunication. Accessed 3 August 2022.

15. Parikh, Jolly, "Scheduling schemes for carrier aggregation in LTE-advanced systems." *International Journal of Research in Engineering and Technology*, vol. 3, 2014, pp. 219–223.

16. Shukair, Mutaz. "How 5G Massive MIMO Transforms Your Mobile Experiences." 24 June 2022.

17. Irram, Fauzia, et al. "Coordinated Multi-Point Transmission in 5G and beyond Heterogeneous Networks." IEEE Xplore, 1 November 2020.

18. Ahmadi, Sassan, Chapter 14 – Enhanced Inter-cell Interference Coordination and Multi-radio Coexistence, LTE-Advanced, Academic Press, 2014, pp. 1029–1068.

19. "Heterogeneous Network (Communication System) – An Overview | ScienceDirect Topics.". (2014) Accessed 3 August 2022. https://www.sciencedirect.com/topics/engineering/heterogeneous-network-communication-system

20. Hadyanto, Dito Pratama, et al. "Device-To-Device Communication in 5G." 2021. Accessed 3 August 2022. https://www.atlantis-press.com/article/125966457.pdf

21. Pana, Vuyo S., et al. "5G Radio Access Networks: A Survey." *Array*, vol. 14, 1 July 2022, p. 100170.

22. Granelli, Fabrizio, Gebremariam, Anteneh, Atumo, Usman, Muhammad, Cugini, Filippo, Stamati, Veroniki, Alitska, Marios & Chatzimisios, Periklis., "Software Defined and Virtualized Wireless Access in Future Wireless Networks: Scenarios and Standards." *IEEE Communications Magazine*, vol. 53, 2015, pp. 26–34. Accessed 3 August 2022.

23. Miyazaki, Toshiaki, Yamaguchi, Shoichi, Kobayashi, Koji, Kitamichi, Junji, Guo, Song, Tsukahara, Tsuneo & Hayashi, Takafumi. "A software defined wireless sensor network."

2014 International Conference on Computing, Networking and Communications, ICNC 2014, 2014, pp. 847–852.

24. Kobo, Hlabishi I., et al. "A Survey on Software-Defined Wireless Sensor Networks: Challenges and Design Requirements." *IEEE Access*, vol. 5, 2017, pp. 1872–1899.

25. "The Role of Network Function Virtualization (NFV) in 5G." *ALLOT.* Accessed 3 August 2022.

26. Bhandari, Shruti & Joshi, Sunil. "Cognitive Radio Technology in 5G Wireless Communications." IEEE Xplore, 1 October 2018.

27. Sasipriya, S. & Vigneshram, R. "An Overview of Cognitive Radio in 5G Wireless Communications." IEEE Xplore, 1 December 2016

28. Arvindpdmn. "5G Quality of Service." Devopedia, 8 April 2021.

29. Abbas, Mohamed. "Quality of Service (QoS) in 5G Networks." 5G HUB, 27 February 2021.

30. Kaabneh, Khalid. "A Survey of QoS in 5G Network for IoT Applications." *International Journal of Science and Applied Information Technology*, vol. 8, no. 6, 2019, p. 159.

31. Rachit, et al. "Security Trends in Internet of Things: A Survey." *SN Applied Sciences*, vol. 3, no. 1, January 2021.

32. Jaber, M., Imran, M. A., Tafazolli, R. & Tukmanov, A., "5G Backhaul Challenges and Emerging Research Directions: A Survey." *IEEE Access*, vol. 4, 2016, pp. 1743–1766.

33. "What Is 5G? How It Works & Why It Matters | Accenture." Accessed 3 August 2022.

34. "What Is 5G? – the Fifth Generation of Mobile Technology." Twi-Global.com, 2019. Accessed 3 August 2022.

35. Attaran, M. "The Impact of 5G on the Evolution of Intelligent Automation and Industry Digitization." *Journal of Ambient Intelligence and Humanized Computing*, 2021. https://doi.org/10.1007/s12652-020-02521-x

36. Sabella, D., Serrano, P., Stea, G., et al. "Designing the 5G Network Infrastructure: A Flexible and Reconfigurable Architecture Based on Context and Content Information." *Journal on Wireless Communications and Networking*, vol. 199, no. 1, 2018. https://doi.org/10.1186/s13638-018-1215-1

37. Nair, M. M., Tyagi, A. K. & Sreenath, N. 2021. The Future with Industry 4.0 at the Core of Society 5.0: Open Issues, Future Opportunities and Challenges. 2021 International Conference on Computer Communication and Informatics (ICCCI), pp. 1–7. doi: 10.1109/ICCCI50826.2021.9402498.

38. Tyagi, A. K., Fernandez, T. F., Mishra, S. & Kumari, S. 2021. Intelligent automation systems at the core of industry 4.0. In Abraham A., Piuri V., Gandhi N., Siarry P., Kaklauskas A., Madureira A. (eds), *Intelligent Systems Design and Applications. ISDA 2020. Advances in Intelligent Systems and Computing*, vol 1351. Cham: Springer. https://doi.org/10.1007/978-3-030-71187-0_1

39. Goyal, Deepti & Tyagi, Amit. 2020. A Look at Top 35 Problems in the Computer Science Field for the Next Decade. doi: 10.1201/9781003052098-40.

40. Tyagi, A. K., Nair, M. M., Niladhuri, S. & Abraham, A. 2020. Security, privacy research issues in various computing platforms: A survey and the road ahead. *Journal of Information Assurance & Security*, 15(1): 1–16.

41. Madhav, A. V. S. & Tyagi, A. K. 2022. The world with future technologies (Post-COVID-19): open issues, challenges, and the road ahead. In Tyagi A. K., Abraham A., Kaklauskas A. (eds), *Intelligent Interactive Multimedia Systems for e-Healthcare Applications*. Singapore: Springer. https://doi.org/10.1007/978-981-16-6542-4_22

42. Mishra, S. & Tyagi, A. K. 2022. The role of machine learning techniques in internet of things-based cloud applications. In Pal S., De D., Buyya R. (eds), *Artificial Intelligence-based Internet of Things Systems. Internet of Things (Technology, Communications and Computing)*. Cham: Springer. https://doi.org/10.1007/978-3-030-87059-1_4

13 6G: Technology, Advancement, Barriers, and the Future

Meghna Manoj Nair and Amit Kumar Tyagi

CONTENTS

13.1 Introduction 239
13.2 Background Work..241
13.3 Problem Definition..242
13.4 Motivation..243
13.5 Progressed Work and Implementation towards Security.............................243
13.6 Popular Critical Challenges and Future Research Directions.....................245
13.7 Conclusion 248
References...248

13.1 INTRODUCTION

Cellular networks, as very commonly known, is a data communication network which facilitates effortless and robust roaming capabilities for complementing the cellular devices. In the initial days, mobile phones connected to such networks were used potentially for sending bare minimum texts and making calls; in the present day, almost every other task and digital chores can be done through smartphones connected to these networks. In fact, they've taken up a primary role of communication in relation to almost every other aspect of daily life [1]. The world has reached a point wherein a minor mishap or glitch in the cellular network has multiple and drastic adverse effects starting from massive losses in the economic sector all the way to disturbances in the financial transactions, inability to attend to emergencies during accidents and attacks, and what not. There are also sufficient cases that throw light on the significance to be given to the security of these cellular networks because of the high dependencies humans have on it [2]. The one thing that can be noticed despite the huge growth and revolution of cellular networks is that there's hardly any importance or initiative taken to accurately and precisely safeguard these networks so as to support and extend the concept to creative and innovative integrations, increased subscribers, more speed/bandwidth, etc. with ease and efficiency.

The 5th generation (5G) network technology is one of the recent and latest works that has been on the rise in last few years and has been very recently

DOI: 10.1201/9781003321668-13

launched in India too. Despite this fact, it's essential to continue looking forward to the communication needs of the future and hence, this work on 6G technology. The main purpose of this chapter is to idealize and provide the foundational aspects of 6G and how it could prove to be revolutionary in the coming years [3]. The main motive of 6G networks is to deliver fast and efficient speed transmission, maximize the capacity and non-proximity, etc. Even though it may be a little early to accurately define this technology, it is very often considered to be the ultimate successor of the 5G networks and cellular technology with a possibility of expanded data rates and increased capacity in terms of bandwidth [4]. This in turn points to very low levels of latency being a necessary requirement for the upcoming wireless technology of networks. In a few more years, it's highly likely that users of such cellular technology are going to be impacted by the huge inflow of data and communication, as a result of which, 6G technology must definitely emphasize on the continue development of wireless technology featuring advanced frequency spectrum in comparison to the previous generations of communication technology [5]. On the whole, it is likely that 6G systems would enable data transmission of around hundreds of GB per second with a combined usage of a millimeter wave and a terahertz wave band. The evolution of cellular communication from its first generation all the way to its fifth generation and proceeding towards the sixth generation is truly astounding. The 1G technology in analog which led to the incorporation of the very first mobile phones in the 1980s supported speed limits of up to 2.8 Kbps with the help of a circuit switch through an analog phone service [6]. With the help of a frequency division multiplexing, it was able to carry out the basic operations and functionalities of a cell phone but offered very little quality for voice calls and consumed large amounts of energy. Then came the 2G digital technology which built its foundation on the global system for mobile communication which was brought about in Finland in the early 1990s. In fact, it was the very first cellular network that attempted to replace the inefficiencies of the previous analog technology such as increased standard of safety and slightly better quality. It also provided features that supported text and media/photo messaging. With this, the third-generation technology was developed with much higher speeds of up to 144 Kbps along with global roaming facilities [7]. Further, it also provided the advantage of connecting to the internet through mobile data or other internet protocol-based networks along with multimedia transmission features. In the late 2000s came the 4G technology with the main goal of achieving excellent quality, maximal capacity, and fantastic user experience with a bandwidth expansion of up to 1 Gbps.

The utilization of this network is done using terminal portability which has a great influence in this level of cellular network. Following the surge of 4G came the 5G technology with a focus on the growing nature of the world wide web and dynamic wireless networks that are ad-hoc in nature. The fact that it provides the opportunity for AI-based integrations is what propelled this concept the furthest. The next up and coming technological concepts, considering that 5G would be economically available across the world in the next few years, is the sixth-generation technology which is the area of focus of this chapter [8]. The major requirements of 6G are shown in Figure 13.1.

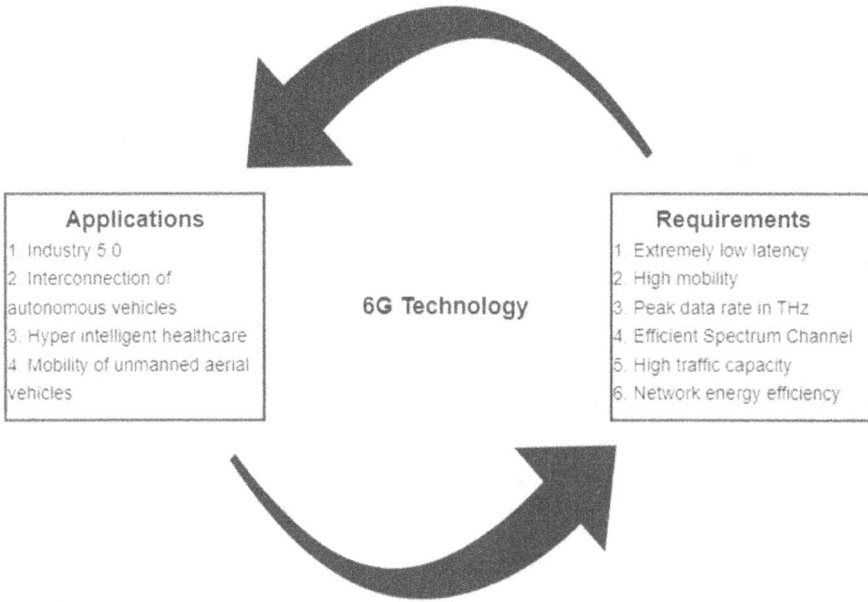

FIGURE 13.1 Major requirements and applications of 6G.

13.2 BACKGROUND WORK

The current works in the field of 6G mainly focus on the prospective technology of 6G in mobile communications, its possible applications, advantages, and so on. The work put forth by the authors of [9] focuses on the possible framework of sixth-generation technology, it's architecture and the communication scenario regarding the same. It also highlights the comparison between 5G and 6G along with the possible issues of the prospective communication technology such as the limited flexibility access to radio, issues regarding network security, the non-uniformity in high-frequency band, and problems in tactile communications. In [10], the work throws light on the vision, requirements, and technological trend of 6G.

The authors believe that the main vision of this revolutionizing concept is to solve the limitations and drawbacks of 5G which consists of system coverage and internet of everything. They've also mentioned the future roadmap of standardization for 6G which dates all the way to 2030s. The authors of [11] emphasizes on the initial point of 6G evolution and the possibility of integrating AI with the same. They've also elucidated on how the three main components of 6G not just focus on human society, information space, and physical world but also incorporates the fourth dimension of the virtual communication-enabling technology. In [11, 12], the research work throws light on the use of 6G communication technology with respect to intelligent healthcare systems. It elucidates and elaborates on the major aspect of this network of communication such as holographic interaction, haptic internet connectivity, and the intelligent framework of medical things/wearables. The works of authors in [12] highlights the future of wireless technology and discusses the networks of 6G as well as 7G, its comparison with the conventional broadband networks, and the major aspects of 7G. The technology has advanced to such an extent that it has helped in evolving from times of using 2G all the way to robotics and automation in 5G. Every subsequent generation of technology in terms of communication would empower major changes and modifications by correcting the various issues in the previous generations.

5G is still noble and in its rudimentary stages but 6G will definitely take over in the coming years. It is expected to boost the deployment of 5G use cases at scale by streamlining and lowering costs, particularly at the business level. At the same time, it will open up new possibilities. Furthermore, 6G will connect the human, physical, and virtual worlds. Consider the notion of the 'Metaverse.' It is one of the 5G use cases that has the potential to disrupt both the traditional and digital spheres. The 'Metaverse' would not only mature into a final form with 6G, but it would also likely integrate with the actual world thanks to AI and machine learning. This is because, according to telecom equipment supplier Nokia Bell Labs, the most striking feature of 6G would be its capacity to perceive the environment, people, and things. The network's sensing ability combined with AI and machine learning will make the network more cognitive. India is running behind schedule on the rollout of 5G, but tables may turn with 6G. This is because the country has already begun the development of 6G. According to Minister of Communication Ashwini Vaishnaw, work towards developing the next generation of communication technology has begun using indigenously developed 6G infrastructure with the aim to launch it either by the end of the year 2023 or early 2024.

13.3   PROBLEM DEFINITION

6G being one of the technologies that's yet to be brought out to the world has quite a few bottlenecks and challenges including those of system coverage, capacity requirements, movement speed of data and its transmission rate, energy efficiency, etc. One of the other pressing concerns is that of the security aspect which is often neglected even though it needs to be given significant importance in scenarios where there's a large influx of data and information. This sixth generation of cellular network technology is likely to take roots by the 2030s and is expected to provide communication efficacies through hyperconnectivity [13]. However, through research, it's essential to highlight the major security aspects of this empowering network technology in order to address the difficulties in relation to privacy preservation, security aspects, and the trust factor of 6G networks. This chapter addresses the security and privacy preservation aspect of 6G technology. The pressing reason for addressing the security aspect of 6G is because of the following four features. First of all, it is likely to provide an opportunity to initiate a platform that offers integrated air, ground, space, and sea-based communication networks. Second, this conceptual implementation would give rise to a novel generation of intelligent and smart services and amenities through AI, Big Data, etc. Third, the combination of terahertz, millimeter wave, and optical communications would help in improving the capacity in terms of network traffic and data speed. Last but not the least, the security and privacy have to be strengthened to ensure that this network of communication technology is easily scalable and preventable from external attacks or breaches. The fourth and most important point is the problem this chapter addresses [14].

13.4 MOTIVATION

Security is of prime concern in the world today especially with the growing dependency of humans on technological devices and equipment that extract so much of information knowingly or unknowingly. Right from the first-generation analog technology, all the way to the fifth generation of network communication technology, there have been quite a few mishaps and glitches in the security and privacy aspects and this has been the motivation for addressing this issue through this chapter. In the early 1980s, with the launch of 1G which mainly used modulations from analog for data transfer, there was absolutely no guarantee or commitment in the field of security and this exposed the system to numerous unencrypted services which were prone to attacks [12, 15]. Similarly, with the initiation of 2G which heavily relied on digital modulations and its protocols along with the GSM standard, there was an added feature of authenticating users for the network service providers to ensure protected transmission and information. However, there was still a number of vulnerability issues in terms of security with 2G because of its linear authentical service instead of the two secure services. With the introduction of 3G in the late 2000s, though there was a hike in terms of the data transmission rate and speed along with internet connectivity facilities, it also made sure to address the security issues faced in 2G by incorporating a two-way validation and key agreement system to stabilize the security. This too did have loopholes that resulted in channel attacks and network threats. For the following fourth-generation technology, there were many security concerns which levered severe damage to the terminal devices or the end nodes in the network leading to tampered hardware, viruses, and operating systems. With regards to the 5G networks which consist of core, backhaul, and access networks, there are chances of connection outages leading to major security concerns. The fact that all generations of network communications possess some or the other security and privacy vulnerability is the motivation for addressing this very issue through this chapter [16, 17].

13.5 PROGRESSED WORK AND IMPLEMENTATION TOWARDS SECURITY

With the evolution of communication network technologies, each advanced level of respective tech generations has tried to address and eradicate the limitations of the previous levels. However, the one bottleneck that has remained consistent throughout is that of the security issue. Figure 13.2 gives a detailed analysis of the security vulnerabilities that have grown or evolved along with the advancement in the respective communication networks [18].

The implementation of 6G technology in the world would call for strict and stringent measures in the field of security and extended network services. However, the most important and highly impactful factor among all belongs to that of the privacy

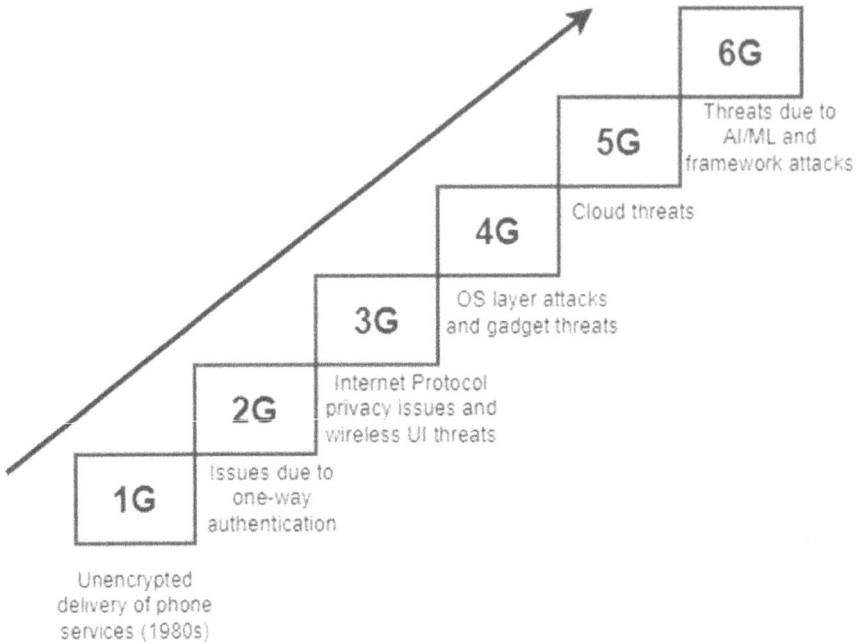

FIGURE 13.2 Security vulnerabilities from 1G to 6G.

or security preservation aspect due to the involvement and integration of advanced framework designs, standardization, policies, etc. Considering the fact that 6G has the capability of being integrated with AI, its security aspect can also be strengthened using the same phenomena. Moreover, it also has the added advantage of the cloud-based and software compatible base from the previous fifth-generation network. The one thing to be noted is that even though these technologies are being enhanced and evolving to be intelligent over the years, the possible attacks and adversaries are also becoming smarter by the day, making it even more challenging to combat the security vulnerabilities. It is equally necessary and important to ensure a trustworthy, reliable, and privacy-preserving environment to safeguard the data during data transmission and to prevent attacks. Though security and privacy are two completely different terms with meanings that lie along different realms, both of them are complementary to each other and are always interlinked. The two parameters that are likely to be useful in terms of casting an impact and measuring the level of security are the key performance indicators (KPI) and the key value indicators (KVI) [19].

One possible way to combat this issue is to utilize one of the growing phenomenon's of blockchain. Blockchain is a distributed ledger-based system to store and record data in a list of blocks which are securely linked and encrypted using hash pointer techniques. The integration of this highly secure and publicly reliable ledger technique could not only ensure security but also simplify management of network services as well as spectrum features. The possibility of developing a safely curated system of a blockchain-based radio access network framework that can handle and deal with the authentication and validation process is the ideal solution. Furthermore, since blockchain is not a centralized system which has its power vested in the hands of a single individual, and since it follows the 51% rule, tampering or breaching the data being transmitted is not practically possible. The major areas and aspects that blockchain would cover in terms of its security safeguarding feature with 6G is efficient and dynamic solutions for resource and spectrum management, compute power and data storage services, and infrastructural handling [18, 19, and 20].

The convergence of communications and sensing is the goal of 6G, which builds on the success of 5G. 6G should be able to train automation systems that cover a wide range of devices, various types of network and communication technologies, and humans through sensing the physical world and human beings. Users should promptly receive the networking services they expect from 6G. Emerging technologies will be embraced, including Internet of Everything, real-time intelligent edges, quantum communication, and molecule communication. As a result, network and information security will be crucial to both individual and societal safety. However, perceiving people and the physical world raises important privacy preservation concerns, which is in tension with trust. Another view of 6G is it is a large-scale heterogeneous network (LS-HetNet) by integrating terrestrial networks, space satellite networks, and marine networks. Such an integrated network can seamlessly support anywhere and anytime networking. But high quality of trust should be offered by LS-HetNets to meet mobile user expectations.

Network resources can be efficiently allocated with high flexibility across different domains in accordance with user demands by integrating with cloud computing and edge computing. However, this calls for trustworthy virtual cooperation between several network operators while maintaining user and operator privacy. ITU-T stipulates that trustworthy networking should be offered in order to prepare for future development. In 6G, reliable networking should provide security and address privacy leakage holistically. In conclusion, it is anticipated that 6G will have appealing features such as reliable and autonomous networking based on efficient sensing to automatically meet user requests by integrating diverse communication and networking technologies. However, these encouraging characteristics present fresh problems with privacy, security, and trust that drive practice and study.

13.6   POPULAR CRITICAL CHALLENGES AND FUTURE RESEARCH DIRECTIONS

This chapter focuses on the main possible issue of 6G in the future which is that of the security aspect. However, there are a number of other challenges and issues apart from security that can be further discussed and researched upon. The very first challenge is the use of terahertz frequency band [21]. Though it would provide expansive bandwidth and speed, it is going to be a herculean challenge to maintain a consistent service. The generations of THz signal is quite difficult as it has stringent requirements in terms of its size, sophistication, and transmission. One of the other possible challenges is the friction faced during underwater communication which is one of the specialty features of 6G [22]. The fact that water currents and waves are ever so dynamic that leads to completely unpredictable environments, leaving behind the only option of acoustic communication in such situations. The 6G technology also calls for heavily designed and efficient transmitter and receiver antenna and it should also have very high integrations [23, 24]. This again is an added challenge as it requires extensive research and development techniques to curate the same. Furthermore, one of the prevailing and predictable issues is that of latency in end-to-end transmissions and reliability factor. In order to perform consistently and seamlessly, robust forward error correction standards and procedures are required along with a parallelized array of channels to distribute the process so as to reduce the latency. High-energy consumptions, overloadable capacity, global coverage, high density or number of nodes in the network per kilometer, overwhelming costs, and non-uniformity are some of the other major challenges that need to be positively overcome in the field of 6G. Figure 13.3 gives a brief overview of the possible issues and challenges in this field. This provides a massive scope for researchers to carry out surveys and develop frameworks to overcome the same through their publications [25].

- From the possibility to the certainty: Due to the unique characteristics of internet protocol, the services offered by mobile internet in the past were rife with ambiguities and instability. These services can readily please subscribers in the 4G age. After all, a little bit of packet loss and network latency won't interfere with customers' ability to watch movies and shop online. However, the expansion of the 5G and 6G networks into all sectors of the economy and across all devices necessitates the provision of low latency and great dependability. This is the rationale behind the introduction of network slicing, MEC, and related technologies in 5G to provide the end-to-end network services capabilities ensured by SLA (Service-level agreement). According to expectations, network services will be more reliable in the 6G era and better able to respond to a variety of scenarios across a wide range of sectors [26].

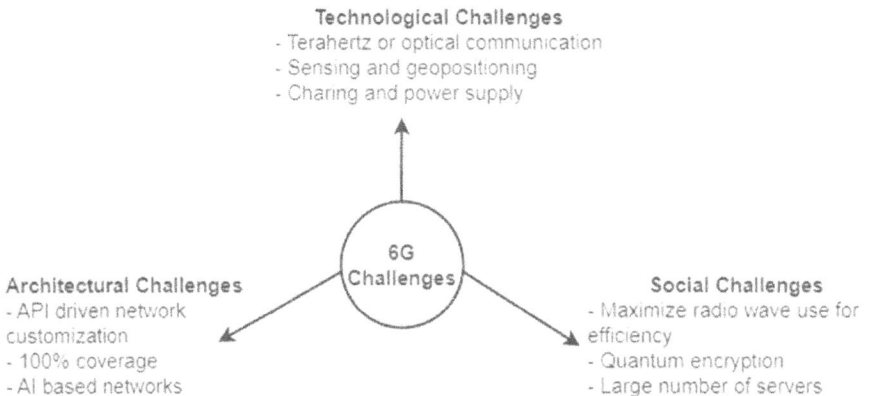

FIGURE 13.3 Challenges of 6G.

- Openness and customization: On the one hand, as we are all aware, the openness and sharing that characterizes the internet is what helps it grow. On the other hand, the ecosystem of mobile communication networks restrains its expansion to some extent by using unique technologies. Moving into the 5G era, mobile networks should actively encourage the integration of CT and IT to support the exploration of more cutting-edge applications in all industries. This will allow many industries to participate in the digital revolution. The 6G era will see an evolution in the ability to be open and customizable, supporting flexible and agile services with API interfaces for industrial clients to fulfil the demands of creating specialized networks and specialized applications [27].
- Artificial intelligence network: AI is now being employed in a variety of sectors, including automatic translation, image and speech recognition, and many more. As network services expand, higher standards for network latency, stability, and user experience are necessary. Another problem is that the more complicated the network, the more difficult it is to maintain and improve network KPIs through regular operation. In order to solve these challenges, network operators and equipment providers are striving to integrate AI into the network to assist network automation and intelligent transformation. However, in order to maximize the usefulness of an AI engine, significant amounts of data and computational power are needed. As a result, the interaction between AI is necessary for the future AI network in the 5G and 6G era [28].
- Hundred percent coverage: With a cell phone nowadays, you can live a convenient and simple life, but more than three billion people globally still do not have access to the internet. The high cost of installing base stations and optical fibre cables as well as the geographical situation contribute to the failure of network construction in remote places. The deployment of the space-earth integration network is required in the 6G era to reach the target of 100% coverage worldwide. In order to construct a space-earth integration network, base stations need be built on platforms in the upper stratosphere and on LEO satellites that can completely supply network signal to certain remote locations. In general, this solution looks at the possibilities of several new applications [29].
- Terahertz communication: The frequency range between 100 GHz and 10 THz is referred to as the terahertz frequency band and will be used in the 6G era. Despite having a large bandwidth, it has never been used. It can, therefore, be used without restrictions. However, it is predicted that terahertz in the 6G era will experience many of the same issues as millimeter wave today, including poor coverage, expensive network deployment, an undeveloped ecosystem of terminals, and other issues that must be addressed by the entire telecom sector [30].
- Perception and location: Mobile operators are currently using the radio spectrum for telecommunication purposes. However, in the 6G era, radio spectrum may be utilized for more than just communications; it can also serve as a sensor and a location-based service, enabling more novel

applications by offering services like communication and location tracing. For instance, to improve and enrich the user experience, radio signals can recognize posture, gesture, and the surrounding environment. By observing the surrounding environments for moisture, temperature, vibrancy, and other elements, you can maintain the steady operation of smart city and all enterprises. Locate new services for exploration [31].

- Make the best use of spectrum: Radio spectrum is an important carrier of innovation in the digital age since it is a valuable resource. Countries design the authorization and distribution systems for spectrum in the era of mobile networks. In the past, this arrangement encouraged network growth, but over time, it led to spectrum waste. As a result, in the 6G future, dynamic spectrum-sharing technology will be researched. The wireless sector is attempting to regulate and distribute the spectrum more intelligently and flexibly by introducing AI, blockchain, and relevant technologies. Massive MIMO is advancing to increase spectrum use efficiency in the meanwhile [32].
- Network security: Network security is essential for the development of the digital economy. Low latency, excellent dependability, wide bandwidth, and network security in particular are components of the 5G value [33–38].

13.7 CONCLUSION

This section concludes the chapter which talks about the technology of 6th-generation network, the security aspect of 6G, and the other possible barriers. We have represented a brief elucidation of the major features that align and showcase 6G communication systems and have proposed a possible solution for the security through blockchain technology. Towards the end of the chapter, we also highlight the various possible issues in the field of 6G apart from the security aspect which span across areas of architectural, technological, and social fields of 6G. In a world that is continuously evolving and improving its technological developments, 6G is just an arm's reach away as we have already entered the phase of 5G technology. It is highly expected that 6G would expand massively and is likely to develop a huge base of users both theoretically and practically. From the networking point of view, 6G would deploy novel architectural frameworks that are intelligent and capable of decision making. On the whole, 6G would definitely be a leap into the next generation of communication networks.

REFERENCES

1. Chowdhury, M.Z., Shahjalal, M., Ahmed, S. and Jang, Y.M. July 20, 2020. 6G wireless communication systems: Applications, requirements, technologies, challenges, and research directions. *IEEE Open Journal of the Communications Society*, 1: 957–975.
2. Jiang, W., Han, B., Habibi, M.A. and Schotten, H.D. February 8, 2021. The road towards 6G: A comprehensive survey. IEEE Open Journal of the Communications Society, 2: 334–366.
3. Saad, W., Bennis, M. and Chen, M. October 15, 2019. A vision of 6G wireless systems: Applications, trends, technologies, and open research problems. *IEEE Network*, 34(3): 134–142.

4. Letaief, K.B., Chen, W., Shi, Y., Zhang, J. and Zhang, Y.J. August 21, 2019. The roadmap to 6G: AI empowered wireless networks. *IEEE Communications Magazine*, 57(8): 84–90.
5. Zhang, Z., Xiao, Y., Ma, Z., Xiao, M., Ding, Z., Lei, X., Karagiannidis, G.K. and Fan, P. July 18, 2019. 6G wireless networks: Vision, requirements, architecture, and key technologies. *IEEE Vehicular Technology Magazine*, 14(3): 28–41.
6. Giordani, M., Polese, M., Mezzavilla, M., Rangan, S. and Zorzi, M. March 18, 2020. Toward 6G networks: Use cases and technologies. *IEEE Communications Magazine*, 58(3): 55–61.
7. Rappaport, T.S., Xing, Y., Kanhere, O., Ju, S., Madanayake, A., Mandal, S., Alkhateeb, A. and Trichopoulos, G.C. June 6, 2019. Wireless communications and applications above 100 GHz: Opportunities and challenges for 6G and beyond. *IEEE Access*, 7: 78729–78757.
8. Huang, T., Yang, W., Wu, J., Ma, J., Zhang, X. and Zhang, D. December 4, 2019. A survey on green 6G network: Architecture and technologies. *IEEE Access*, 7: 175758–175768.
9. Nawaz, F., Ibrahim, J., Junaid, Muhammad A.A., Kousar, M. and Parveen, S.T. 2020. A review of vision and challenges of 6G technology. *International Journal of Advanced Computer Science and Applications*, 11(2).
10. Chen, S., Liang, Y.C., Sun, S., Kang, S., Cheng, W. and Peng, M., 2020. Vision, requirements, and technology trend of 6G: How to tackle the challenges of system coverage, capacity, user data-rate and movement speed. *IEEE Wireless Communications*, 27(2): 218–228.
11. Zhang, P., Niu, K., Tian, H., Nie, G., Qin, X., QI, Q. and ZHANG, J., 2019. Technology prospect of 6G mobile communications. *Journal on Communications*, 40(1): 141–148.
12. Nayak, S. and Patgiri, R. 2021. 6G communication technology: A vision on intelligent healthcare. In *Health Informatics: A Computational Perspective in Healthcare* (pp. 1–18). Singapore: Springer.
13. Wang, M., Zhu, T., Zhang, T., Zhang, J., Yu, S. and Zhou, W. August 1, 2020. Security and privacy in 6G networks: New areas and new challenges. *Digital Communications and Networks*, 6(3): 281–291.
14. Porambage, P., Gür, G., Osorio, D.P., Livanage, M. and Ylianttila, M. June 8, 2021. 6G security challenges and potential solutions. In 2021 Joint European Conference on Networks and Communications & 6G Summit (EuCNC/6G Summit) (pp. 622–627). IEEE.
15. Nguyen, V.L., Lin, P.C., Cheng, B.C., Hwang, R.H. and Lin, Y.D. August 30, 2021. Security and privacy for 6G: A survey on prospective technologies and challenges. *IEEE Communications Surveys & Tutorials*, 23(4): 2384–2428.
16. Lu, Y. September 4, 2020. Security in 6G: The prospects and the relevant technologies. *Journal of Industrial Integration and Management*, 5(3): 271–289.
17. Abdel Hakeem, S.A., Hussein, H.H. and Kim, H. March 2, 2022. Security requirements and challenges of 6G technologies and applications. *Sensors*, 22(5): 1969.
18. Hewa, T., Gür, G., Kalla, A., Ylianttila, M., Bracken, A. and Liyanage, M. March 17, 2020. The role of blockchain in 6G: Challenges, opportunities and research directions. 2020 2nd 6G Wireless Summit (6G SUMMIT): 1–5.
19. Nguyen, T., Tran, N., Loven, L., Partala, J., Kechadi, M.T and Pirttikangas, S. March 17, 2020 Privacy-aware blockchain innovation for 6G: Challenges and opportunities. 2020 2nd 6G Wireless Summit (6G SUMMIT): 1–5.
20. Maksymyuk, T., Gazda, J., Volosin, M., Bugar, G., Horvath, D., Klymash, M. and Dohler, M. October 6, 2020. Blockchain-empowered framework for decentralized network management in 6G. *IEEE Communications Magazine*, 58(9): 86–92.
21. Elmeadawy, S. and Shubair, R.M. November 19, 2019. 6G wireless communications: Future technologies and research challenges. In 2019 international conference on electrical and computing technologies and applications (ICECTA) (pp. 1–5). IEEE.
22. Akyildiz, I.F., Kak, A. and Nie, S. July 21, 2020. 6G and beyond: The future of wireless communications systems. *IEEE Access*, 8: 133995–134030.
23. De Alwis, C., Kalla, A., Pham, Q.V., Kumar, P., Dev, K., Hwang, W.J. and Liyanage, M. April 7, 2021. Survey on 6G frontiers: Trends, applications, requirements, technologies and future research. *IEEE Open Journal of the Communications Society*, 2: 836–886.

24. Shahzadi, S., Iqbal, M. and Chaudhry, N.R. June 25, 2021. 6G vision: Toward future collaborative cognitive communication (3c) systems. *IEEE Communications Standards Magazine*, 5(2): 60–67.

25. Latva-aho, M., Leppänen, K and Clazzer, F., Munari A. Key drivers and research challenges for 6G ubiquitous wireless intelligence. Report, available at: http://jultika.oulu.fi/files/isbn9789526223544.pdf

26. Arunkumar, T. and Kalaiselvi, L. July 2014. Latest technology of Mobile communication and future scope of 7.5 g‖. *International Journal of Engineering & Technology Research*, 2(4): 23–31.

27. Gawas, A.U. 2015. An overview on evolution of mobile wireless communication networks: 1G–6G. *International Journal on Recent and Innovation Trends in Computing and Communication*, 3(5): 3130–3133.

28. Gill, J. and Singh, S. 2015. Future prospects of wireless generations in mobile communication. *Asian J. Comp. Sci. Technol*, 4(2): 18–22.

29. Zong, B., Fan, C., Wang, X., Duan, X., Wang, B. and Wang, J., 2019. 6G technologies: Key drivers, core requirements, system architectures, and enabling technologies. *IEEE Vehicular Technology Magazine*, 14(3): 18–27.

30. Yang, P., Xiao, Y., Xiao, M. and Li, S. 2019. 6G wireless communications: Vision and potential techniques. *IEEE Network*, 33(4): 70–75.

31. Khutey, R., Rana, G., Dewangan, V., Tiwari, A. and Dewamngan, A. 2015. Future of wireless technology 6G & 7G. *International Journal of Electrical and Electronics Research*, 3(2): 583–585.

32. Kalbande, D., Haji, S. and Haji, R. June, 2019. 6G-Next Gen Mobile Wireless Communication Approach. In 2019 3rd International conference on Electronics, Communication and Aerospace Technology (ICECA) (pp. 1–6). IEEE.

33. Nair, M.M., Tyagi, A.K. and Sreenath, N. 2021. The Future with Industry 4.0 at the Core of Society 5.0: Open Issues, Future Opportunities and Challenges. 2021 International Conference on Computer Communication and Informatics (ICCCI), pp. 1–7. doi: 10.1109/ICCCI50826.2021.9402498.

34. Tyagi, A.K., Fernandez, T.F., Mishra, S. and Kumari, S. 2021. Intelligent automation systems at the core of industry 4.0. In Abraham A., Piuri V., Gandhi N., Siarry P., Kaklauskas A., Madureira A. (eds), *Intelligent Systems Design and Applications. ISDA 2020. Advances in Intelligent Systems and Computing*, vol 1351. Cham: Springer. https://doi.org/10.1007/978-3-030-71187-0_1

35. Goyal, Deepti and Tyagi, Amit. 2020. A Look at Top 35 Problems in the Computer Science Field for the Next Decade. 10.1201/9781003052098-40.

36. Tyagi, A.K., Nair, M.M., Niladhuri, S. and Abraham, A. 2020. Security, privacy research issues in various computing platforms: A survey and the road ahead. *Journal of Information Assurance & Security*, 15(1): 1–16.

37. Madhav, A.V.S. and Tyagi, A.K. 2022. The world with future technologies (Post-COVID-19): open issues, challenges, and the road ahead. In Tyagi A.K., Abraham A., Kaklauskas A. (eds), *Intelligent Interactive Multimedia Systems for e-Healthcare Applications*. Singapore: Springer. https://doi.org/10.1007/978-981-16-6542-4_22

38. Mishra, S. and Tyagi, A.K. 2022. The role of machine learning techniques in internet of things-based cloud applications. In Pal S., De D., Buyya R. (eds), *Artificial Intelligence-based Internet of Things Systems. Internet of Things (Technology, Communications and Computing)*. Cham: Springer. https://doi.org/10.1007/978-3-030-87059-1_4

Index

A

Accelerometers, 144
Amazon Web Services (AWS) 108
AML models 14
Application service layer 159
Artificial general intelligence 1, 2
Artificial narrow intelligence, 1, 1
Artificial super intelligence 1, 2
Authentication and Key Agreement (AKA) 74

B

Baseband unit (BBU) 227
Beam division multiple access (BDMA) 224–225
Big Data 2, 5, 12–14, 19–21, 32, 38, 44, 53–54,
  68, 77, 123, 133, 140, 145, 162, 167,
  169, 197, 220, 222, 236, 242
Blockchain 2, 5, 10–12, 14, 17, 19, 21–22, 25,
  44, 108–109, 139, 218, 229, 244–245,
  248, 249
Blood sample reader (BSR) sensor 205
Body Area Networks (BANs) 108

C

Centralized Radio Access Network (CRAN) 227
Chronic obstructive pulmonary disease (COPD) 201
Cloud Computing 121, 125, 165, 167–169, 172,
  184, 227, 245
Cognitive radios (CRS) 227
Component carriers (CCs), 225
Cyber-physical system (CPS) 26

D

Deep neural network (DNN) 162
Deep reinforcement learning (DRL) 162
Deep-learning algorithms (DL) 162
Denial of service (DoS) 86
Distributed denial of service (DDoS) 86

E

Edge intelligence (EI) 161
Edge-of-Things (EoT) 2
Electronic Healthcare Records (EHRs) 2, 12
eMBB (enhanced Mobile Broad Band) 171
Empirical risk minimization (ERM) 203
Extra Tree (ET) 207

F

Frequency Division Duplexing (FDD) 225
Fuzzy-based sustainable, Interoperable, and
  Reliable Algorithm (FISRA) 24

G

Global positioning system (GPS) 180
Gradient boosting decision tree (GBDT) 207
Gradient boosting machines (GBM)
Graphical user interfaces (GUIs) 62
Gyroscopes 144

H

H2H (Hospital-to-Home) 175
Haptic Technology 121, 134, 141, 163
Hospital emergency smart band (HESB) 62
Hospital-to-home (H2H) 221, 205
Human–computer interaction (HCI) 134, 163
Hypertension 152
Human activity recognition (HAR) 143

I

Inertial measurement units (IMU)150
Information and Communication Technology
  (ICT) 10
Infrastructural handling 245
Innovative Internet of Medical Things
  (IIoMT) 134
Intelligent Internet of Medical Things (IIoMT) 35
Intelligent wearable devices (IWD), 23, 35,
  205, 221
International Telecommunication Union (ITU) 218
Internet layer 159
Internet of bio-nano things (IoBNT) 52
Internet of Everything (IoE) 25, 129, 133,
  168, 172
Internet of Medical Things (IoMT) 23, 26, 35
IoMT (Internet of Medical Things) 171
IoNT (Internet of Nano-Things) 175–176
IoT European Research Cluster (IECR) 10

K

Key performance indicators (KPIs) 235
Key value indicators (KVI) 244
K-Nearest Neighbour (KNN) 45, 199, 203

L

Large-scale heterogeneous network (LS-HetNet) 245
Logistic regression (LR) 207
LSTM 52, 151

M

Machine-learning algorithms; Decision Tree,
    Naive Bayes, Random Forest 117
mMTC (massive Machine Type
    Communication) 171
Management and orchestration (MANO) 235
Medical and healthcare services
METASTART 61, 68
Mobile edge computing (MEC) 27
Mobile Healthcare (mHealthCare) 72, 90–92,
    100, 104–106, 117, 118
Mobility management (MM) 235
Multiple-input-multiple-output (MIMO) 204

N

Natural language processing (NLP)
Networking layer 159
Neural information processing systems (NIPS) 202
Non-orthogonal multiple access (NOMA) 204

O

Object group localization designs (OGL) 219
Oncology 6, 32

P

Parkinson 3
Personal Health Information (PHI) 72
Plethysmography theory 3
Principal component analysis (PCA)

Q

QoE (Quality of Experiences) 175
Quality of life (QoL) 165
Quantum decision tree (QDT) 207
Quantum Gaussian Naïve Bayes (QGNB) 207
Quantum K-nearest neighbour (QKNN) 207
Quantum random forest (QRF) 207

R

Radio resource management (RRM) 235
Random Forest (RF) 199, 202
Registered Medical Practitioners (RMPs) 71
Reinforcement learning 162
RFID (radio frequency identification) 7, 10, 61,
    68, 125, 151, 153–154, 156, 229

S

Self-organized things (SoT) 219
Sensor layer 159
Smart glasses 125
Smart healthcare system 172
Software-defined wireless sensor networking
    (SD-WSN) 227
Spartan acute respiratory syndrome coronavirus
    (SARS-CoV-2) 200
START (simple triage and rapid treatment) 61
Stanford Research International (SRI), 6
Structural risk minimization (SRM) 203
Structures of increased reality (ARS) 59
Subscriber Identity Module (SIM) 74
Subsidiary component carriers (SCC) 225
SUMEX-AIM 6
Support Vector Machine (SVM) 46, 199, 202

T

Time Division Duplexing (TDD) 225

U

UI (User Interface) and UX (User Experience) 94

V

Virtual/Augmented Reality (VR and AR) 24
Virtualization of Network Function
    (NFV) 227
Visible light communication (VLC) 28, 52,
    172, 176

W

World Health Organisation (WHO) 47

For Product Safety Concerns and Information please contact our EU
representative GPSR@taylorandfrancis.com
Taylor & Francis Verlag GmbH, Kaufingerstraße 24, 80331 München, Germany

www.ingramcontent.com/pod-product-compliance
Lightning Source LLC
Chambersburg PA
CBHW060352220326
41598CB00023B/2889